A Student Guide to Health

VOLUME 1

Health Basics
Georganna Leavesley

VOLUME 2

Nutrition and Physical Fitness
Alice C. Richer

VOLUME 3

Sexual Health and Development
Georganna Leavesley and Yvette Malamud Ozer

VOLUME 4

Alcohol, Tobacco, and Other Drugs
Nancy A. Piotrowski and Yvette Malamud Ozer

VOLUME 5

Mental and Emotional Health
Yvette Malamud Ozer and Nancy A. Piotrowski

A Student Guide to Health

Understanding the Facts, Trends, and Challenges

VOLUME 3

Sexual Health and Development

Georganna Leavesley
and Yvette Malamud Ozer

Yvette Malamud Ozer
Set Editor

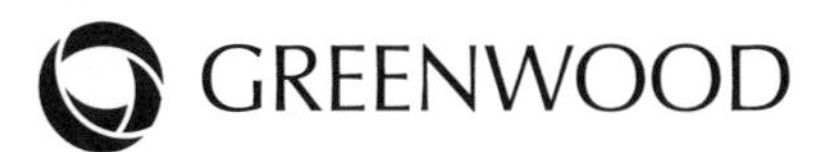

AN IMPRINT OF ABC-CLIO, LLC
Santa Barbara, California • Denver, Colorado • Oxford, England

Library of Congress Cataloging-in-Publication Data

A student guide to health : understanding the facts, trends, and challenges /
Yvette Malamud Ozer, set editor.
v. cm.
Includes bibliographical references and index.
ISBN 978-0-313-39305-1 (hard back : alk. paper) —
ISBN 978-0-313-39306-8 (ebook)
1. High school students—Health and hygiene—United States. 2. Health education (Secondary)—United States. I. Malamud Ozer, Yvette.
RA777.L43 2012
613.071'2—dc23 2012019221

ISBN: 978-0-313-39305-1
EISBN: 978-0-313-39306-8

16 15 14 13 12 1 2 3 4 5

This book is also available on the World Wide Web as an eBook.
Visit www.abc-clio.com for details.

Greenwood
An Imprint of ABC-CLIO, LLC

ABC-CLIO, LLC
130 Cremona Drive, P.O. Box 1911
Santa Barbara, California 93116-1911

This book is printed on acid-free paper ♾
Manufactured in the United States of America

Disclaimer: This book discusses treatments (including types of medication and mental health therapies), diagnostic tests for various symptoms and mental health disorders, and organizations. The authors have made every effort to present accurate and up-to-date information. However, the information in this book is not intended to recommend or endorse particular treatments or organizations, to substitute for the care or medical advice of a qualified health professional, or to be used to alter any medical therapy without a medical doctor's advice. Specific situations may require specific therapeutic approaches not included in this book. For those reasons, we recommend that readers follow the advice of qualified health care professionals directly involved in their care. Readers who suspect that they may have specific medical problems should consult a physician about any suggestions made in this book.

This set is dedicated to Becca, Harley, and all the young people who contributed their viewpoints and energy to this project. All of you help me keep it real and remind me why I do what I do.

—*Yvette Malamud Ozer*

Contents

Introduction: Sexual Health and Development, ix

Chapter 1: Development **1**

The Human Reproductive System, 1
Circumcision, 14
Changes: The Transition from Child to Adult, 18
Puberty, 19
Menstruation, 20
Social, Emotional, and Cognitive Changes, 24
Sexual Orientation, Gender Identity, and LGBTQI, 34
Resources, 53
References, 58
Glossary, 61

Chapter 2: Relationships and Environmental Influences **67**

Types of Relationships, 67
Sexual Behavior, 84
Relationship Issues, 99
Abusive Relationships, 101
Rape, 109
Sexual Harassment, 114
Resources, 118
References, 123
Glossary, 125

Chapter 3: Safe Sex **129**
Abstinence, 129
Contraception, 132
Safe Sex, 146
Legal Issues Pertaining to Sexual Activity, 149
HIV/AIDS, 152
Sexually Transmitted Diseases, 155
Tests for STDs and HIV, 163
Resources, 164
References, 166
Glossary, 170

Chapter 4: Pregnancy and Parenting **177**
Pregnancy, 177
Labor and Childbirth, 194
Infant Nutrition, 201
Parenting, 204
Childhood Health Care, 207
Baby Care, 209
Child Care, 218
Other Responsibilities for Parents, 220
Resources, 221
References, 224
Glossary, 227

About the Authors, 231
Index, 233

Introduction
Sexual Health and Development

Sexual function is basic to survival, as sexual activity is necessary to create offspring. Without offspring, the human species would cease to be. Therefore, we have an interest and a drive for sexual activity to ensure that our species will survive. Gender and sexuality are important aspects of our identity. Our view of ourselves as males or females helps define many of our social roles, interests, and abilities.

Our confidence in relationships with others may be influenced by how sexually attractive we feel. For some people, whether they are desired as a sexual partner affects their overall desirability as a person. People in close loving relationships often see sexual activity as a way to express and experience their love for each other. Many people enjoy and pursue sexual activity as something very important to their satisfaction with life.

During the teen years sexual characteristics are emerging, and attitudes toward relationships and sexual activity are forming. This volume contains information about sexual development and sexual orientation. Chapters discuss relationships, sexual activity, safety in sexual behaviors, birth control, and sexually transmitted diseases. The final chapter discusses pregnancy and parenting.

Acknowledgments

I would like to thank my coauthor, Dr. Georganna Leavesley, who also authored volume 1. I am extremely grateful to Dr. Leavesley for also contributing to volume 5, reviewing materials along the way, and providing valuable input and support throughout the project. I very much appreciate the contributions of Rebecca Malamud Ozer, Harley Hosford, Amber, and all the teens and young adults who shared their opinions and ideas on topics covered in this volume. This volume is dedicated to my partner Richard Ozer, who supports and encourages me and makes me happy every day.

—*Yvette Malamud Ozer*

I am very grateful to my coauthor and editor, Yvette Malamud Ozer, for making working on this project such a rewarding and pleasant experience. Her feedback and guidance were invaluable, and she seemed to be constantly on the job of producing an excellent product. Her gifts, wisdom, and dedication are remarkable. I dedicate this volume to my family and friends, who have taught me the incredible value of intimate relationships.

—*Georganna Leavesley*

CHAPTER 1

Development

This chapter provides background to the discussion of human development by reviewing the human reproductive system and then discussing the physical, social, and emotional changes associated with puberty. Basic female and male anatomy are addressed, as are issues of male and female circumcision. **Intersex** conditions are described within the context of puberty and development. The social, emotional, and cognitive changes associated with puberty are examined within a context of **self-image** and **self-esteem**. An overview of adolescent developmental processes is provided, including tasks of individuation and increasing independence and intimacy. **Sexual orientation**, **gender identity**, and homophobia are addressed, as are **coming out**.

The Human Reproductive System

Before discussing sexual development, it is a good idea to review some basic human anatomy. Knowing the correct names and functions of body parts will help the reader make sense of discussions about puberty and human sexuality.

Humans have two sexes: male and female. Females (girls and women) and males (boys and men) have different reproductive systems. **Genitals** are another name for the reproductive organs. The word "genitals" comes from the Latin root *genitus*, which roughly means "to beget" (or to give birth). In humans, both the male and the female reproductive systems are needed for reproduction. The male and female reproductive systems function in ways that nourish and transport the egg or the sperm. Both egg and sperm are needed to create a new individual (a baby). Pregnancy and reproduction will be discussed more in chapter 4 of this volume.

The Female Reproductive System

In females, the reproductive system is located entirely in the **pelvis**. The pelvis is the lowest part of the abdomen (belly). The **vulva,** which means "covering," is the **external** part of the female reproductive organs. External means "outside," while **internal** means "inside." The vulva is located between the legs and covers the opening to the vagina. Just above the top of the vaginal opening is a fleshy area called the **mons pubis.** The **labia** (which means "lips") are two pairs of skin folds or flaps that surround the vaginal opening. The outer pair is referred to as the labia majora (major). After puberty, the labia majora are covered with pubic hair and hide the rest of the vulva. The inner labia (labia minora, or minor) are inside the labia majora and go from the hood of the **clitoris** to below the opening of the vagina. The labia are sensitive and can swell when a woman is sexually aroused. Labia vary in shape, size, and color depending on a woman's skin color and other individual differences.

The clitoris is a small sensory organ located toward the front of the vulva where the folds of the labia join. The clitoris varies in size from smaller than a pea to the size of a small finger. The clitoris is extremely

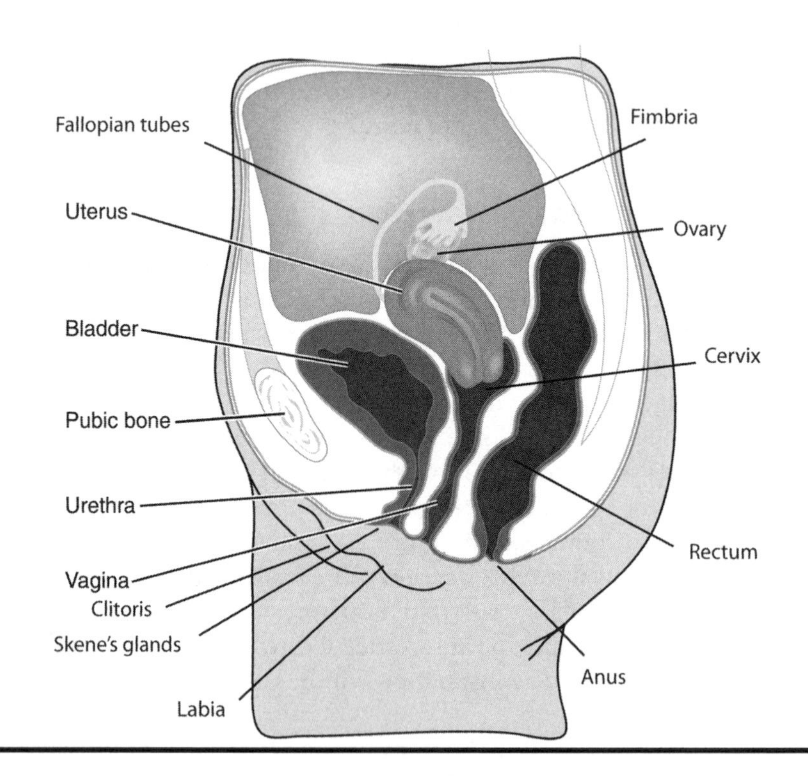

FIGURE 3.1.1 **TYPICAL FEMALE REPRODUCTIVE SYSTEM.** *(Shutterstock.com)*

sensitive, although this varies from one woman to the next. When a woman is sexually aroused, the clitoris swells and becomes stiff. Openings to the **urethra** and vagina are located between the labia. The urethra is a tube or canal that carries urine from the bladder to the outside of the body. After girls are sexually mature, the outer labia and mons pubis are covered with pubic hair.

The internal female reproductive organs are the uterus, **fallopian tubes**, **ovaries**, and vagina. The vagina is a hollow tube. It runs from the vaginal opening to the uterus. The muscular walls of the vagina allow it to expand and contract. This ability means that the vagina can be narrow enough to hold a slender tampon or stretch wide enough to give birth to a baby. The walls of the vagina are lined with mucous membranes. The mucous membranes protect the vagina and keep it moist. The vagina has several roles. It is used during sexual intercourse, it allows blood to flow out of the body during **menstruation** (the period), and it is the pathway that a baby takes out of its mother during childbirth.

The **hymen** is a membrane that partially covers the vaginal opening. Sometimes the hymen stretches, tears, or bleeds a little after a woman's first sexual experience. However, some girls or women have hymens that are torn before they ever have sex. This can happen through strenuous physical activity or using tampons. The hymen varies from person to person. Some girls are born without much of a hymen, while in others it covers more of the vaginal opening.

The uterus (or womb) is a hollow muscular organ in the female pelvis. The uterus is about the size of a pear. It expands during pregnancy as the embryo develops. **Endometrium,** a thick mucous membrane that serves as an environment for the embryo, lines the uterus. Some of the uterine lining is discarded through menstruation and exits the body through the vagina. Menstruation is described more fully later in this chapter.

The uterus narrows at its base to a passage to the vagina, called the **cervix**. The word "cervix" is related to the term "cervical," a medical term referring to the neck. The cervix is thus the neck of the uterus. This opening to the uterus is mostly closed, but there is a small passageway for menstrual flow to leave the uterus and for **semen** to enter the uterus. In the delivery of a baby the cervix expands, or widens, to permit the baby to exit the uterus by way of the vagina.

The ovaries produce **ova** (eggs). Eggs are stored in the ovaries until they mature and are released during the reproductive cycle. **Estrogen** and progesterone (female **hormones**) are produced by the ovaries. The ovaries also release small amounts of **androgens** (male hormones). The ovaries are located on either side of the uterus at the end of the fallopian tubes.

Fallopian tubes attach to the uterus, on each upper corner, and travel to the ovaries. The end of the fallopian tube near the ovary is trumpet-shaped and rimmed by **fimbria**. Fimbria are fingerlike structures that catch up the ova or ovum when released by the ovary. The ova travels through the tube, moved along by tiny hairlike structures known as **cilia.** Fertilization usually takes place as the egg travels toward the uterus. The fertilized ovum will continue into the uterus and settle into the uterine lining to begin development into an embryo. When there is no fertilization, the ovum is later discarded when the lining of the uterus is shed as part of the **menstrual cycle**.

Annual female health checkups are discussed in chapter 3, "Prevention," in volume 1. Descriptions of the female reproductive anatomy are provided in table 3.1.1.

TABLE 3.1.1 **FEMALE REPRODUCTIVE ANATOMY**

Female Part	**Description and Function**
Uterus (womb)	• Consists of muscular walls, a lining (endometrium), and cervix • Houses and protects embryo/fetus
Cervix	• Bottom section of the uterus • Produces fluids to help sperm travel • Produces a mucous plug to keep germs out during pregnancy
Vagina	• A stretchy collapsed tube (like a deflated balloon) • Allows passage of sperm, shed endometrium during menstruation, and baby during birth • Produces fluids to cleanse and lubricate itself and to help sperm travel • Provides sensation
Ova	• Egg cell (singular: ovum) • Carry chromosomes
Ovaries	• Place for ova to be stored and mature • Produce sex hormones (estrogen, progesterone, androgens)
Fallopian tubes	• Allow passage of ova toward uterus and sperm from uterus
Cilia	• Hairlike structures that line the fallopian tubes and sweep an ovum down the fallopian tube
Fimbria	• Fringe-like or fingerlike outer ends of fallopian tube • Guide mature ovum into fallopian tube after release from ovary

(*continued*)

TABLE 3.1.1 **FEMALE REPRODUCTIVE ANATOMY** (*Continued*)

Female Part	**Description and Function**
Skene's glands	• Area of firm tissue toward the front wall of the vagina, surrounding the urethra • Responds to pressure, sometimes causing orgasm; sometimes produces fluid • Also known as Graffenberg spot (G-spot)
Hymen	• Membrane partly covering vaginal opening
Vulva	• Consists of labia majora, labia minora, and clitoris • Protects openings of urethra and vagina • Provides sensation
Labia	• Two pairs of skin folds or flaps that surround the vaginal opening • Outer labia (labia majora) have pubic hair • Inner labia (labia minora) are inside the labia majora and go from hood of the clitoris to below opening of vagina
Clitoris	• Made up of shaft, internal branches (crura), glans, and hood • Glans, located at front of vulva where the labia meet, and about the size of a pearl • Provides sensation
Clitoral hood	• Protects the glans of the clitoris • When not erect, mostly covers the clitoris (like a cap) • Provides sensation
Urethra	• Below clitoris, above vaginal opening • Allows passage of urine

Source: Adapted from Reis (2011).

Breasts

All mammals (humans, cows, dogs, cats, and others) have breasts. Breasts are glands that produce milk. They are made up of fat, blood vessels, nerves, and milk ducts. In women, breasts enlarge and develop during puberty. Breasts allow women to feed (nurse) babies.

Breast development usually starts with a small tender lump under the nipple. This happens to both boys and girls. Breasts are more developed in women, but some men may also have enlargement of breasts. About

Breasts are made up of fat, blood vessels, nerves, and milk ducts. *(Shutterstock.com)*

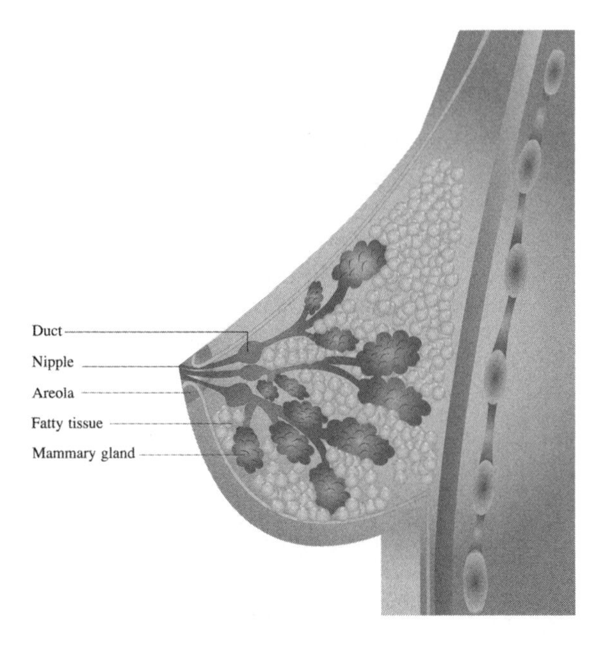

half of males develop breast tissue during puberty; this is called **gynecomastia.** Gynecomastia is caused by hormones. It is completely normal and is usually temporary, going away after puberty. Gynecomastia can be associated with some diseases, medications, or drugs, such as steroids or marijuana. Extra fat in the chest area can look like breasts; this is called pseudogynecomastia (not true gynecomastia).

In girls, breasts start to develop early during puberty. It can take 4 or 5 years for breasts to reach their full adult size. Breast size varies greatly between individuals. It is normal for one breast to be larger than the other. Big differences in breast size usually even out by young adulthood (ages 16 to 20). However, adult women may have one breast that is a different size or shape than the other.

Breasts can be tender or sore. Breasts can be sore when they start to develop (both in boys and girls). Breast sensitivity varies in different people. Breast tenderness does not necessarily mean that there is something wrong. In girls and women, sore breasts are common near the beginning of the menstrual period. Sore breasts can also be an early sign of pregnancy. Monthly breast soreness usually disappears after the menstrual period begins. Aching breasts may also be relieved by wearing a supportive bra, getting enough sleep, and eating a healthy diet. It may help to avoid salty foods and caffeine (found in cola, coffee, some teas, and chocolate). It's a good idea to consult a doctor or other health professional if there is discharge from either breast or if breast pain continues or is severe.

TABLE 3.1.2 **HOW TO DO A BREAST SELF-EXAMINATION**

A breast self-examination (BSE) can be done monthly to reduce the risk of breast cancer. BSE only takes a few minutes and involves inspecting and feeling the breasts to check for changes, lumps, or discharge (liquid) from the nipple. Breast cancer is very rare in teens and young women. To do a BSE:

1. **LOWER & LIFT:**	Examine breasts in front of mirror, first with arms at sides, then with arms raised over head.
2. **LOOK:**	Look for changes in size, shape, contour, dimpling, pulling, redness, or scaling of the skin on breast or nipple. Then with arms slightly raised, examine each underarm (armpit).
3. **LIE:**	Lie on back with pillow under right shoulder.
4. **TOUCH:**	Use pads of left three middle fingers to feel for lumps in right breast. Use dime-sized circular motions.
5. **CIRCLE:**	Circle breasts, beginning at the nipple, using firm, smooth pressure and moving in larger and larger circles until you reach outer edge of the breast. Begin with a soft touch and constantly increase pressure. Use three levels of pressure: light to feel tissue closest to skin's surface, medium to feel a little deeper, and firm to feel tissue closest to the chest and ribs.
6. **UP & DOWN:**	Feel up and down breasts, first with a soft touch, then increase pressure. Feel for changes from top to bottom and side to side. Cover entire breast and don't miss any tissue.
7. **REPEAT:**	Move pillow under left shoulder. Repeat steps 4–6 using right hand on left breast.

Source: Bright Pink (2011).

A health care practitioner should be alerted if any problems are found in self-examination. The practitioner can then decide what, if any, treatment is needed. Breast pain (unless related to the menstrual cycle), swelling or heat in the breast, or a lump in the armpit may be signs of an infection in the breast and should be reported to a health care practitioner (Hirsch 2010b). Breasts are also examined by the health care practitioner at a yearly physical exam. As adults, women may also be advised to have regular mammograms (an x-ray procedure to look for abnormalities in the breasts).

WHAT PEOPLE ARE SAYING **TEEN OPINIONS ON PLASTIC SURGERY**

Should teens be allowed to get plastic surgery, such as breast implants or nose jobs?

- "Plastic surgery is an incredible invention . . . when it's used for what it's meant to. If my face ever gets burned off because I was in a house fire or a car accident, I will be extremely grateful that plastic surgery exists to be able to give me my old face back. Or another, real-life example, my nose was brutally broken and now I have a deviated septum. And in a year, after my face stops growing, through plastic surgery they are going to give me a nose job [septoplasty] so that I can breathe out of my right nostril again. But people spending fortunes to make their nose smaller to try and fit into our perfectionist society when their 'not perfect' original nose looked better with the rest of their face anyway? No." GBH, age 17, California
- "If there is a medical reason to perform 'plastic' surgery, then I support it wholeheartedly. I cannot understand any healthy person going under the knife, if doing so because of vanity and insecurities over their appearance—it's just weird and unnatural to me. The idea of someone allowing their child to make permanent physical changes is just wrong—like I said, a legitimate medical reason is a completely different matter. I think there should be an age requirement for plastic surgery, except in extreme situations such as an accident leaving significant scarring or disfiguration, or health reasons such as breast reduction to reduce back stress. If teens are allowed to get plastic surgery at a young age, they are more likely to become dependent on the surgeries to boost their own self-image later in life." ES, age 20, California
- "No, because it may be something you regret when you become more mature. Also, your body's not done growing and any adjustments may end badly." PW, age 16, Virginia
- "I believe they should be able to, because some teens suffer from low self-esteem that only surgeries like these can correct; however, there should be an age requirement to have these things done." KK, age 19, Kentucky

? Did You Know?

Women can have cosmetic surgery to change their breast size. Dissatisfaction with smaller breasts may be related to society's emphasis on the attractiveness of larger breasts. Exercises or creams advertised to make breasts larger do not work. Breast augmentation surgery is the only way to increase breast size after natural development is complete (Hirsch 2009). Breast augmentation surgeries implant artificial materials or use tissue from other parts of the body. Women who have had surgery to remove cancerous breast tissue or have breast injuries may have reconstructive surgery to restore the breast to its former appearance.

Some women may feel that their breasts are too large. Very large breasts may attract unwelcome attention, and some girls and women may have physical discomfort or health problems related to large breast size. The weight of breasts can cause a stooped posture and lead to back or shoulder pain. Bra straps can cut into the shoulders when breasts are very heavy. When breasts are extremely large, skin problems can occur where the breast lies on the skin of the lower chest. Breast reduction makes breasts smaller by removing breast tissue. The nipple, supporting nerves, blood supply, and other tissues are left intact. The skin is sewn back together, leaving incisions underneath the breast where they will be less visible.

Women who plan to breast-feed infants must consult with the surgeon about whether it is possible to preserve the ability of the breast to provide breast milk. If this is not possible, the woman may choose to delay surgery until after she feels that her breast-feeding days are over.

The Male Reproductive System

The male reproductive system includes external structures (the **penis**, **scrotum**, testicles, and **epididymides**) and internal organs (the prostate gland, vas deferens, and seminal vesicles). The external organs are located at the front of the body, in the groin area. The internal reproductive organs lie within the pelvic cavity. The urethra, a tube that carries urine from the bladder to the outside of the body, is also a part of the reproductive process.

Sperm, the male sex cell for reproduction, are tiny cells that act to fertilize the female's egg and form an embryo. The head of the sperm cell contains genetic (heredity) material, and the sperm has a tail that moves

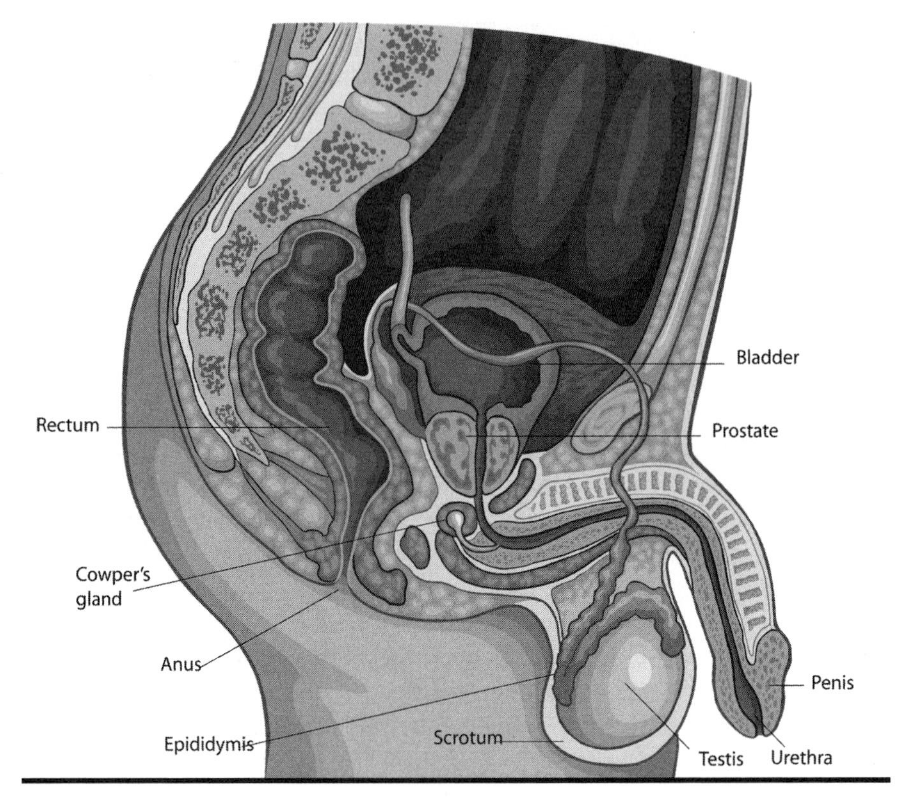

FIGURE 3.1.2 **TYPICAL MALE REPRODUCTIVE SYSTEM.** *(Shutterstock.com)*

to propel the sperm toward the egg for fertilization. Sperm cells are produced by the testicles (or testes). Testicles also produce and release male hormones: **testosterone** and androgens. The testicles are located in the scrotum (a muscular sack on the outside of the body that holds the testes and other reproductive structures). The scrotum adjusts in size to hold the testes closer to the body when cold and farther away when the area is heated. These adjustments help keep the sperm cells within the scrotum at a temperature that promotes healthy sperm production. Restrictive clothing may also keep the testicles and sperm too close to the heat of the body. Loose underwear and roomier pants are sometimes recommended to increase the chances of reproduction.

The epididymis is connected to the tubes within the testicles where sperm are formed. It is a group of ducts (or tubes) where sperm are held and mature. Sperm are also stored within the **vas deferens** (or **ductus deferens**), which begins at the end of the epididymis that is farthest from the testicle. The inner lining of these structures puts out glycogen that helps keep the sperm cells alive. The sperm cells travel, by means of rhythmic contractions, through the epididymis and vas deferens. During this process, the sperm cells become more mature and become capable of moving on their own.

The **prostate gland** supplies fluids that make up part of the semen. This gland lies between the urinary bladder and the **rectum** (the part of the large intestine closest to the anus). The inner zone of the prostate gland sends out fluids that provide moisture for the urethra (a tube that carries urine and semen). The outer zone produces seminal fluid to carry the sperm into the female during sex. The prostate gland releases its fluids directly into the urethra. The sperm are combined with semen, a thick fluid that carries the sperm and helps them live longer.

When the male is sexually aroused (excited), the epididymides contract and send sperm cells into the vas deferens. During **ejaculation** (when semen is ejected from the penis during sex), the sperm are released from the vas deferens and travel along toward the prostate gland and the urethra. Just before reaching the prostate gland, the **seminal vesicles** (saclike structures that produce a sugar-rich fluid that provides energy for the sperm) join with the vas deferens and form an ejaculatory duct that empties the semen to the urethra (Cleveland Clinic 2011). The urethra carries the semen through the penis, and the semen spurts forth from the tip of the penis. During vaginal sex the semen is sent out into the vagina, where the sperm make their way to the cervix and into the uterus and fallopian tubes in search of the ova to fertilize.

The penis is the external organ used for sexual intercourse. The penis has three parts: the root where it attaches to the abdomen, the shaft (the cylindrical-shaped body), and the **glans** (head) of the penis. The glans of the penis is covered at birth with a hood of skin (**foreskin**) that can be pulled back. Some males have this skin removed in a process called **circumcision.** The body of the penis is formed of columns of spongy tissue filled with blood vessels. This tissue fills with blood when the male is sexually excited. The full blood vessels cause the penis to get larger, harder, and erect. This erect condition aids in inserting the penis into the vagina for sex (InnerBody 2011).

Erections are a normal occurrence in males. The erection usually goes away on its own over time or after ejaculation. An erect penis results in the flow of urine being blocked, which prevents urine mixing with the semen during ejaculation. In teenagers, the erections may occur at embarrassing moments or without any known cause. These responses are considered normal, and guys do not have control over how the penis responds. Some males have erections in their sleep and may ejaculate during the night (called **nocturnal emissions** or wet dreams). Most men have three to four erections during their sleep (Dowshen 2010).

Penis length may vary a good bit among males. Penises vary in thickness and shape as well. The size of the **flaccid** (soft, not erect) penis varies more between mature males than the size of the erect penis, which is more similar across men (Dowshen 2008). Male reproductive anatomy is summarized in table 3.1.3.

Measures to protect the testicles include wearing protection during sports and avoiding twisting the testicles. A sharp sudden pain in the testicles could indicate a **testicular torsion** (the testicle becoming twisted inside the scrotum). This can be a serious condition; a health care practitioner should be consulted immediately (Planned Parenthood 2011). The skin on the scrotum and the penis should be observed for sores, itchiness, or bumps. These could be due to jock itch, sexually transmitted disease, or a simple scratch. (See chapter 3, "Prevention," in volume 1, for more information about skin health.) Any concerns should be discussed with a health care practitioner.

It is a very painful experience to get hit in the testicles. This area of the body has many nerve endings that sense pain, a built-in reason for the male to protect this region of his body and his reproductive ability. Most blows to the testicles recover in a short time, but at the moment of getting hit the guy may feel nauseated by the extent of the pain. Ice packs to the area and taking pain medication may be helpful. If there is serious swelling, a puncture to the scrotum or testicle, or fever, medical care must be sought immediately. Testicular torsions or ruptures require emergency treatment within six hours, or permanent damage may result (Figueroa 2010).

Yearly physical examinations by the health care practitioner should include looking at and feeling the testicles. The practitioner looks for abnormalities and checks that the sex organs are developing properly. Having someone feel and examine the penis or testicles may seem awkward or strange. Practitioners are very used to seeing genitals as a part of working in health care. Some guys may get an erection during the exam, but the practitioner will have seen this reaction before, and it is not a cause for apology (Figueroa 2009).

The health care practitioner may press against the groin while asking the patient to turn his head and cough. The downward pressure of the cough may reveal a hernia in the groin or scrotum. An **inguinal hernia** is a weakness in the muscular wall of the lower abdomen that allows a portion of the internal organs to slip through. This condition may require treatment or surgery.

TABLE 3.1.3 **MALE REPRODUCTIVE ANATOMY**

Male Part	**Description and Function**
Testes (testicles)	• Produce sperm and sex hormones (androgens, testosterone) • Made of several hundred feet of tightly coiled tubes
Epididymis (plural: epididymides)	• Allows maturation of sperm
Cilia	• Hairlike structures lining the epididymides • Sweep sperm cells through the epididymides
Semen	• Helps sperm live longer and travel better
Sperm	• Carry chromosomes (strings of genes) or DNA instructions that are used if the sperm cell fertilizes an egg cell
Spermatic cords	• Suspend the testis • Supply blood to and carry sperm from the testis • Provide sensation
Vas deferens (sperm ducts)	• Provide storage for and allow passage of sperm • Lead into abdomen, where they widen into storage sacs behind the bladder
Seminal vesicles	• Contribute fructose (sugar) to semen to nourish sperm
Prostate gland	• Produces most of the fluid that makes up semen
Cowper's gland (bulbourethral glands)	• Produces preejaculate, a fluid that protects the sperm by cleansing the urethra of acid
Urethra	• Tube inside the penis; allows passage of urine and semen
Penis	• Made up of shaft, glans, and sometimes foreskin • Allows passage of urine and of semen • Provides sensation
Foreskin	• Protects the glans of the penis • Provides sensation
Scrotum	• Muscular sac that holds the testes • Controls temperature, provides sensation

Source: Reis (2011).

TABLE 3.1.4 **HOW TO PERFORM A TESTICULAR SELF-EXAM**

Guys need to keep an eye on their sexual health. A testicular self-exam (TSE) should be done every month. Testicular cancer is not common but can strike males at any age. Catching it early can preserve the function of the testicles for sex and for reproduction.

Perform TSE after a warm bath or shower. The heat causes the scrotal skin to relax, making it easier to find anything unusual. TSE is simple and only takes a few minutes:

- Examine each testicle gently with both hands. Place the index and middle fingers underneath the testicle while the thumbs are placed on the top.
- Roll the testicle gently between the thumbs and fingers. It is normal for one testicle to be larger than the other.
- The epididymis is a cord-like structure on the top and back of the testicle. Do not confuse the epididymis with an abnormal lump.
- Feel for any abnormal lumps on the front and side of the testicle. These lumps are usually painless and about the size of a pea.
- Consult a health care practitioner about any lumps or anything else unusual.

Source: Men's Health Network (2011).

Circumcision

Male Circumcision

Circumcision refers to the removal of the foreskin of the penis, usually shortly after birth. The foreskin covers the glans (tip) of the penis. About 60 percent (6 out of every 10) of boys in the United States are circumcised shortly after birth. This means that 40 percent (4 out of 10) are not circumcised (Planned Parenthood 2011). Sometimes uncircumcised boys and men are referred to as uncut, and circumcised boys and men are referred to as cut. Circumcision does not change how the penis functions—mostly it changes its appearance. Boys and men who are uncircumcised may need to pull back the foreskin of the penis when they urinate, to put on a condom, or to wash themselves.

Circumcision is not medically necessary. Some parents choose to have their sons circumcised for religious beliefs, cultural or social reasons, or

? Did You Know?

- Male circumcision is almost universal among Jewish and Muslim populations throughout the world. It is widely practiced among Coptic Christians in Egypt and Orthodox Christians in Ethiopia.
- Among ethnic groups who do not practice circumcision for religious reasons, male circumcision rates are high among the Xhosa of South Africa, the Yao of Malawi, and the Lunda and Luvale of Zambia.
- The United States has the highest rate of male circumcision in the Western world: about 60 percent of newborn males in the United States are circumcised.
- Throughout the world, male circumcision rates are correlated with higher socioeconomic status.

Source: DeLaet (2009).

concerns about hygiene (cleanliness) or appearance. There has been some controversy about circumcision. People used to think that it was necessary to prevent infections. However, as long as an uncircumcised male washes his penis and underneath the foreskin, there should be no risk of infection. Whether a penis is circumcised or uncircumcised, keeping it clean is important. People also used to think that circumcision decreased the risk of penile cancer (cancer of the penis), but there is no evidence to support this (Gowen 2003).

Female Circumcision

Female circumcision is sometimes referred to as female genital mutilation (FGM). Unlike male circumcision, which usually refers to a single procedure (removal of the foreskin of the glans), FGM can involve several different procedures involving removal of part or all of the external female genital organs. FGM has been classified by the World Health Organization into four types: removal of all or a portion of the clitoris (type 1), clitoris and labia minora (type 2), and clitoris, labia majora, and labia minora, with suturing of the remaining tissue leaving only a small hole for urination, menstruation, and childbirth (type 3). This procedure is known as fibulation. Type 4 includes all other FGM procedures, including piercing, cutting, scraping, scarring, or burning the genital tissue (McGargill 2009). As with male circumcision, FGM is not performed for reasons of medical necessity.

FGM is performed for cultural or religious reasons. Some of the beliefs underlying FGM practices include the belief that the clitoris is poisonous and that if a man touches it he will die, that FGM practices promote better hygiene, that female appearance after FGM is more beautiful, that daughters with FGM will be more marriageable, and that FGM promotes chastity (McGargill 2009). In societies that condemn FGM practices (such as in the United States), FGM is viewed as a means of social control by which men maintain social positions of power over women. In the United States, people tend to emphasize that FGM can be psychologically traumatic and physically damaging. Some of the effects, depending on what type of FGM is performed, may include loss of sensation, inability to experience pleasure during sex, or inability to achieve orgasm.

In some cases FGM may be performed in unsanitary conditions with crude instruments and may result in infection, permanent injury, psychological trauma, or death. In other situations FGM is performed under more sanitary conditions and may be performed with anesthesia (numbing) or analgesia (pain medication). FGM is performed on female infants, girls, and women. It is often part of a rite of passage as a girl passes into adulthood.

FGM has historically been practiced among certain sects of Christians, Muslims, and Jews. Currently FGM is mostly practiced in Africa and among predominantly Muslim populations. Countries with the highest rates of FGM (over 80 percent) include Egypt, northern Sudan, Mali, and Ethiopia. Other countries with high rates of FGM include Burkina Faso, Mauritania, Chad, and Kenya. Rates of female circumcision vary by level of education, with the lowest rates among younger and more highly educated women (DeLaet 2009). There are also high rates of FGM among girls and women who emigrate from these countries to the United States. According to the African Women's Health Center 2000 census, over 225,000 women in the United States were at risk of FGM, over 62,000 of them under the age of 18. An estimated 130 million women worldwide have undergone FGM (McGargill 2009).

There has been a great deal of controversy about FGM, which has been referred to as a form of child abuse and also as a type of violence against women. In 1993 the United Nations (UN) General Assembly declared FGM as violence against women (UN Resolution 48/104). In 1997 a joint statement between UNICEF, the World Health Organization, and the UN Population Fund (UNFPA) called for a reduction and eventual eradication of FGM within three generations. The UN High Commissioner for Refugees and the Office of the High Commissioner for Human Rights have also condemned FGM as a human rights violation (DeLaet 2009). Several countries have made it illegal to practice FGM. In some countries, people who practice FGM on minors (girls) can be arrested for child abuse, with the minor child being taken into protective custody.

Male Circumcision as a Human Rights Issue?

There has been worldwide pressure to end FGM, which is often seen as child abuse, violence toward women, a means by which men continue to control women, and a violation of basic human rights. However, some people also describe male circumcision as genital mutilation and a violation of human rights. After all, male circumcision is also done on children who do not consent to the procedure, and it is done for reasons that are not medically necessary. Most people agree that infant males who are circumcised may feel pain during the procedure—especially if no anesthesia (numbing) or analgesia (pain relief) is used. Most boys and men do not remember the pain and don't claim long-term physical or psychological damage from the procedure. However, there are risks with male circumcision, including hemorrhage, lacerations, infection, urinary retention, or accidental amputation of the tip of the penis. Occasionally more invasive forms of male circumcision are practiced, mostly in South Arabia and among some Australian Aborigines.

Critics of male circumcision claim that it has the potential for long-term physical and emotional harm and that it violates human rights in the same ways as female circumcision. Other people take the perspective that FGM has a greater risk of long-term physical and emotional health consequences than male circumcision and violates human rights in a way that male circumcision does not.

While FGM is illegal in many places, some similar procedures are legal. For example, female genital reshaping (labiaplasty or labia reduction) is an elective surgical procedure that is not medically necessary. Labiaplasty is associated with risks of nerve damage and discoloration. Some people find it a contradiction that there is such opposition to FGM as an abusive human rights violation, very little opposition to male circumcision, and promotion of elective cosmetic procedures such as labiaplasty. None of these procedures (FGM, male circumcision, and female genital reshaping) is medically necessary, and all have risks of long-term physical or emotional harm (DeLaet 2009; McGargill 2009).

Changes: The Transition from Child to Adult

The teenage years are a time of great change. Several terms are used to refer to this period of life: teenager, adolescence, and puberty. These terms do not all mean quite the same thing. A teenager is someone who is between the ages of 13 and 19. Puberty refers to the period when a person is physically changing from a child to an adult. Adolescence comes from the Latin word *adolescere*, which means "to grow up." In the United States, adolescence is the period from puberty until a person achieves full adult responsibilities. Often adolescence lasts through a person's mid to late 20s (Haffner 2008). As life spans have lengthened, young people may take more time to decide what they want to do with their lives. Other factors that have increased the duration of adolescence in recent decades include an economy with high rates of unemployment combined with high costs of living. These factors may make it more difficult for young people to get jobs or to afford to move out on their own, so many continue to live longer with their parents.

Individual Differences

The transition from child to adult involves many changes—physical, emotional, cognitive (intellectual), and social. Change varies a great deal from one individual to another. Since people develop at different rates, people of the same age may have developed differently in terms of physical, emotional, and social maturity. Physical, social, and emotional development may occur at different rates in one individual. For example, while a 15-year-old girl may be well along in her physical development toward adulthood, emotionally she may be more like a younger child and socially may be just beginning to experiment with adolescent social interactions. Likewise, a 16-year-old boy may be slower in his physical development than other boys his age but may be socially on a par with his peers and emotionally more mature than others his age.

Stages of Adolescence

While there are many differences between individuals, adolescence can be divided into three stages. Age estimates for these stages are approximate. Early adolescence occurs in girls ages 9–13 and boys ages 11–15. Middle adolescence occurs in girls ages 13–16 and in boys ages 14–17. Late adolescence usually begins in girls ages 16–18 and in boys around age 17 or 18.

? **Did You Know?**

Throughout history, people from many cultures have marked life transitions with rites of passage. There are rituals to celebrate births, weddings, and graduations. Different cultural and religious rites of passage are used to mark the coming of age: the transition from childhood to adulthood. Some are traditional, such as Quinceañera, a Latin American celebration of a girl's 15th birthday to mark the transition from childhood to womanhood. At a Débutante Ball (coming-out party), a young woman is presented to society as eligible to marry. Other rites of passage are more modern, such as a sweet-16 party to celebrate a teen's 16th birthday. A bar or bat mitzvah is a Jewish ritual that welcomes a teen as an adult member of the congregation. Some cultures have spirit quests or ceremonies involving rigorous feats of stamina and endurance to signify a young person's readiness for adulthood. Some cultures have special ceremonies with rituals to mark a young woman's menarche (first period) as a sign of transitioning into adulthood.

Puberty

Puberty is a stage of physical development. The beginning of puberty is signaled by the first physical changes and adult growth. Puberty ends when a human being is physically mature and capable of sexual reproduction. Boys begin and end puberty an average of two years later than girls. So while girls will be going through early adolescence between the 4th and 8th grades, boys will more likely be going through early adolescence between 6th and 10th grades. Some teenagers (boys and girls) do not physically mature until their junior or senior year of high school. The physical changes of puberty can occur quickly, in as little as one year, or can take as long as five years.

Physical Changes during Puberty

Boys and girls grow rapidly during early adolescence. This growth spurt occurs over a 2- or 3-year period. Girls have their growth spurt an average of 2 years before boys. Girls grow the most around age 12, while boys grow the most at age 14. Girls grow most the year before their first period. Both boys and girls gain weight as well as height during the growth spurt.

During puberty, both boys and girls also develop secondary sexual characteristics. Secondary sexual characteristics include development of underarm and pubic hair and deepening of the voice. They also include development of sweat glands in the underarm and genital regions. These sweat glands are responsible for body odor (see also the section on hygiene in chapter 3, volume 1).

What Triggers Puberty?

When a person reaches a certain age, the brain releases a growth hormone that starts the changes of puberty. This growth hormone is called gonadotropin-releasing hormone, or GnRH. Hormones are chemical substances that act like messengers in the body. GnRH causes the pituitary gland to release two puberty hormones into the bloodstream. The pituitary is a small gland that sits below the brain. Both boys and girls have these puberty hormones: luteinizing hormone (LH) and follicle-stimulating hormone (FSH).

Puberty in Males

In males (boys and men), LH and FSH signal the testes to start producing testosterone and sperm. Testosterone is the hormone responsible for most of the changes in males during puberty. Sperm is necessary for males to reproduce.

Puberty in Females

In females (girls and women), the ovaries have contained eggs since birth. FSH and LH stimulate the ovaries to produce estrogen. Estrogen is a hormone that causes girls to mature. Estrogen also prepares the female body for pregnancy.

Menstruation

Menstruation (having a period) is the monthly discharge of blood and other matter from the uterus. Blood from the uterus passes through a small opening in the cervix and leaves the body through the vagina. Starting to have periods is one of the signs of a girl going into puberty and moving toward adulthood. Because it is a sign of maturing, many girls are anxious for their periods to begin. Other girls may find this new experience a scary thought. A girl's period begins 2 to 2.5 years after her breasts start to develop (Gavin 2010). **Menarche** is the term for the start of having periods. The first period may happen between ages 8 and 15; 12 is the average age for periods to begin (Women's Health 2009).

The menstrual cycle includes monthly hormonal changes, **ovulation**, and periods. The typical menstrual cycle is 28 days. In the first part of this cycle, the level of estrogen put out by the ovaries increases. The estrogen signals the uterus to thicken its lining of blood and tissue. An ovary will respond to the estrogen level by starting to mature an egg (ovum). Around day 14 of the cycle, ovulation occurs (the ovary releases the matured egg).

If the egg is fertilized (by sperm from a male), it settles into the uterine lining, and estrogen levels remain high to support the growth of an embryo. If the egg is not fertilized, the egg breaks apart in the uterus, and the estrogen level drops. The lower estrogen level will signal the uterus to shed its lining. The cycle of changing hormone levels, ovulation, and shedding uterine lining will repeat (unless the woman is pregnant) every month from puberty to **menopause**. Menopause is a time (around age 50) when women stop ovulating and having periods (Women's Health 2009).

Periods vary in amount, length, and frequency among females. This is especially true in the first two years of menstruating (Gavin 2010). A typical period lasts three to five days. It is also normal for a period to be as short as two days or as long as seven days (Women's Health 2009). The amount of blood coming from the vagina may be small to heavy and may vary over the course of the period. The length of time and amount of flow in periods may not be the same every month. The space between periods (cycle) may vary as well, especially when menstruation first starts.

Irregular periods do not come with a dependable timetable. The hormones (estrogen or thyroid) may not function in a typical pattern. Ovulation may not occur every month in some women. Sometimes, irregular periods are the result of stress or a change in lifestyle. Irregularity in periods may decrease as the girl matures or may continue into adulthood. Some girls become irregular or stop having periods because of too much exercise, not eating enough, or low body weight. Other women may have excess amounts of male hormones that interfere with the menstrual cycle. A health care practitioner may be consulted about problems with irregular periods (Hirsch 2010c). Girls who have sex should suspect a pregnancy if their period is more than a few days late in coming.

Women who do not have a predictable menstrual cycle can watch for signs that their period is about to begin. They may notice back discomfort, swelling of breasts, or moodiness. Skin problems or overall **bloating** (puffiness) may occur. Girls may also be signaled that a period is coming by **menstrual cramps** (muscle contractions) in the lower abdomen (Hirsch 2010c).

More than half of women who menstruate have cramps during the first few days of their periods (Hirsch 2010a). Menstrual cramps occur in the uterus and are felt in the lower part of the abdomen or sometimes in the woman's back. The cramp may be a dull ache or a sharp pain. Sometimes the discomfort is so intense that the girl is nauseated. Over-the-counter medicine for pain may relieve cramps. Taking a warm bath or placing a hot water bottle on the abdomen may also be helpful. Exercise may also play a role in reducing or avoiding cramps.

Premenstrual syndrome (PMS) refers to emotional and physical changes in women just before their monthly period begins. Girls and women who have PMS may be more irritable or depressed. They may have trouble concentrating and may be tired or stressed out. Food cravings or skin breakouts, headaches and backaches, and problems with sleeping may also be seen. These symptoms may be present for one to two weeks before the menstrual period.

Not all girls and women have PMS. PMS may be caused by hormone levels, sensitivity to changes and discomforts, and lifestyle or eating habits. Eating a balanced diet with plenty of fruits and vegetables and

TABLE 3.1.5 **WHEN TO SEEK MEDICAL ADVICE ABOUT YOUR PERIODS**

Consult a health care professional about your period if:

- Breasts haven't started to grow by age 13.
- Menstruation has not started within 3 years after breast growth began, or by age 15.
- Periods suddenly stop for more than 90 days or become very irregular after having had regular monthly cycles.
- Period occurs *more* often than every 21 days (3 weeks) or *less* often than every 35 days (5 weeks).
- You are bleeding for *more* than 7 days (1 week) or more heavily than usual or using more than one pad or tampon every 1 to 2 hours.
- Bleeding between periods.
- Severe pain during periods.
- You suddenly get a fever and feel sick after using tampons.

Source: Adapted from Women's Health (2009).

reducing intake of salt and preservatives may reduce PMS. Daily exercise and stress-reduction methods may also be helpful. Avoiding caffeine and getting lots of sleep may help as well (Hirsch 2010a). A health care practitioner should be seen for severe cases of PMS that interfere with day-to-day life.

Girls and women use various products to absorb the menstrual blood coming from the vagina. Some use **pads**, and others use **tampons**. Women sometimes use both these items. A pad (**sanitary napkin**) is an absorbent item worn on the outside of the vaginal area. Most pads are disposable, but some pads are made of layers of absorbent cloth and are reused after laundering. A **panty liner**, which is a thin pad that covers the crotch of underwear, may be used when menstrual flow is very light or to prevent staining from leaks from a tampon. A tampon is a cylinder-shaped column of absorbent material placed inside the vagina to absorb menstrual blood. It is discarded after use. Information about how to use and insert tampons can be found at the Center for Young Women's Health website, listed in the resources section at the end of this chapter.

Other products may be used during menstruation, such as sea sponges, folded cloths, cotton wool, or **moon cups**. A moon cup is a cup or barrier worn inside the vagina during menstruation to collect menstrual fluid.

Some girls prefer to use a pad when they first begin menstruation. Some cultures believe that using a tampon is not appropriate for virgins. Tampons are found to be more convenient for many girls because they do not interfere with swimming or water sports and may be seen as less messy than pads. Tampons are also more compact to carry than pads and are not bulky under clothing. There may also be less menstrual blood odor from tampons than pads.

Cleanliness is important for girls during their periods. Regular bathing can reduce odor from the menstrual blood. Used sanitary supplies (pads or tampons) should be wrapped up to reduce visibility and odors and placed in a trash can. Flushing of pads, tampons, or the applicators used to insert tampons is not recommended. Clogged toilets and costly plumbing problems may result from flushing these products.

Many girls are embarrassed for anyone to know they are having a period. Most girls are very disturbed if they start their period and have blood on their outer clothes that others can see. If this happens, it is best to remain calm, have some tampons or pads on hand in a purse or backpack, and get a change of clothes as quickly as possible. People know that girls have periods, and most will be sympathetic if they see a girl who has had a mishap with menstruation.

Pads should be changed before they become soaked with blood to prevent leaks and to increase absorbency. A tampon should be changed every four to eight hours. Tampons come in different levels of absorbency, and the lowest level that will work for one's flow should be used. Bacteria may grow in the vaginal area from pads or tampons that are not changed often enough. These bacteria (*streptococcus* and *staphylococcus*) may cause infections and serious health problems.

Toxic shock syndrome (TSS) is an illness in which the body reacts to toxins from bacterial infections. It is sometimes linked to tampons but can also be related to using barrier birth control methods (diaphragms and cervical sponges). Symptoms of TSS include high fever; a drop in blood pressure; a rash on the body; muscle aches and headache; severe redness of the vagina, eyes, mouth, or throat; and vomiting or diarrhea. As the syndrome progresses, the person may have confusion, seizures, and organ failure. TSS is a medical emergency, as the infection affects the entire blood supply and body. A health care practitioner must be consulted immediately (Hirsch 2011).

Social, Emotional, and Cognitive Changes

The changes of adolescence don't occur all of a sudden; they are usually gradual. Sometimes people go back and forth: a person may think or act more like an adult one day and feel or behave more like a child the next day. These changes can be confusing or can cause anxiety for changing adolescents or the people around them. Friends and family members may act differently around a changing adolescent. Family and friends may not know how to react to the changing adolescent. Despite all the challenges and changes, the majority of teenagers adjust and cope well with adolescence (Haffner 2008).

Emotional and Cognitive Changes

There is a great deal of growth and change during adolescence. Besides the physical changes that can be seen throughout puberty, there are cognitive (thinking) and emotional (feeling) changes that may be less apparent. Puberty is accompanied by changes in hormone levels, which can influence mood. Changing hormone levels can contribute to mood swings. A teen may be happy and upbeat one minute, followed by feelings of being down, sad, angry, irritable, or depressed. This is not unusual for this time of life.

Major growth and changes in the brain are also occurring during this time, which is associated with improved abilities to selectively pay attention, solve problems, and organize complicated tasks. Abilities to regulate emotions and manage behavior also improve during adolescence. Changes in the brain allow typical teens to better read nonverbal social cues, such as tone of voice, facial expressions, and body language. There is also an increased appreciation of interpersonal relationships, which goes along with a tendency to be less dependent on parents and family and more involved with peers and friends (Yurgelun-Todd 2007).

Just as with physical changes in puberty, emotional and cognitive changes occur at different rates for different people. For example, one 15-year-old may be physically very mature while having little interest in social relationships. Another 15-year-old may be physically immature while having more advanced planning and problem-solving skills and well-developed emotional regulation abilities. Everyone matures at their own rate. There are also many individual differences. Just as adults have the different abilities to solve problems, pay attention, and manage their emotions, teens also have individual differences.

Self-Image and Self-Esteem

Self-image is the idea or conception that one has about oneself. Teens have a self-image that is shifting and developing. Adolescents and young adults often experience an identity crisis as they struggle to figure out who they are as individuals and what social role best fits with their self-image. This is related to the transition from being a child—whose identity is largely shaped by family—to an independent adult. Teens and young adults are still in the process of discovering their interests, abilities, and social roles in relation to peers (Reevy, Malamud Ozer, and Ito 2010). Self-esteem is the value that one places on oneself—whether one feels good or bad about oneself as a person. Along with self-image, self-esteem may fluctuate during adolescence.

Adolescents tend to be very concerned about their physical appearance. Teenagers may focus more on the appearance of their clothes, hair, skin, and body shape than they did as children. They may feel that they are too fat or too thin or may worry that their clothing is not fashionable. Society may promote body image ideals, suggesting through media images that males should be big and strong, while females should be thin and beautiful. These pressures can result in distorted body images. People who see themselves as heavier than what is portrayed in magazines and on television may develop eating disorders. More girls develop eating disorders, but boys may also have eating disorders related to body image. Distorted body image may also contribute to substance misuse. For example, boys or men may use steroids or growth hormones in attempts to gain muscle mass and get bigger. Both boys and girls may use stimulants (e.g., diet pills, methamphetamine) to get or stay thin (Reevy, Malamud Ozer, and Ito 2010).

It is common for adolescents to be **self-conscious,** which means being intensely aware of oneself. Someone who is self-conscious may be embarrassed or anxious that others are looking at or judging her or him. A self-conscious person may be self-critical or have self-doubt. Adolescents may become preoccupied about other people's opinions of them. It is typical for adolescents to be more concerned about their peers' opinions than about those of their families. As teenagers' self-image and sense of identity develop, they may be more confident and less concerned about physical appearance. Self-image and self-esteem are discussed further in chapter 1, "Environment and Mental Health," in volume 5.

In addition to cosmetic breast surgery (breast augmentation), young people who are dissatisfied or critical of their bodies are getting other types of cosmetic surgery, including nose jobs (to change the size and shape of the nose) and cheek or chin implants. Some young people are also undergoing cosmetic procedures such as collagen injections (to make lips appear plumper), permanent makeup, and Botox injections. Botox involves injections of botulin toxin, a poison that paralyzes the muscles. By paralyzing certain facial muscles, Botox may temporarily leave a smoother, more wrinkle-free appearance. While most teens don't have visible wrinkles—which increase naturally with aging and exposure to the sun—some teens are so concerned with their appearance that they undergo costly and sometimes dangerous cosmetic procedures. Botox, for example, may have side effects such as bruising, allergic reactions, or paralysis of the wrong muscle group. A research study found that Botox may dampen or interfere with the ability to experience emotion in certain situations (Neal and Chartrand 2011).

Body Modifications

Media portrayals of what is considered fashionable as well as peer pressure to present oneself like others in one's peer group may prompt some teens to dress in certain ways or have certain hairstyles. Some teens may also want to get body art or modifications, such as tattoos or piercings. Some states have regulations that do not allow minors (individuals under 18 years of age) to get tattoos or piercings or to get them without parent or guardian permission.

Tattoos

A tattoo is a puncture wound, made by penetrating the skin with a needle and then filling the wound with ink. The tattoo is usually made into a design and may be many colors or just one color. The ink is injected into a deep layer of skin (the dermis) so that the ink design will stay even after natural periodic shedding of the outer skin (epidermis).

A tattoo should be done by a qualified professional in a clean tattoo studio. People should not attempt to tattoo themselves (or a friend) at home. Infection and other complications are much likelier if a tattoo is not done by a professional. Anyone getting a tattoo should be up to date on immunizations (for example, tetanus and hepatitis). If you have health conditions such as asthma, allergies, skin conditions, diabetes, problems with the immune system, infections, or are pregnant, you should check these issues with a health care professional before deciding to get a tattoo. If you are prone to getting keloid scars (the overgrowth of scar tissue from a wound), you should not get a tattoo.

After making sure that the tattoo artist is qualified and the tattoo studio is clean, you should make sure the equipment and tools are clean. Clean equipment, proper procedures, and aftercare all help reduce the chance of infection or other complications. The tattoo professional should provide instructions about taking care of a tattoo until it's healed (Van Vranken 2009).

It's a good idea to think carefully before getting a tattoo. One thing to think about is the body part. It may hurt a lot to get a tattoo on a

WHAT PEOPLE ARE SAYING **TEEN OPINIONS ON BODY MODIFICATIONS**

Many states don't allow people under a certain age to get tattoos and some types of body piercings. Should there be an age requirement?

- "Yes, I agree with the age requirement because it's permanent. And when you're young you shouldn't make those stupid mistakes. Maybe ear piercings are okay without permission." GBH, age 17, California
- "I think there should be an age requirement because teenagers are often impractical in their choice of tattoos and piercings and can be irresponsible when caring for a new tattoo or piercing." KG, age 19, Texas
- "I believe there should be an age requirement. I know that there were tattoos and piercings I wanted to get when I was 14 or 15 that I know I would definitely regret having now." KK, age 18, Louisiana
- "Parental consent is what is needed here. Getting a tattoo at a young age can stretch and not have the desired effect as you grow; you can also find that you don't want that piercing anymore also as you develop more (personal experience with eyebrow piercings)." HH, age 20, California

FIGURE 3.1.3

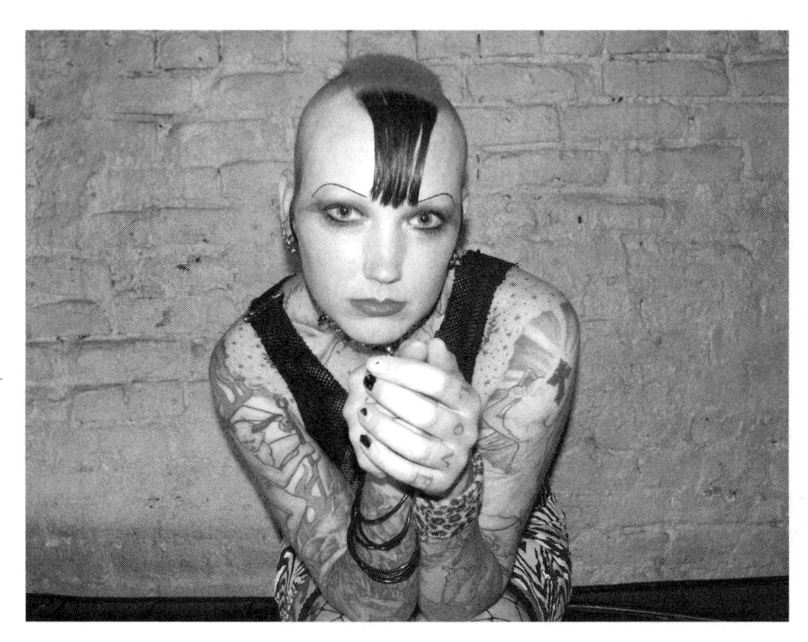

Some state regulations do not allow minors to get tattoos or piercings. *(Cora Reed / Dreamstime)*

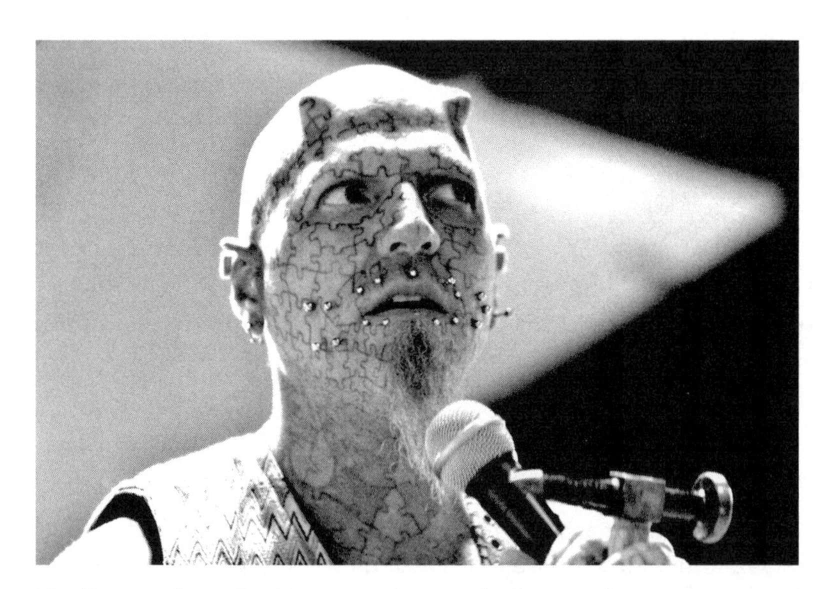

The Enigma (born Paul Lawrence) is a sideshow performer, actor, and musician who has undergone extensive body modification, including horn implants, ear reshaping, multiple body piercings, and a full-body jigsaw puzzle tattoo. *(Candace Beckwith / Dreamstime.com)*

particularly sensitive body part. Also think about what the body part may look like in 15 or 20 years. For example, some people get tattoos around an upper arm, which might look terrific on a young man with great biceps or a young woman with slender firm arms. However, it's useful to notice whether one's older relatives have body types that sag, loosen up, or tend to get flabby in certain areas. Before deciding to get a tattoo in a certain body region, imagine how that tattoo would look on an older relative.

It's also good to keep in mind that tattoos are not temporary. You are stuck with a tattoo unless you go to great lengths to have it removed, such as laser tattoo removal (a long and sometimes painful process). After breaking up with a boyfriend or girlfriend, you might regret having a tattoo of his or her name. You might think twice about getting that flame tattoo on your forehead (which seemed like a funny idea at the time) when getting ready for a job interview.

Piercings

Piercings may be done in different parts of the body, including ears, nose, eyebrows, lips, tongue, belly button, and genitals. The piercer cleans the body part to be punctured, punctures it with a sterile (clean) needle, and inserts a piece of jewelry into the puncture hole. Numbing medication (anesthesia) is not usually used during piercings, so the procedure may hurt considerably.

A piercing should always be done by a professional piercer who is licensed by the Association of Professional Piercers (APP). Not all states require piercers to be licensed. A licensed professional may be more likely to have adequate training, use appropriate procedures and instruments in a clean and sterile environment, and provide follow-up instructions and care. These may help reduce the chances of infection or other serious complications of piercing. It is important to always have piercings and other body modifications done by a professional in a sterile setting and never to attempt to pierce oneself or a friend at home. It is important to follow instructions for cleanliness and self-care after getting a piercing. Healing times vary, depending on the body part pierced and how quickly an individual is able to heal.

Piercing complications may include bacterial infection, bleeding, scarring, nerve damage, or allergic reaction to the jewelry. There is also a risk of contracting HIV, hepatitis B, hepatitis C, or other infectious diseases. Ear lobe piercings have a relatively low risk, but ear cartilage piercings can have infections and healing problems resulting in scarring that deforms the ear. Keloid (hypertrophic) scars can also permanently deform pierced body parts. Infection is a common complication of mouth, nose, and genital piercings (Chang 2010). Tongue piercings can result in damage to the

? Did You Know?

Carroll, Riffenburgh, Roberts, and Myhre (2002) conducted a survey of 552 teenagers and found that:

- 26.9 percent reported having a piercing in a location other than their earlobe.
- 1.2 percent had their nipples pierced, and 0.8 percent reported having their genitals pierced.
- Girls were more likely than boys to have an intimate body piercing.

Brooks, Woods, Knight, and Shrier (2003) conducted a study with 210 Massachusetts teens (average age 16) and found that:

- 10 percent of teens with a piercing and 10 percent with tattoos reported that they did not use a sterile needle during the procedure, and 2 percent of adolescents reported sharing a needle.
- 10 teens reported scarring or branding.
- 9 percent of teens were unhappy that they obtained a body modification.

Sources: Brooks, Woods, Knight, and Shrier (2003); Carroll, Riffenburgh, Roberts, and Myhre (2002).

teeth. Tongue, lip, and cheek piercings may cause gum problems (Moser 2006; Van Vranken 2008).

Social and Emotional Changes

Sexuality educator Debra Haffner (2008) describes five developmental tasks that adolescents accomplish as they grow up. Haffner refers to these as the five I's of adolescent development: intellect, independence, identity, integrity, and intimacy. Developmental tasks are tasks that typically must be accomplished to successfully mature from a child to an adult. As with physical growth, everyone grows at his or her own pace. An individual might mature quickly in one area (such as identity) and slower in another (such as intimacy or independence). Table 3.1.6 describes each of the five I's as people mature from childhood through adolescence and into adulthood.

With all of these developmental changes, one needs to consider differences in culture and family. Some cultures place less emphasis on independence and individual goals. Instead, identity, goals, and values are

TABLE 3.1.6 **THE FIVE I'S OF ADOLESCENT DEVELOPMENT**

Child → Teen	Teen → Adult
Intellect	
• *Thinks concretely:* Difficulty planning ahead, problem solving, anticipating consequences of own actions • Less ability to see a situation from another's perspective	• *Thinks abstractly:* Can think through the consequences of one's own actions • *Social cognition and empathy:* Better able to see situation from another's perspective
Independence	
• *Dependent:* Lives at home; financially dependent on parents; parents help or take care of cooking, cleaning, shopping • Parents provide comfort and help child develop emotional management skills	• *Independent:* May live in own home or with roommates; can support self financially; can take care of self • *Emotionally and psychologically independent:* Has abilities to soothe and comfort self and manage emotions
Identity	
• *Family shapes child's identity:* Culture, religion, educational and career ideas, politics	• Young adult develops own interests and identity in educational and career goals, religion, politics • Adult has own gender identity and sexual self-concept (including sexual orientation)
Integrity	
• Child learns and often shares the family's values	• Young adult develops own sense of ethics, values, and what is right, just, or fair • Young adult explores values and sense of integrity; this may change his or her ideas about religion and politics
Intimacy	
• Intimacy is experienced in context of family (parents, siblings, and extended family)	• Teens experiment with romantic relationships and develop mature capacity for intimacy

Source: Adapted with permission from Haffner (2008).

shaped by what is best for the family or community rather than emphasizing individual desires and feelings. In some families and cultures, it is not considered typical for young adults to move out on their own immediately after high school. Instead, many generations live in one house, and family roles, responsibilities, and expectations are oriented toward what is expected in that family or culture. Economic forces and financial realities will also shape the path toward independence and adulthood. For example, when jobs are scarce, it may make sense for young people to continue living with their families after high school while they pursue educational or career goals.

Some developmental changes fall into one of these areas, but many have elements of more than one. As teens become more independent, they develop a sense of autonomy and self-sufficiency. Autonomy means being more self-directed. For example, parents often arrange playdates for their children, and young children's friends are often determined by who their parents associate with or what other kids live nearby. As teens start maturing and developing their own identities, they start to seek out friends with similar interests. Teens start to transition from a child's perspective (when parents and family are most important) to a peer orientation (when peers are most important). This means that teenagers hang out more with peers their own age and have more choice about who their friends are. Teens are more autonomous—they don't need their parents to arrange friends or activities or tell them what clothes to wear. More mature teens and young adults choose their own friends and develop their own preferences for clothing, music, and activities.

Because teens are more oriented to peers than to family, teens are also more easily influenced by their peers. If a teen's peer group tends to get in trouble with the law or at school, the teen is more likely to also get in trouble. Peers who belong to groups in which drinking, drug use, or risk-taking behaviors are tolerated or promoted may be influenced to join in these behaviors. However, adolescence is also a period of developing a sense of one's own integrity. If a teen decides that the behaviors of a peer group are not in line with his or her values, the teen will likely find a different peer group, one with values that are similar to his or her own.

One's identity describes the values or groups with which one **identifies**—feels a similarity in values or kindred spirit with. A teen may identify with a certain religion, culture, ethnicity, sexual orientation, **gender**, and social set. In any high school, there may be several social sets or cliques. Some kids may be part of groups or social sets that are into certain types of music, sports, science and math, or drinking. One person can identify with several groups and ideas at the same time (for example, a

Christian Latina girl who believes in abstinence until marriage, no drugs, and likes math and science). Although adolescents are strongly motivated to find where they fit in, identity is more than just a list of groups. It is important to feel a sense of belonging or fitting into certain groups, but it is also important to consider the whole person. Individuals are a collection of influences from their families (genetics, shared history, ethnicity, values), cultural groups, and the societies in which they live.

Other influences on identity include standard of living (income, wealth or poverty), parents' occupations and education level, and advantages and challenges within the community (crime, violence, unemployment, gangs). An individual's identity may also include physical appearance and abilities, learning style, and ways of feeling, behaving, and coping with life. Identity may include how many friends a person has, whether the person has a best friend, how comfortable the person feels in social situations, and whether the person feels a sense of fitting in with her or his family. A person's self-image and identity may change if there is a family member who uses drugs or has a mental or physical disability. Identity may be influenced by experiencing homelessness, abuse, violence, or a natural disaster.

As a teenager becomes more autonomous and independent and more interested in peers, it is natural for relationships with family members to change. For example, maybe you used to be very close to your siblings, but as a teenager you may no longer want to spend time playing with a younger brother. You may prefer different types of activities and may want to hang out with friends your own age. You may also feel embarrassed to be seen with a parent or younger sibling in public. As teens explore their developing **sexual identity**, they may desire more privacy. This can cause some friction with parents. It can be especially difficult for a parent to adapt if a parent has been involved in every aspect of a child's life. It may be challenging for the parent to back off and give the teenager space and privacy.

Roles within a family may change as teens mature. If a child always depended on a parent to take care of household chores (or tell the child what to do and when), the teenager may begin to take more responsibility for the family and chores around the house. For example, teens who learn to drive and have access to a car may be asked to do grocery shopping, pick up a younger sibling from school, or babysit. Teenagers may also be expected to get jobs to help pay for their own clothes or contribute to the family. Teens may need to negotiate with family members to find a reasonable balance between taking on more responsibility at home and pursuing their own interests and activities. As teens develop their own interests, values, and feelings around religion, they may need to discuss expectations for things the family has traditionally done together, such as attending church or going on family outings or vacations.

As teens start to explore romantic relationships and intimacy, their friendships may change. They may be more interested in hanging out with groups of teens and less interested in spending time with a best friend. Or, they may experience conflict if their best friend doesn't spend as much time with them because they're always spending time dating. Adolescence is a continuous process of making adjustments, especially as teenage interests change at different rates and often go off in different directions. Teens and parents will need to negotiate boundaries around privacy and dating. There may be clear rules and boundaries such as curfews for younger teens who are just starting to date. More mature teens and their parents will need to discuss what is acceptable in a family in terms of spending the night away from home, curfews, rules around drinking and driving, and privacy.

Sexual Orientation, Gender Identity, and LGBTQI

Sexual Orientation

Sexual orientation describes the sex of the person one is attracted to. There are a range of sexual orientations, including **heterosexual**, **homosexual**, and **bisexual**. *Hetero* is the Greek prefix for "other," *homo* is the Greek prefix for "same," and *bi* is the Greek prefix meaning "two." Heterosexual means that one is romantically and physically attracted to people of the opposite sex, such as when boys are attracted to girls. Homosexual means that one is attracted to people of the same sex (such as when girls are attracted to each other). Bisexual (also known as bi) means that one is attracted to people of the same sex and people of the opposite sex.

Some people believe that there is a spectrum of sexual orientation, ranging from completely heterosexual to 100 percent homosexual, with bisexual right in the middle. This theory suggests that most people are not 100 percent heterosexual or homosexual and that most people fall somewhere in between. For example, the Heterosexual-Homosexual Rating Scale (also known as the Kinsey Scale) developed by Alfred Kinsey and his colleagues (Kinsey, Pomeroy, and Martin 1948, 636–659) rates people on a range from 0 (exclusively heterosexual) to 6 (exclusively homosexual). Later they added another category for asexuality (someone who is not sexually active or is not sexually attracted to other people). Kinsey and colleagues found that people's sexual orientation may be flexible or fluid, changing over time. A person may be completely heterosexual at one time in her or his life and bisexual or homosexual at another point. Table 3.1.7 shows the Kinsey Scale.

TABLE 3.1.7 **THE KINSEY HETEROSEXUAL-HOMOSEXUAL RATING SCALE**

0	Exclusively heterosexual
1	Predominantly heterosexual, only incidentally homosexual
2	Predominantly heterosexual, but more than incidentally homosexual
3	Equally heterosexual and homosexual (**bisexual**)
4	Predominantly homosexual, but more than incidentally heterosexual
5	Predominantly homosexual, only incidentally heterosexual
6	Exclusively homosexual
x	Asexual

Source: Adapted from Kinsey, Pomeroy, and Martin (1948).

Do People Choose Their Sexual Orientation?

Most medical professionals and researchers now agree that people do not choose their sexual orientation. Sexual orientation is a complicated mixture of biology, psychology, and environmental factors. Some people disagree; they think that people are attracted to a **gay** lifestyle or choose to be gay. These people may believe that with enough willpower or the right kind of treatment, someone can change his or her sexual orientation. Usually these people focus on changing from a homosexual to a heterosexual orientation. However, more and more evidence shows that physiological factors, such as genes, hormones, and prenatal development, influence sexual orientation. Sexual orientation is not a choice.

Homophobia

Sometimes one's family, religion, culture, or the media convey attitudes that are homophobic. **Homophobia** is fear of or discrimination against homosexuals. Family members may be more or less accepting and understanding of sexual orientation. Some people believe that homosexuality is a choice or a lifestyle. These people may not understand about different sexual orientations. **Heterosexism** is presuming that everyone is heterosexual and that anyone who isn't is strange, morally flawed, or somehow

WHAT PEOPLE ARE SAYING **TEEN OPINIONS ON SEXUAL ORIENTATION**

Do you think sexual orientation is a choice or a lifestyle, or do you think a person's sexual orientation is already set at birth?

- "I think sexual orientation is biological." KG, age 19, Texas
- "I believe it is an orientation you are born with, mostly because I don't understand why anyone would make their own life so hard by *choosing* to be gay." KK, age 19, Kentucky
- "Sexuality is a continuum, and everyone falls in between the two extremes. It isn't a lifestyle, it isn't a choice, and there is little evidence that it is biological in origin—it's just who you happen to be, and if you prefer one type of genitalia over the other then that's your preference." ES, age 20, California
- "You're born with it. The stereotypes come with being part of the culture and wanting to fit in. It's part of being in a group. There's no real gay or straight though. Just lots of in-between." GBH, age 17, California

different than the norm. Just as homophobia may be behind hate crimes and more blatant and obvious discrimination against LGBT (**lesbian**, gay, bisexual, or **transgender**) people, heterosexism may underlie more subtle types of discrimination. For example, assuming on school forms that a student has two parents, one father and one mother, is a form of heterosexism. This does not consider a student with same-sex parents (two mothers or two fathers). Also, asking a boy if he has a girlfriend (or a girl if she has a boyfriend) is making an assumption that "normal" boys will be attracted to girls (and vice versa); this attitude doesn't allow LGBT people to just be themselves without feeling a need to explain or make excuses for who they are.

Sometimes an LGBT individual will be pressured by family or a religious congregation to deny or change sexual orientation. Interventions designed to change someone's sexual orientation to heterosexuality are known as **reparative therapy** or orientation change therapy. Reparative therapies use many techniques, including aversive conditioning, hypnosis, prayer, camps, peer therapy, and electric shocks. Many of the organizations that support change therapy programs or camps are sponsored or run by religious groups that oppose homosexuality. There are even 12-step programs for people who want to change their sexual orientation (Homosexuals Anonymous). While some people who complete reparative therapies claim that they have changed their sexual orientation, many people who undergo the therapy develop confused roles and identities or develop other mental health or substance use problems. Some people who have attempted to deny or change their sexual orientation have suffered harm, including lowered self-esteem, depression, or suicide attempts.

When people's sexual orientation clashes with their family values or religious beliefs, they may experience fear, distress, or conflict about their sexual orientation. People who experience internal conflict because they feel same-sex attraction but believe that they should be heterosexual may speak or behave in homophobic ways. This is known as internalized homophobia. Internalized homophobia may result in denial of one's own feelings, attempts to assert or prove one's masculinity (for men) or femininity (for women) or demonstrate heterosexual behavior, or self-hatred. Internalized homophobia can be a serious problem and may lead to:

- Acceptance of discriminatory behavior or abusive treatment
- Distrust, loneliness, isolation
- Impaired sexual functioning
- Unsafe sex
- Addictions
- Eating disorders
- Lack of self-worth
- Domestic violence
- Mental health issues
- Suicide

Research on the effectiveness of reparative therapy is inconclusive. Many people consider reparative or orientation change therapies to be coercive and unethical. In fact, the ethical codes of many professional therapy organizations such as the American Psychological Association and the National Association of Social Workers specifically prohibit therapists from performing reparative therapy. In some states, a therapist who advocates for or practices change therapies can lose his or her professional license.

Homosexuality used to be considered a mental health disorder in the United States but no longer is. In 1973, the American Psychiatric Association removed homosexuality from its official list of mental health disorders, the *Diagnostic and Statistical Manual of Mental Disorders* (*DSM*). Other professional organizations such as the American Psychological

Association and American Medical Association have also issued statements affirming that homosexuality and bisexuality do not constitute mental illness or emotional instability (Advocates for Youth 2008).

In a community that is extremely accepting of LGBT individuals and families, a teen might feel pressured to be gay in order to fit in with family or friends. A teen may be attracted to stereotypes of gay people as depicted on television or in movies. However, just as someone who is homosexual cannot magically change her or his sexual orientation, a heterosexual person cannot just decide to be homosexual. The term "metrosexual" has been used to describe heterosexual men or boys who spend a lot of time and money on shopping, clothes, and personal appearance. The term has sometimes been used to refer to boys or men who reject a traditional masculine gender role, sometimes adopting stereotypically homosexual fashions or mannerisms.

People may have different motivations for wanting to have a particular sexual orientation. For example, a girl or woman who has a history of negative experiences with men—such as having been sexually abused—might feel uncomfortable or afraid of men and might feel more comfortable being intimate within a lesbian relationship. Someone with this experience may try to persuade other girls or women that they would be happier in a lesbian relationship.

Gender Identity

Gender identity is the gender that one identifies with. Gender identity is not necessarily the same as sex. **Biological sex** is generally determined at birth. Most boys have male anatomy; they are biologically male, and their biological sex is male. Most girls are biologically female. However, gender is not a biological sex. Rather, gender is a sense of one's maleness or masculinity, one's femaleness or femininity. Masculinity is a feeling or sense of being male. Femininity is a feminine feeling, a sense of being female.

The Masculinity-Femininity Spectrum

Masculinity and femininity occur along a spectrum, or range (see figure 3.1.4). For example, some girls feel extremely feminine and may like many typically girly things, while others may be more like tomboys—girls who tend to like activities or clothes that boys typically enjoy. Similarly, there may be extremely masculine boys and boys who identify less with the extreme. Toward the center of the spectrum is androgyny. Androgyny is the quality of being or feeling neither specifically masculine nor feminine.

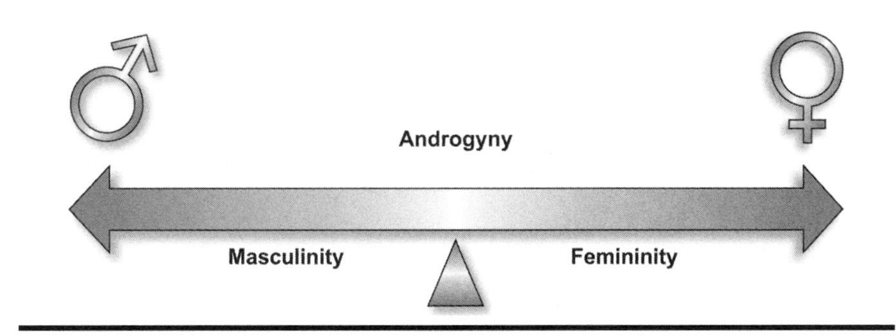

FIGURE 3.1.4 **MASCULINITY-FEMININITY SPECTRUM.**
(Yvette Malamud Ozer, 2012)

Gender Roles and Socialization

Individuals are socialized to a gender by society, culture, and their parents. There are certain expectations that go along with being a boy or a girl, including what colors people think are appropriate for boys (blue) and girls (pink), toys, clothes and shoes, hairstyles, activities, and behaviors. Boys may be expected to be active and loud and play with trucks. Girls might be expected to play with dolls, enjoy quieter activities, and wear jewelry and makeup. Boys and girls may be expected to display different feelings. Typical gender roles may suggest that it is okay for girls to cry but not okay for boys or that it isn't okay for girls to express angry feelings. These are all types of gender roles and expectations.

Gender roles and stereotypes may also influence academic performance. For example, if children are told that girls are not good at math and teachers don't expect girls to be good at math, some girls may not even try to do well in math. Because so many people—parents, teachers, children—believe this myth that girls are not good at math, fewer girls believe in themselves, and some end up not doing as well as boys in math. This means that fewer women specialize in math and the sciences in college, and fewer women have careers in these areas. Fewer women represented in math- and science-related careers keeps the stereotype going. Although there have been some improvements in recent years—more girls and women being encouraged to pursue studies and careers in math and the sciences—the stereotype persists. There are other gender roles and stereotypes, such as what boys' and girls' abilities are, what careers they should pursue, and who should be responsible for which household chores and child-rearing tasks.

Sometimes gender roles can cause confusion or distress or can limit someone's goals or ideas about themselves and their future. For example, some girls may perform poorly in school because they have been told that attractive girls are not smart (or smart girls are not attractive). Parents or peers may feel that pink is an inappropriate color for boys or men to wear. Gender roles and stereotypes may influence a teen's self-image, self-esteem, and choices about what to wear, what activities to pursue, and how to behave.

Transgender

Most people's gender identity—their feeling of masculinity or femininity—matches their biological sex, or anatomy. However, there are individuals who are born with a biological sex that does not match their gender identity. A person with a gender identity that is not the same as their biological sex is transgender. Transgender individuals typically feel as if they have been born in the wrong kind of body. A transgender individual may be born into a female body but feel male. This person might feel uncomfortable, as if the body is all wrong—it should be a male body. The person's biological sex is female, but gender identity is male.

Some transgender individuals have felt different since they were children; other people start to feel different or uncomfortable about their gender around puberty. This discomfort can cause confusion and emotional conflict. This may be especially true if there are strong family or cultural expectations around gender roles. Some transgender individuals decide to physically change their bodies to match their gender identity. This can be done by taking hormones or through surgery. Physically transitioning to another gender can be a long, expensive, and complicated process. Some people choose not to change their bodies physically but to dress and live their lives in line with their gender identity, including changing their names. This can be especially complicated for someone who has been raised or has been living as one gender, then transitions to another gender in the same family, school, job, or community. Friends, family members, and coworkers may not know how to respond to someone who has a new name and appearance.

People who are born as biological males and have a female gender identity are sometimes referred to as male-to-female (**MTF**), while people born biologically female who have a male gender identity are known as female-to-male (**FTM**). Gender identity is not the same as sexual orientation. A transgender person may be heterosexual, homosexual, or bisexual, depending on whether the person is romantically attracted to men or women. Dressing in clothes usually associated with people of the opposite gender is known as cross-dressing. Not everyone who cross-dresses is

? **Did You Know?**

Transgender Tips

- *If you don't know what pronouns to use, ask. Politely and respectfully.* Respect transgender individuals' gender by referring to them by their chosen name and using the appropriate gender pronoun. Don't refer to someone as having had a different gender in the past (e.g., "when you used to be a man") because many transgender people feel that they have always been their true gender. Don't refer to a transgender person using derogatory terms such as "trannie" or "shemale."
- *Don't make assumptions about a trans person's sexual orientation.* Gender identity is different from sexual orientation, which describes whom one is attracted to. A transgender person may identify as gay, straight, bisexual, pansexual, or asexual.
- *Don't assume that a transgender person takes hormones, has had surgery, or plans to have surgery.* Some transgender individuals choose to use medical technology to change their bodies. Others wish to be recognized as their gender of choice without surgery or hormones.
- *Don't be afraid to ask, except . . .* It's fine to ask some questions. Most people are okay answering questions that aren't too personal. It's not okay to ask someone about genitals, surgeries, or former names.
- *Respect a transgender person's privacy.* Just because someone has come out to you as transgender doesn't mean that it's okay for everyone to know. **Outing someone** who has not given you permission is not okay.
- *Don't just say you're an ally!* A lot of people like to say that they're LGBT allies without doing the work. People need to examine their own gender stereotypes and **transphobia** and be willing to stand up and advocate for trans people.

Source: Adapted from Lurie (2009); WikiHow (2011).

transgender. Some people just like to dress up. A transvestite is someone who cross-dresses for emotional gratification or sexual reasons. Transgender individuals are more likely to cross-dress because it is in line with their gender identity, not for any type of sexual gratification.

Health experts have many theories about what may cause someone to be transgender. It may be a combination of factors such as biology, psychology, and the environment. As with sexual orientation, being transgender is not a personal choice.

? Did You Know?

In 1998, a transgender woman named Rita Hester was murdered because of her gender identity. Her murder is still unsolved. Each year on November 20, many communities around the world mark the day by organizing activities and candlelight vigils to remember the many people who have been killed because of fear or hate of their gender identity.

According to statistics from the International Transgender Day of Remembrance (TDoR) website, in 2008 at least 45 people were murdered worldwide because of their actual or suspected gender identity. TDoR knows of 151 people murdered in 2009 and 22 murdered in 2010.

Source: International Transgender Day of Remembrance (2010).

Transgender Challenges and Support

Transgender people face many challenges, including how to come out (reveal their gender identities to friends and families). Transgender people may face discrimination in housing and employment and may experience bullying at school. People who are uncomfortable or don't understand transgender identity may feel angry and may reject a transgender person. Transgender teens may experience bullying, rejection, or unfair treatment from teachers, friends, or family members. These conflicts may make a transgender teen feel isolated, anxious, or depressed.

There are different types of support for transgender people. Some communities have advocacy and support groups for transgender individuals. Some organizations that began as groups of family, friends, and allies of gay people have expanded to include support for all **sexual or gender minority** individuals. For example, some high schools have GSAs (gay-straight alliances), which support transgender individuals. PFLAG (Parents, Family, and Friends of Lesbians and Gays) also promotes the health of transgender individuals.

Intersex

Intersex describes a variety of conditions in which a person is born with reproductive or sexual anatomy that doesn't appear to fit typical definitions of male or female. A person might look male on the outside (have genitals that appear male) while having some female anatomy on the inside. Someone might be born with chromosomes that don't match their outward appearance.

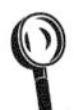

CASE STUDY **INTERVIEW WITH AMBER: TRANSGENDER DISCRIMINATION AND SOURCES OF SUPPORT**

Please share a little background about yourself:

I'm currently 24 years old, and I work as a software engineer for a California company. I went to college in southern California and graduated in 2010 with a BS degree. Before that, I went to high school in Indiana. I started presenting as female during my final year of college.

Have you experienced discrimination because of your transgender status?

For the past few months I've been involved in a lawsuit against a government agency and an employee of that agency who had misused my personal information to harass me due to my trans status. That lawsuit was recently settled, with part of the settlement being a stipulation for better employee training. It's been a somewhat grueling process, but in the end, it was worth it. The takeaway lesson here is that if you are treated wrongly, speaking up about it is not worthless, nor hopeless—you can help make things better for everyone.

How have you been affected by typical gender roles, beliefs, and expectations?

I didn't really wind up running into any significant amount of trouble with gender roles until around high school. High school was when more general societal beliefs started to take over—the social interactions and expectations kick themselves up a notch when you hit that general grade range, and I wound up just trying to tune it out as best I could. I kept to the friends who I enjoyed being with, most of whom also didn't really put much stock in the clique-y atmosphere.

What sources of support have you found most valuable?

A few close, accepting friends in college have gone a long way. At the end of the day, knowing that I had someone I could go to who would be willing to listen helped immensely.

School LGBT groups have also been useful for the simple purpose of realizing that I'm not alone. It can seem really, really lonely when it feels like no one else can relate, but in reality there are often people who can, you just haven't realized it yet.

What advice would you give to a high school student who is trans or is an ally?

- **To those who are trans:** Yes, it can be really scary to tell your friends that you're trans. Do it anyway. Seriously. They will be more supportive than you think, especially those closest to you. Having people who you don't have to hide yourself from is so amazingly wonderful and will make your life so much better.
- **To those who would be allies:** If you really want to make things better on a personal level, start with the small things: if someone makes a bigoted joke, call them on it. If someone messes up pronouns, remind them (politely).

People inherit chromosomes from both parents. Most boys are born with one X chromosome and one Y chromosome, which combine to make an XY (typically male) chromosome. Most girls have two X chromosomes (one from each parent), which combine into an XX chromosome or **karyotype**. A karyotype is a picture of the chromosomes in a cell; it refers to the number, position, and size of the chromosomes in a cell. A typical girl would have 22 pairs of matched chromosomes plus two X chromosomes, with a karyotype of 46,XX.

Usually people with XY chromosomes are exposed to hormones and other processes before and after birth that cause them to grow into boys. Most people with XX chromosomes develop into girls. Some of the developmental changes don't kick in until puberty, at which time the body produces more hormones and undergoes rapid changes, leading to sexual maturity. Because many changes don't take place until puberty, a person doesn't find out about being intersex until puberty. For example, a person may be born looking like a girl and be raised as a girl. Then at puberty, male hormones start changing the appearance of the person to that of a boy.

Types of Intersex Conditions

There are many different intersex conditions and terms, some of which are described in the following sections. More information can be found at the Intersex Society of North America website listed in the resources section at the end of this chapter.

5-Alpha-Reductase Deficiency

A deficiency in 5-alpha-reductase (5ARD), an enzyme, allows a baby to develop as a girl. However, at puberty, testosterone production increases and causes **virilization** (developing masculine characteristics).

Androgen Insensitivity Syndrome (AIS)

In an individual with complete AIS, the body's cells are unable to respond to androgen (male hormones). A newborn AIS infant has genitals of normal female appearance, undescended or partially descended testes, and usually a short vagina with no cervix. At puberty, the testes are stimulated by the pituitary gland and produce testosterone, which is converted back to estrogen in the bloodstream, causing breast growth. Most AIS women have little or no pubic or underarm hair. AIS women do not menstruate (have periods) and are **infertile** (cannot get pregnant).

Aphallia

Aphallia means being born without a penis in a person with otherwise typical male anatomy.

Clitoromegaly

Clitoromegaly describes a larger-than-expected clitoris. The most common cause is probably congenital adrenal hyperplasia (CAH).

Congenital Adrenal Hyperplasia (CAH)

CAH, the most prevalent cause of intersex among people with XX chromosomes, is the only intersex condition that presents a medical emergency for newborns. The adrenal glands have difficulty making cortisone (a steroid) and produce high levels of virilizing hormones. This causes an XX baby to have a larger-than-average clitoris, a clitoris that looks like a penis, or labia that looks like a scrotum. Masculinization continues after birth and may cause the person to develop dense body hair, a receding hairline, a deep voice, and prominent muscles. Metabolic problems may upset sodium balance. CAH effects can be counteracted with cortisone, but cortisone has side effects and long-term health risks.

In XY individuals, CAH does not cause ambiguous genitalia but does require medical attention because of health problems. If untreated, CAH may cause boys to have puberty much earlier than other boys. This can interfere with them growing taller, and they may end up as very short adults. Because of early puberty, boys with CAH may have strong sexual thoughts and desires much earlier than other children their age.

Hypospadias

Hypospadias is a very common condition in which the urethral meatus ("pee-hole") is located along the underside of the penis instead of at the tip.

Klinefelter Syndrome

Men with Klinefelter syndrome inherit an extra X chromosome from one parent. Their karyotype is 47,XXY. Boys with Klinefelter are usually born with male genitals that look like other boys, although the testes are small and quite firm. At puberty, they may not virilize very strongly—they may not develop much body hair or may experience breast development. The ejaculate contains no sperm.

Micropenis

Micropenis is a term used by doctors to describe a typical penis that is very small.

MRKH (Mayer Rokitansky Kuster Hauser Syndrome)

MRKH is also known as Mullerian agenesis, vaginal agenesis, and congenital absence of vagina. In MRKH ovaries are present, but the uterus is absent, misshapen, or small. The vagina is absent. MRKH is associated with kidney and spine anomalies in a minority of individuals. MRKH is usually diagnosed between the ages of 15 and 18, after a young woman has not had her first period (Center for Young Women's Health 2009).

Ovotestes

Ovotestes (formerly called true hermaphroditism) are sex glands (gonads) that contain both ovarian and testicular tissue. A person might be born with two ovotestes, with one ovary and one ovotestes, or some other combination. If the ovotestes contain testicular tissue, there is an increased risk of gonadal cancer. Some people with ovotestes look fairly typically female, some look typically male, and some have genital development that is somewhere in between.

Partial Androgen Insensitivity Syndrome (PAIS)

PAIS in 46,XY individuals typically results in ambiguous genitalia. There may be a large clitoris or a small hypospadic penis. PAIS may cause infertility in some men with typical male genitals.

Swyer Syndrome (XY gonadal dysgenesis)

A person with Swyer syndrome is born without functional gonads (sex glands). Instead the person has gonadal streaks, which are minimally developed gonad tissue in place of testes or ovaries. A child born with Swyer looks like a typical female. She will not enter puberty or develop most secondary sex characteristics without hormone replacement therapy.

Turner Syndrome

People with Turner syndrome have only one functional X chromosome, sometimes referred to as 45,XO or 45,X karyotype. The typical female karyotype is 46,XX. With Turner syndrome, female sex characteristics are present but underdeveloped compared to typical females. Women with Turner syndrome may have short stature, lymphedema (swelling of hands and feet), a broad chest and widely spaced nipples, a low hairline, low-set ears, and infertility.

Virilization

Virilization is the process by which someone develops male or masculine characteristics such as a deep voice and facial hair. Androgens or male hormones usually cause virilization.

How Common Are Intersex Conditions?

Since not everyone agrees on what counts as an intersex condition and since not everyone who has an intersex condition is identified, it is hard to estimate how common intersex conditions are. One study estimates that 1 in 100 (1 percent) of people have bodies that differ from the standard male or female bodies. Table 3.1.8 shows some other approximations for various intersex conditions.

Treatment of Intersex Conditions

Some intersex people are born with genitals that don't appear to fit what people think of as typical. For example, a boy might be born with a very

TABLE 3.1.8 **ESTIMATED FREQUENCY OF INTERSEX CONDITIONS**

Intersex Condition	Estimated Number
Late onset adrenal hyperplasia	1 in 66 individuals (1.52%)
Hypospadias	1 in 770 (0.13%) to 2,000 (0.05%) births
Klinefelter (XXY)	1 or 2 in 1,000 births (0.1–0.2%)
Not XX and not XY	1 in 1,666 births (0.06%)
Vaginal agenesis	1 in 6,000 births (0.02%)
Androgen insensitivity syndrome (AIS)	1 in 13,000 births (0.01%)
Classical congenital adrenal hyperplasia (CAH)	1 in 13,000 births (0.01%)
Ovotestes	1 in 83,000 births
Idiopathic (no discernable medical cause)	1 in 110,000 births
Partial androgen insensitivity syndrome (PAIS)	1 in 130,000 births
Complete gonadal dysgenesis	1 in 150,000 births

Source: Blackless et al. (2000).

small penis, or a girl might be born with a very large clitoris. If doctors are uncomfortable or unsure whether the child is a boy or a girl, the doctor might try to persuade the parents to do surgery to make the child's genitals look more like typical boy or girl genitals. Historically (especially in the United States), many people who were born with genitals that didn't look typical were given cosmetic surgery as infants and children. Many people who were subjected to these surgeries as infants and children have experienced serious side effects and life problems as a result of the surgeries. After growing up, some people realized that they did not feel like the gender that was imposed on them. However, after having been subjected to surgeries and hormones, they have few options to remedy the situation. Other people have had physical problems, including infections, constant pain, sexual dysfunction, and lack of ability to enjoy sex or have an orgasm. The most humane approach when a baby is born with ambiguous genitals is to raise the baby as a boy or a girl but not to perform any unnecessary cosmetic surgery on an infant or child. Only surgery that is medically necessary for the health of the child should be performed. Then, after puberty, the intersex individual will be able to choose if he or she wants to undergo surgery. It is best for people to be able to consider all the options—including possible risks and benefits—and make an informed decision for themselves (Intersex Society of North America 2008).

Intersex versus Gender Identity or Sexual Orientation

Intersex is not the same as transgender. People who are transgender have a gender identity that does not match the biological sex of the body with which they were born. For example, a transgender man may have been born with a typical female body and may choose to have surgery or take hormones so that his physical body will match his gender identity. Intersex people, on the other hand, have anatomy that is not typically male or female. Intersex people are noticeably externally physically different from typical males and females. Transgender individuals have an internal feeling of their body not matching their gender identity. There are some similarities, in that both intersex and transgender people may take hormones or have surgery to change their physical appearance or function. But they make these changes for different reasons. An intersex person is not automatically any particular sexual orientation. An intersex individual may be heterosexual, homosexual, bisexual, or asexual (Intersex Society of North America 2008).

Puberty in Intersex Individuals

Depending on what intersex condition an individual has, puberty may follow the pattern of typical boys or girls, or there may be some differences.

? Did You Know?

In Greek mythology, Hermaphroditus was the child of Aphrodite and Hermes. Born a boy, Hermaphroditus was transformed into a being with male and female characteristics by the water nymph Salmacus. Hermaphroditus has been depicted in Greek and Roman art as a female figure with male genitals and is sometimes considered a minor god of bisexuality and fertility.

Intersex people born with a combination of male and female genitals, or ambiguous genitals, have historically been referred to as hermaphrodites. This is misleading, as it implies that someone is both fully female and fully male. Use of the word "hermaphrodite" to refer to intersex people is stigmatizing. It is preferable to use the term "intersex" when referring to a group of people with intersex conditions or to use the name of a specific intersex condition. When describing someone, it is best to describe the person first rather than referring to the person's gender, sexual orientation, ethnicity, or other characteristic or group membership.

Source: Intersex Society of North America (2008).

Some individuals may not realize that they have an intersex condition until puberty—their parents may not know either. Some intersex individuals may not develop some secondary sexual characteristics, such as genital and underarm hair. Some may have delayed development of breasts or deepening of the voice. Others may experience puberty very early, leading to sexual development and hair growth and a strong sex drive years before their peers experience these things. This can lead to teasing by peers and misunderstanding by adults. Developmental changes in intersex conditions may also affect growth, with some individuals ending up extremely short and some growing up to be extremely tall. Some girls with intersex conditions may not menstruate (have periods).

Some intersex individuals may be infertile (unable to reproduce). Infertility may be a source of sadness, stress, or grief for some people who want to have their own children. Depending on the intersex condition an individual has, how the person's parents and doctors have handled the intersex condition, and many other factors, intersex people have to deal with a variety of challenges. People who have intersex conditions with medical complications or who were given surgery as infants or children may have to contend with pain or physical problems. Some people with intersex conditions have to take medications such as hormones or steroids their whole lives. People whose appearance is different from typical males and females may feel shame or embarrassment, especially if they've had to keep their condition secret their whole lives. People who look different may be teased, harassed, or bullied. This can get particularly difficult in schools when kids have to share bathrooms or change and take showers in locker rooms. It can be helpful for intersex individuals and their families to seek support from other people who are dealing with similar issues. There are some organizations that provide support or advocate for people with a variety of intersex conditions and some organizations that support people with specific conditions (for example, Turner syndrome or CAH). The resources section lists several of these organizations.

Coming Out

Coming out is a process in which an **LGBTQI** (lesbian, gay, bisexual, transgender, **queer** or **questioning**, intersex) person discloses his or her sexual orientation or gender identity to family, friends, or the community (at school or work). Someone who has not come out (disclosed) his or her sexual orientation or gender identity is referred to as **in the closet**. The coming-out process can be accompanied by fear, anxiety, and stress. It can be especially challenging in a community or family that is not tolerant or understanding of LGBT people or issues or where there is blatant homophobia or heterosexism. It may be difficult if the LGBT person is a member of a religion or family that views homosexuality or nontypical gender as a sin, a form of mental illness, or a moral weakness.

A person who is considering coming out is already feeling vulnerable about revealing her or his true identity to others. It may seem scary to publicly come out in a school where LGBT people are teased or bullied. It can be very threatening to come out in a community where LGBT people have been subjected to hate crimes or discrimination.

What if parents don't understand and try to invalidate an LGBT person's reality? For example, a parent might tell a teen that he is just going through a phase, that he doesn't really know what he wants, or that he'll grow out of it. What if members of one's peer group don't understand and no longer want to be friends or do things together? Adolescents may already be questioning their own religious and spiritual beliefs as part of developing their own identities and values, a natural part of growing up. Teens may fear their emerging feelings about sexuality and attraction; they may be concerned that coming out may be upsetting. It may be upsetting to the family to challenge several family values, beliefs, or expectations at the same time about religion, sexual orientation, gender identity, or politics.

When deciding when to come out, a teen must also consider whom to come out to. It might make sense to discuss the issue with a close friend who is tolerant and nonjudgmental and accepts people for who they are.

It may also help to be a member of a community that is accepting and supportive of LGBT people. Some religious congregations make a point of being welcoming and inclusive of LGBT people. Some schools have GSAs—clubs that support LGBT students, families, and their allies. Certain teachers, school counselors or school psychologists, or other school personnel make it known that they are supportive of LGBT people. Teachers and other school staff may display a Safe Space sticker to indicate that they are available to support LGBT students. Safe Space stickers vary, but they are usually rainbow-colored and shaped like inverted triangles.

LGBT students may become stressed, depressed, or suicidal because of bullying, teasing, discrimination, and hate crimes. This can be exacerbated by feelings of loneliness, isolation, and rejection by friends or family. The Trevor Project works to reduce rates of suicide among LGBT teens and to provide support for teens who are thinking of coming out or have recently come out. The Trevor Project, listed in the resources section at the end of this chapter, provides resources for teens and provides crisis intervention services, including a 24-hour crisis lifeline, a text messaging service to chat with volunteers, and ways to connect with other youths.

What the Heck Does LGBTQI Stand For?

Various initialisms are used to represent identities or orientations on the spectrum of sexual orientation and gender identity. Whereas an **acronym** combines the first letters of several words into a single pronounceable word (such as "radar" or "snafu"), an **initialism** is an abbreviation formed from the initial letters of each word in a phrase. Some of the initialisms that represent the sexual orientation–gender identity spectrum are LG, GLBT, LGBT, LGBTQI, and LGBTQQIA. So what do all these letters stand for? L stands for lesbian, G for gay, B for bisexual, T for transgender or transsexual, Q for queer or questioning, I for intersex, and A for asexual or ally (Advocates for Youth 2008; GLSEN 2009).

LGB: Sexual Orientations

The first two letters in this part of the initialism stand for lesbian (L) and gay (G), both same-sex sexual orientations. The B stands for bisexual, another sexual orientation.

T: Gender Identity

T stands for transgender. Transgender is a gender identity rather than a sexual orientation. Someone who is transgender has a gender identity that is different from her or his original biological sex. Some people who are transgender transition to the gender with which they identify through use of hormones and/or sexual reassignment surgery.

People who refer to themselves as **genderqueer** may consider their gender to be fluid (changing) or consider themselves genderless (without gender). The terms "genderqueer" and "**pansexual**" may also apply to someone who is attracted to people across the gender spectrum, including people who are male, female, trans, or androgynous.

Q: Questioning or Queer

The word "queer" used to be a derogatory and insulting term referring to LGBT people. More recently, some people in the LGBT community have reclaimed it as a term of pride. A queer family may be a family with LGBT parents or children. Some people still feel that the term is derogatory, similar to terms like "dyke" or "fag."

Questioning describes the identity of a person who is unsure of his or her sexual orientation or gender identity.

I: Intersex

The letter "I," which stands for intersex, is sometimes included in the LGBTQI initialism. However, intersex is neither a sexual orientation nor a gender identity. The term "intersex" is used for a variety of conditions in which a person is born with reproductive or sexual anatomy that doesn't appear the same as typical male or female anatomy. Genitals or features may be ambiguous (not clearly male or female), or the intersex individual may have a combination of male and female characteristics. Intersex conditions may affect chromosomes, genitals, or secondary sexual characteristics.

A: Asexual or Ally

The "A" that sometimes appears in the LGBTQIA initialism can stand for asexual, or it can stand for ally. Asexuality refers to a person who is not sexually active or someone who is not sexually attracted to other people. Some adults who are not sexually attracted to other people describe their sexual orientation as asexual or describe themselves as not having any sexual orientation. Because of differences in rates of maturity and hormone levels, it is typical for some teens to have a great deal of sex drive (libido) and other teens to have very little or none. Most teens who do not engage in sexual activities because of little or no sex drive or attraction would probably consider themselves abstinent rather than asexual.

The term "ally" represents someone who is an ally, friend, or supporter to a person or people who fall somewhere on the LGBTQI spectrum. Some schools have gay-straight alliances (GSAs) that welcome allies or supporters of LGBTQI individuals. A school with an active GSA with lots of allies can help create a more welcoming and inclusive environment.

There are many advocacy and support groups for families, friends, and allies of LGBTQI individuals. Some of these include PFLAG, COLAGE, and Our Family Coalition. See the resources section for more organizations that support LGBTQI individuals, their families, and allies.

Allies are important to improving tolerance and acceptance of LGBTQI people in schools, workplaces, and the community. It is not only important for an LGBTQI student to feel safe and welcomed in school. There may also be students who have LGBTQI parents or siblings as well as LGBTQI teachers or other school personnel. Groups that advocate for LGBTQI rights in society are attempting to create a safe society that is free of discrimination where hate crimes and bullying based on gender identity or sexual orientation are not tolerated.

Resources

Websites, Help Lines, and Hotlines

About Kids Health. How the Body Works: Sexual Differentiation
Interactive explanations and diagrams of sexual differentiation, including genital development, male and female genital anatomy, puberty in boys and girls; descriptions of several intersex conditions: http://www.aboutkidshealth.ca/HowTheBodyWorks/Sexual-Differentiation.aspx?articleID=6850&categoryID=XS-nh3

AIS Support Group
Support group and resources for people with Androgen Insensitivity Syndrome (AIS), an intersex condition: http://www.aissg.org/

Asexual Visibility and Education Network (AVEN)
An informational resource for people who are asexual and questioning: http://www.asexuality.org/home/overview.html

Bright Pink
Breast Self Exam: http://www.bebrightpink.org/programs/support-community/breast-self-exam-email-reminder/

Center for Young Women's Health (Children's Hospital Boston)
A Guide to Using Your First Tampon: http://www.youngwomenshealth.org/tampon.html

Coalition for Positive Sexuality (CPS)
A site for teens who are sexually active or thinking about having a sexual relationship; information about decision making, contraception, STDs, and pregnancy: http://www.positive.org/

COLAGE
National movement of children, youths, and adults with one or more LGBTQ parent(s); builds community and works toward social justice through youth empowerment, leadership development, education, and advocacy: http://www.colage.org/about/

Community United Against Violence (CUAV)
A multicultural antioppression organization working to end violence against and within diverse LGBT and questioning communities: www.cuav.org/

Gender Equity Resource Center
LGBT Resources; definition of terms: http://geneq.berkeley.edu/lgbt_resources_definiton_of_terms#asexual

GLSEN (Gay, Lesbian, & Straight Education Network)
Safe Space programs for schools, including free downloadable Safe Space posters and stickers. Resources for LGBT students, their allies, and their families, including support to create a school GSA: http://www.glsen.org/

Go Ask Alice! Columbia University
Health Q&A Service. Information about alcohol and other drugs, fitness and nutrition, emotional health, general health, sexuality, sexual health, and relationships: http://www.goaskalice.columbia.edu/

Human Rights Campaign (HRC): Transgender Day of Remembrance
Information about the national Transgender Day of Remembrance to mark the passing of transgender or those perceived to be transgender individuals who have been murdered because of hate: http://www.hrc.org/issues/transgender_day_of_remembrance.asp

I Wanna Know! American Sexual Health Association (ASHA)
Information about sexual health, relationships, LGBT, pregnancy, and parenthood: www.iwannaknow.org

International Transgender Day of Remembrance
Information about transgender day of remembrance events; statistics about murders and hate crimes against transgender people: http://www.transgenderdor.org/

Intersex Society of North America (ISNA)
http://www.isna.org

Frequently Asked Questions: http://www.isna.org/faq/

Lou Sullivan Society (FTMSF)
Serving the female-to-male (FTM) transgender community: http://www.ftmi.org

Love Is Not Abuse
Information, resources, and quiz to test one's knowledge about teen dating violence: http://loveisnotabuse.com/

Love Is Respect
National Dating Abuse Helpline, a community with support, resources, and information to understand dating abuse: http://www.loveisrespect.org/

MRKH Organization, Inc.
Resources and support for women with MRKH (aka Mullerian agenesis, vaginal agenesis, congenital absence of vagina), an intersex condition: http://www.mrkh.org/

National Dating Abuse Helpline
1-866-331-9474

TTY: 1-866-331-8453

National Gay and Lesbian Task Force (NGLTF)
LGBT issues, public policy, and advocacy: http://thetaskforce.org/

National Transgender Advocacy Coalition (NTAC)
Information on transgender rights, issues, resources, and advocacy: http://www.ntac.org/

Our Family Coalition
Promotes the rights and well-being of LGBT families through education, advocacy, social networking, and grassroots community organizing: http://www.ourfamily.org/

PFLAG (Parents, Families, and Friends of Lesbians and Gays)
A resource for families and friends of LGBT individuals: http://community.pflag.org/

Planned Parenthood
Info for Teens: http://www.plannedparenthood.org/info-for-teens/our-bodies-33795.htm

Sex, Etc.
Sex education by teens and for teens; overseen in part by the Center for Psychology at Rutgers University and in service for 30 years: http://www.sexetc.org/topic/emotional_health

Sex Info SF
A sexual health text messaging program for San Francisco youths: http://www.isis-inc.org/sexinfo.php

Sexuality Information and Education Council of the United States (SIECUS)
A nonprofit with access to accurate information on sex and sexual health: http://www.siecus.org/

TeensHealth from Nemours
Information for teens in English and Spanish about the body, the mind, physical and emotional health, relationships, drugs and alcohol, sexuality, and many other topics from the Nemours Foundation, which provides children's health information and care: http://teenshealth.org/teen/

Teen Source
Sexual health for youths to encourage informed decision making: http://www.teensource.org/

Teens in Charge (Chinese Community Health Resource Center)
Health topics in English, Chinese, and simplified Chinese. Topics include dating and relationships, diseases, emotional and sexual health, addiction and substance misuse, nutrition and fitness, and general health: http://www.teensincharge.org/en/health-topics

The Trevor Project
Suicide prevention and resources for LGBT youths, including a 24-hour crisis intervention phone line and suicide prevention resources: http://www.thetrevorproject.org/

866-4-U-TREVOR (1-866-488-7386)

Turner Syndrome Society of the United States
Support and resources for girls and women with Turner syndrome: http://www.turnersyndrome.org/

We Are Talking/Teen Health (Palo Alto Medical Foundation)
Health information for teens: http://www.pamf.org/teen/

Youth Resource
Information on sexual health for gay, lesbian, bisexual, transgender, and questioning youths: http://www.amplifyyourvoice.org/youthresource

Videos and Films

Ensler, Eve. 2006. *Beautiful Daughters*. LOGO TV: http://www.logotv.com/video/beautiful-daughters/1623325/playlist .jhtml. *A 46-minute video in which four transgender women confront the issues they face and how being cast in "The Vagina Monologues" allows them to address these issues in front of a mass audience.*

Gender Identity Project (GIP). *Transgender Basics*. LGBT Community Center, New York: http://www.gaycenter.org/gip/transbasics/video. *A 20-minute educational film on the concepts of gender and transgender people. Two providers from the Center's Gender Identity Project (GIP) discuss basic concepts of gender, sexual orientation, identity and gender roles. Three transgender community members share their personal experiences of being trans and genderqueer.*

Ward, Phyllis. 2000. *Is It a Boy or a Girl? A Discovery Channel Documentary on Medical Management of Children with Ambiguous Sex Anatomy*. Great Falls, VA: Discovery Channel. Cable broadcast. Broadcast March 26: http://www.isna.org/videos/purchase. *A one-hour documentary describing medical management of children with intersex conditions.*

Further Reading

Basso, Michael. 2003. *The Underground Guide to Teenage Sexuality*. 2nd ed. Minneapolis: Fairview.

Beam, Cris. 2011. *I Am J*. New York: Little, Brown. *Young adult novel about transgender teen.*

Corinna, Heather. 2007. *S.E.X.: The All-You-Need-to-Know Progressive Sexuality Guide to Get You through High School and College*. New York: Marlowe.

Eugenides, Jeffrey. 2002. *Middlesex: A Novel*. New York: Picador. *A novel about Callie, an intersex individual who starts life as a girl and starts developing male characteristics at age 14.*

Fausto-Sterling, Anne. 2000. *Sexing the Body: Gender Politics and the Construction of Sexuality*. New York: Basic Books.

Fine, Cordelia. 2010. *Delusions of Gender: How Our Minds, Society, and Neurosexism Create Difference*. New York: Norton.

Gowen, L. Kris. 2003. *Making Sexual Decisions: The Ultimate Teen Guide*. Lanham, MA: Scarecrow.

Hasler, Nikol. 2010. *Sex: A Book for Teens; An Uncensored Guide to Your Body, Sex, and Safety*. San Francisco: Zest Books.

Hirsch, Larissa. 2009. "Breast and Pelvic Exams." TeensHealth from Nemours. March. http://kidshealth.org/teen/sexual_health/girls/obgyn.html?tracking=T_RelatedArticle#.

Pascoe, C. J. 2007. *Dude, You're a Fag: Masculinity and Sexuality in High School.* Berkeley: University of California Press.

Rademeyer, Carol-Ann. 2007. "Intimate Body Jewelry in Women: A Piercing Inquiry." http://www.instituteofmidwifery.org/MSFinalProj.nsf/a9ee58d7a82396768525684f0056be8d/d6b2d59c5c2d20798525739400424ec0?OpenDocument.

Russell, Stephen T. 2010. "Contradictions and Complexities in the Lives of Lesbian, Gay, Bisexual, and Transgender Youth." *Prevention Researcher* 17(4): 3–6.

Rye, B. J., and Maureen T. B. Drysdale. 2009. *Taking Sides: Clashing Views in Adolescence.* New York: McGraw-Hill/Dushkin.

Taverner, William, and Ryan McKee. 2011. *Taking Sides: Clashing Views in Human Sexuality.* New York: McGraw-Hill/Dushkin.

U.S. Department of Health and Human Services. 2007. *Teen Survival Guide: Health Tips for On-the-go Girls.* http://www.womenshealth.gov/pub/TeenSurvivalGuide.pdf.

Weston, Carol. 2004. *Girltalk: All the Stuff Your Sister Never Told You.* 4th ed. New York: Harper Perennial.

References

Advocates for Youth. 2008. "Frequently Asked Questions about Sexual Orientation and Gender Identity." http://www.advocatesforyouth.org/lessonplans/index.php?option=com_content&task=view&id=606&Itemid=66.

Blackless, Melanie, Anthony Charuvastra, Amanda Derryck, Anne Fausto-Sterling, Karl Lauzanne, and Ellen Lee. 2000. "How Sexually Dimorphic Are We? Review and Synthesis." *American Journal of Human Biology* 12: 151–166. doi:10.1002/(SICI)1520-6300(200003/04)12:2<151::AID-AJHB1>3.0.CO;2-F.

Bright Pink. 2011. "Breast Self Exam." http://www.bebrightpink.org/programs/support-community/breast-self-exam-email-reminder/.

Brooks, Traci L., Elizabeth R. Woods, John R. Knight, and Lydia A. Shrier. 2003. "Body Modification and Substance Use in Adolescents: Is There a Link?" *Journal of Adolescent Health* 32(1): 44–49. doi:10.1016/S1054-139X(02)00446-9.

Carroll, Sean T., Robert H. Riffenburgh, Timothy A. Roberts, and Elizabeth B. Myhre. 2002. "Tattoos and Body Piercings as Indicators of Adolescent Risk-Taking Behaviors." *Pediatrics* 109(6): 1021–1027. doi:10.1542/peds.109.6.1021.

Center for Young Women's Health. 2009. "MRKH: A Guide for Parents and Guardians." Children's Hospital Boston. http://www.youngwomenshealth.org/mrkh_parent.html.

Chang, Louise. 2010. "Genital Piercings." WebMD. March 11. http://www.webmd.com/sex/genital-piercings.

Cleveland Clinic. 2011. "The Male Reproductive System." http://www.cchs.net/health/health-info/docs/2300/2376.asp.

DeLaet, Debra. 2009. "Framing Male Circumcision as a Human Rights Issue? Contributions to the Debate over the Universality of Human Rights." *Journal of Human Rights* 8(4): 405–426. doi:0.1080/14754830903324795.

Dowshen, Steven. 2008. "Is My Penis Normal?" TeensHealth from Nemours. August. http://kidshealth.org/teen/sexual_health/guys/penis.html#cat20016.

Dowshen, Steven. 2010. "Is It Normal to Get Erections?" TeensHealth from Nemours. May. http://kidshealth.org/teen/sexual_health/guys/normal_erections.html#cat20016.

Figueroa, T. Ernesto. 2009. "Testicular Exams." TeensHealth from Nemours. April. http://kidshealth.org/teen/sexual_health/guys/testicles.html#.

Figueroa, T. Ernesto. 2010. "Testicular Injuries." TeensHealth from Nemours. September. http://kidshealth.org/teen/sexual_health/guys/testicular_injuries.html#.

Gavin, Mary L. 2010. "All about Menstruation." TeensHealth from Nemours. October. http://kidshealth.org/teen/sexual_health/girls/menstruation.html#.

GLSEN. 2009. *Safe Space Kit: Guide to Being an Ally to LGBT Students.* New York: Gay, Lesbian and Straight Education Network. http://www.glsen.org/binary-data/GLSEN_ATTACHMENTS/file/000/001/1511-4.pdf.

Gowen, L. Kris. 2003. *Making Sexual Decisions: The Ultimate Teen Guide.* Lanham, MA: Scarecrow.

Haffner, Debra W. 2008. *Beyond the Big Talk: A Parent's Guide to Raising Sexually Healthy Teens from Middle School to High School and Beyond.* New York: Newmarket.

Hirsch, Larissa. 2009. "Can I Make My Breasts Larger?" TeensHealth from Nemours. May. http://kidshealth.org/teen/sexual_health/girls/larger_breasts.html#cat20015.

Hirsch, Larissa. 2010a. "Coping with Common Period Problems." TeensHealth from Nemours. September. http://kidshealth.org/teen/sexual_health/girls/menstrual_problems.html#.

Hirsch, Larissa. 2010b. "How to Perform a Breast Self-Examination." TeensHealth from Nemours. May. http://kidshealth.org/teen/sexual_health/girls/bse.html?tracking=T_RelatedArticle#.

Hirsch, Larissa. 2010c. "Irregular Periods." TeensHealth from Nemours. September. http://kidshealth.org/teen/sexual_health/girls/irregular_periods.html#.

Hirsch, Larissa. 2011. "Toxic Shock Syndrome." TeensHealth from Nemours. January. http://kidshealth.org/teen/sexual_health/girls/tss.html#cat20015.

InnerBody. 2011. "Male Reproductive System." http://www.innerbody.com/image/repmov.html.

International Transgender Day of Remembrance. 2010. "Statistics and Other Info." http://www.transgenderdor.org/?page_id=192.

Intersex Society of North America. 2008. "Frequently Asked Questions." http://www.isna.org/faq/conditions.

Kinsey, Alfred, Wardell Pomeroy, and Clyde Martin. 1948. *Sexual Behavior in the Human Male*. Philadelphia: W. B. Saunders.

Lurie, Samuel. 2009. "Action Steps for Being a Trans Ally." http://www.tgtrain.org/steps.html.

McGargill, Patricia. 2009. "Female Genital Mutilation." *On the Edge* 15(2) (Summer). http://www.iafn.org/displaycommon.cfm?an=1&subarticlenbr=336.

Men's Health Network. 2011. "Testicular Self-Examination." http://www.menshealthnetwork.org/library/tca.pdf.

Moser, Rod. 2006. "Ear and Other Piercings." WebMD. May 16. http://blogs.webmd.com/all-ears/2006/05/ear-and-other-piercings.html.

Neal, David T., and Tanya L. Chartrand. 2011. "Embodied Emotion Perception: Amplifying and Dampening Facial Feedback Modulates Emotion Perception Accuracy." *Social Psychological & Personality Science*, April 21. doi:10.1177/1948550611406138.

Planned Parenthood. 2011. "Info for Teens: Your Penis and Testicles." http://www.plannedparenthood.org/info-for-teens/our-bodies/your-penis-testicles-33817.htm.

Reevy, Gretchen M., Yvette Malamud Ozer, and Yuri Ito. 2010. *Encyclopedia of Emotion*. Santa Barbara, CA: Greenwood.

Reis, Elizabeth. 2011. *F.L.A.S.H.: A Curriculum in Family Life and Sexual Health*. Department of Public Health, Seattle and King County, WA. www.kingcounty.gov/health/flash.

Van Vranken, Michele. 2008. "Body Piercing." TeensHealth from Nemours. November. http://kidshealth.org/teen/your_body/body_art/body_piercing_safe.html.

Van Vranken, Michele. 2009. "Tattoos." TeensHealth from Nemours. November. http://kidshealth.org/teen/your_body/body_art/safe_tattooing.html.

WikiHow. 2011. "How to Respect a Transgender Person." May 29. http://www.wikihow.com/Respect-a-Transgender-Person.

Women's Health. 2009. "Menstruation and the Menstrual Cycle." October 21. http://www.womenshealth.gov/faq/menstruation.cfm#top.

Yurgelun-Todd, Deborah 2007. "Emotional and Cognitive Changes during Adolescence." *Current Opinions in Neurobiology* 17(2): 251–257. doi:10.1016/j.conb.2007.03.009.

Glossary

acronym: Combination of the first letters of several words into a single pronounceable word (such as radar or snafu); acronyms are a type of initialism.

androgen: Male sex hormone (such as testosterone).

biological sex: The sex that one is born with, usually based on genitalia, anatomy, and chromosomes.

bisexual: Romantic or sexual attractions to partners of the same and different genders.

bloating: Puffiness, swelling, or inflammation; may occur just before or during menstruation.

cervix: The neck of the uterus.

cilia: Tiny hairlike structures.

circumcision: Removal of foreskin.

clitoris: A small sensory organ in females, located toward the front of the vulva where the folds of the labia join.

coming out: The process of disclosing one's sexual orientation or gender identity to others. Someone who has not come out is considered in the closet.

ductus deferens: *See* **vas deferens.**

ejaculation: The ejection of semen from the penis during sex.

endometrium: A thick mucous membrane lining the uterus that serves as an environment for the embryo.

epididymides (sing., epididymis): A group of ducts (or tubes) where sperm are held and mature; connected to the tubes within the testicles where sperm are formed.

estrogen: A sex hormone secreted chiefly by the ovaries, placenta, adipose tissue, and testes; stimulates the development of female secondary sex characteristics and promotes the growth and maintenance of the female reproductive system.

external: Outside.

fallopian tubes: Pair of tubes in the female that transport the ova (eggs) from the ovaries to the uterus.

fimbria: Fringes or fingerlike structures at the entrance of the fallopian tubes that catch up the ovum when released by the ovary.

flaccid: Soft, not erect.

foreskin: A hood of skin covering the glans of the penis.

FTM: Female-to-male; someone who is born biologically female who has a male gender identity.

gay: A male who is attracted to people of the same gender.

gender: A sense of masculinity (maleness) or femininity (femaleness). A social construction; may or may not match one's biological sex.

gender identity: An internal sense of self based on gender; the gender with which one identifies. One's gender identity may not be consistent with one's birth sex.

genderqueer: People who consider their gender to be fluid (changing), consider themselves genderless (without gender), or are attracted to people across the gender spectrum.

genitals: Sexual or reproductive organs.

glans: Head of the penis or clitoris.

gynecomastia: Development of breast tissue in males; caused by hormones.

heterosexism: Presumption that everyone is heterosexual and that anyone who isn't is strange, morally flawed, or somehow different than the norm.

heterosexual: Sexual attraction to people of the opposite sex.

homophobia: Fear of or discrimination against homosexuals; may extend to fear or hatred of other LGBTQ people.

homosexual: Term previously used to describe same-sex sexuality. Associated with historical perspective of medical disease or psychiatric disorder; term is now mostly considered a pejorative when used to describe or label someone.

hormones: Cells secreted by glands; hormones circulate in body fluids and stimulate activity in other cells in the body.

hymen: A membrane that partially covers the vaginal opening.

identifies: Feels a similarity in values, a kindred spirit, or shared identity.

in the closet: When someone has not disclosed his or her sexual orientation or gender identity to others. The person's sexual orientation or gender identity is not generally known; he or she has not yet come out.

infertile: Unable to sexually reproduce.

inguinal hernia: A weakness in the muscular wall of the lower abdomen that allows a portion of the internal organs to slip through.

initialism: An abbreviation formed from the initial letters of each word in a phrase, such as LGBT; some initialisms are also acronyms.

internal: Inside.

intersex: A variety of conditions in which a person is born with reproductive or sexual anatomy that doesn't appear to fit typical definitions of male or female.

karyotype: A picture of the chromosomes in a cell; refers to the number, position, and size of the chromosomes in a cell.

labia: Two pairs of skin flaps surrounding the vaginal opening. The outer pair is called the labia majora (major), and the inner pair is the labia minora (minor).

lesbian: A female who is attracted to people of the same gender.

LGBTQI: Initialism that represents several sexual orientations and gender identities: lesbian, gay, bisexual, transgender, queer or questioning, and intersex.

menarche: The start of having menstrual periods; usually occurs between ages 8 and 15.

menopause: A time (around age 50) when women stop ovulating and having periods.

menstrual cramps: Dull, cramping, or throbbing pains in the lower abdomen.

menstrual cycle: Includes monthly hormonal changes, ovulation, and menstrual periods.

menstruation: Having a period; the monthly discharge of blood and other matter from the uterus.

mons pubis: Fleshy area located just above the top of the vaginal opening.

moon cup: A cup or barrier worn inside the vagina during menstruation to collect menstrual fluid.

MTF: Male-to-female; someone who is born biologically male and has a female gender identity.

nocturnal emissions: Ejaculation during sleep; wet dreams.

outing someone: When one person discloses another's sexual orientation or gender identity without permission.

ova: Female egg cells (gametes).

ovaries: Produce ova (eggs) in the female.

ovulation: Releases of matured ovum (egg) from the ovary.

pad: Sanitary napkin used during menstruation.

pansexual: Someone who is attracted to people across the gender spectrum. Similar to genderqueer.

panty liner: A thin pad that covers the crotch of underwear; may be used when menstrual flow is very light or to prevent staining from leaks from a tampon.

pelvis: The belly, the lowest part of the abdomen.

penis: External male organ used for sexual intercourse and urination.

premenstrual syndrome (PMS): Emotional and physical changes that may occur in women just before the beginning of their monthly menstrual period.

prostate gland: A gland located near the base of the male urethra; secretes fluid for semen.

queer: Used to describe LGBTQ people. Generally considered appropriate when used among LGBTQ persons (within the group). Still considered pejorative or distasteful by many.

questioning: An identity of a person who is uncertain or exploring his or her sexual orientation and/or gender identity.

rectum: Part of the large intestine closest to the anus.

reparative therapy: Interventions designed to change someone's sexual orientation to heterosexuality; also referred to as conversion therapy or orientation change therapy.

sanitary napkin: An absorbent pad worn on the outside of the vaginal area to absorb menstrual fluids.

scrotum: A muscular sack on the outside of the male body that holds the testes and other reproductive structures.

self-conscious: Being intensely aware of oneself; may be accompanied by embarrassment or anxiety.

self-esteem: The value that one places on oneself; whether one feels good or bad about oneself as a person.

self-image: The idea or conception that one has about oneself.

semen: A thick fluid that carries sperm.

seminal vesicles: Saclike structures that produce a sugar-rich fluid that provides energy for the sperm.

sexual identity: The personal labels that people choose to describe themselves (e.g., heterosexual, lesbian, gay, bisexual, queer, questioning).

sexual or gender minority: An umbrella term used to be broadly inclusive of people based on marginalized sexual or gender identities.

sexual orientation: An internal motivation or set of feelings, desires, and attractions to others based on their gender.

tampon: A cylinder-shaped column of absorbent material placed inside the vagina to absorb menstrual blood.

testicular torsion: A painful and potentially serious condition in which the testicle becomes twisted inside the scrotum.

testosterone: A hormone (androgen) usually associated with males and the development of male secondary sexual characteristics, such as facial hair and a deep voice. Both males and females have some level of testosterone. In males, testosterone is produced by the testes.

toxic shock syndrome (TSS): An illness in which the body reacts to toxins from bacterial infections.

transgender: A person who has a gender identity that is different from his or her birth sex.

transphobia: Fear of or discrimination against transgender individuals.

urethra: Canal that carries urine from the bladder to the outside of the body; in males, also carries semen.

vas deferens: A sperm-carrying duct; begins at the end of the epididymis farthest from the testicle.

virilization: A process that causes a person to develop masculine characteristics, such as a deep voice and facial hair.

vulva: The external part of the female reproductive organs.

CHAPTER 2

Relationships and Environmental Influences

The first part of this chapter discusses different types of relationships, including family, friends, casual relationships, and intimate or romantic relationships. In the context of intimate or romantic relationships, this portion covers dating, **sex** with partners, and **commitment**. The text describes some characteristics of healthy relationships and how to tell if a relationship is unhealthy. Several types of unhealthy or dangerous situations are discussed, including abuse, sexual assault, and **sexual harassment**.

The second part of the chapter discusses how different aspects of the environment influence body image, sexual behavior, **sexual orientation**, and relationships. The environment in this case does not mean the physical environment, such as natural resources or the climate, but instead refers to the social environment, which includes influences such as family, culture, social norms (customs), peer groups, and the media, including television, movies, music, and the Internet.

Types of Relationships

There are many different types of relationships, including family, friends, intimate or romantic relationships, and casual or other acquaintances. Healthy relationships with family and friends are also discussed in chapter 1, "Environment and Mental Health," in volume 5.

Family

Family consists of parents, siblings (brothers or sisters), and other relatives. A family is a group of people who are related by blood, marriage, or adoption. Family may include grandparents, cousins, aunts, and uncles.

Family can also include stepparents, stepsiblings, and half siblings as well as parents' partners, boyfriends, or girlfriends.

People first learn about relationships in their families. Ideally, family members demonstrate love, trust, and good communication. However, real-world families don't always model perfect relationships or communications. Family members may have communication problems; there may be friction, arguments, anger, or lack of trust. In the real world, families are hardly ever perfect. Things can be especially difficult during a separation or divorce. Understanding something about how to communicate and how to cope with arguments or misunderstandings can help improve relationships within a family.

If a family is dealing with challenges such as divorce, unemployment, homelessness, poverty, or violence, it can be hard for family members to cope. It is important to remember that children are not responsible for causing adult problems. Even though the burden of these problems affects all family members, children—even almost-grown children, such as teenagers—are not responsible for fixing the problems. Teenagers can best help by taking care of themselves. It's great if teenagers can make efforts to communicate effectively and demonstrate that they care about family members. Ways to support family members may include helping around the house and expressing care and concern for family members.

This may be especially challenging in families where there is abuse or **domestic violence**. In such families, it is most important to stay safe. It can also be challenging to maintain healthy boundaries. Teens may be able to find their own support from other family members, friends, and caring adults at school and in the community.

Friends

A friend is someone one cares about or feels affection for, someone one enjoys talking to or being around. The reasons that people become friends (or stay friends) change as people get older. Younger children may be friends because they go to the same school or live in the same neighborhood or because their parents arrange activities for them together. As kids get older, they begin hanging out with people their own age who have similar interests.

Shared interests in activities, music, food, or fashion may draw people into friendships. In high school, people with similar interests—sports, academics, music interests, and other activities—may sort themselves into peer groups. Sometimes people form close-knit cliques that exclude other people. Changing friendships and peer groups is a natural part of growing up. That doesn't mean it's easy. People can feel betrayed if longtime friends develop different interests or can feel excluded or pressured by different peer groups or cliques. Some people may feel that they need to dress or behave in certain ways to be accepted by a peer group. Things can seem really tough, especially in high school. Sometimes teens are picked on, ostracized, bullied, or teased. Fortunately, some people who bully or tease others grow out of these behaviors. Having good friends and other support in high school (family, other adults, and supportive people outside of school) can help teens who are bullied survive high school.

True friendship is **mutual**—each person can count on the other. Like other relationships, healthy friendships involve trust, mutual caring and support, and communication. True friends should be able to say that they disagree about something and still be friends. In healthy friendships, friends support and encourage each other, cooperate, and compromise and are considerate. If one friend hurts the other's feelings, direct and clear communication (including an apology if necessary) may help smooth things over.

Casual Relationships

A casual relationship is one with an acquaintance—someone other than a family member, friend, or intimate partner. This could include teachers, professionals (such as a doctor or counselor), other adults, or peers such as other students in school. These may be peers you are friendly with, other students in class, or just people you pass in the hallway or see on the streets.

It's important to maintain healthy relationships with acquaintances, because most other relationships (including intimate partners and friendships) begin with casual relationships. It's also generally a good idea to remain on positive terms with people, even those who aren't close friends. This can involve something as simple as saying hello or being polite or friendly when interacting with someone. Relationships that may seem unimportant at one point may become important later on.

Intimate Relationships

There are different types of intimate relationships, including intimate friendships and romantic or sexual relationships. Intimacy isn't just physical; it is also a sense of emotional **closeness** to another person. For example, some intimate friends confide in each other, sharing their deepest feelings and beliefs. They are not intimate in a physical or sexual way. Other relationships can be physically intimate without being sexual. For example, some people may fix each other's hair or feel comfortable undressing in front of each other without having a sexual relationship. Other relationships are physically intimate in a romantic or sexual way. Taking the time to get to know someone, become friends, and develop some emotional intimacy may lead to a more meaningful and stable romantic relationship.

Dating

Dating describes an activity (going out on a date with someone) and also describes a type of romantic relationship. Dating is a way to get to know someone better, engage in new social behaviors as a couple or small group, and explore one's identity within an intimate relationship. Dating can be a way to get to know someone without making a commitment to a deeper, longer-term relationship. Sometimes dating leads to a committed relationship, but not always.

Dating can be casual, a way to go out and have fun with other people. Dating can also be a way to figure out if someone is a suitable partner for a romantic or intimate relationship. There are several types of dating, including casual or serious dating, blind dates, double dating, speed dating, and online dating. Dating preferences and practices will vary depending on a person's family upbringing, culture, and individual personality.

Casual Dating

Casual dating is when someone may be dating several different people. It is a way to go out and have fun, get to know different people, and try a variety of activities without committing to an exclusive or long-term relationship. People who date casually may be looking for a partner to eventually commit to, may be looking for sexual relationships, or may just want to socialize with different people.

Blind Dating

Blind dating is when two people who don't know each other are set up to go on a date by someone else, usually a mutual friend or family member. In some cultures, it is considered more appropriate for two people to be introduced through an arranged meeting.

Double Dating and Group Dating

Double dating is when two or more couples go out together. Group dating is when a group of people with similar interests go out together. When a group of people go to an activity together (for example, a concert, party, or sports event), it may not be entirely clear whether it is a group date or just a bunch of friends having fun together. Some people prefer the ambiguity of this type of situation—not knowing if it is a date or not. This leaves open possibilities for intimate, or romantic, interactions without having to commit to them. Other people prefer to know whether they're going on a date, whether they're expected to pair off as couples, or whether it's more casual—just a group of people friends having fun together.

Speed Dating

Speed dating is usually set up by a club, organization, or dating service. At a speed dating event, people quickly get to know one person, then move on to the next person. People usually spend 5 or 10 minutes with one person before moving on. Speed dating is a way to meet many people in a short time. People who find that they have common interests or are attracted to each other typically go out on a longer one-on-one date sometime after the speed dating event.

Online Dating

With online dating, people meet and get to know each other over the Internet. This can be done through a chat room, a forum, a dating service, or e-mail. Sometimes people exchange photos online. People who are interested in pursuing more intimate relationships may make arrangements to meet in person.

Online dating can be a good way to meet many different people without spending a lot of time and money on in-person dates. However, online dating does have some drawbacks. One is that people may not really know whom they're talking to. The Internet allows people to portray themselves as they'd like to be seen, not necessarily as they actually are. For example, on the Internet a person might describe himself as tall, athletic, funny, and friendly. You might not realize until after meeting this person that he is actually not so tall, doesn't like sports, has a strange sense of humor, and is more interested in being physically friendly (just wants to have sex) than actually friendly.

Serious Dating

Serious dating is when two people make a decision to only date each other and consider themselves a couple. This usually means a commitment—each person commits to being with the other. When people decide to have a committed relationship, they may hope that it will lead to a long-term relationship.

Commitment

Commitment is a social contract, or agreement between people, involving loyalty and trust. When people are in a committed relationship they

WHAT PEOPLE ARE SAYING **TEEN OPINIONS ABOUT ONLINE DATING**

What do you think about online dating? What are some of the risks and benefits?

- "Online dating is like a lot of stuff the net provides. There's a wall between people. People who do online dating are playing it safer and can be robbed of the initial experience of getting to know each other for real." GBH, age 17, California
- "It can be good for some people, but not appealing to me. You could end up meeting your soul mate, or be put in a very uncomfortable situation." JW, age 16, Texas
- "It depends on your definition of online dating. If you mean being in a romantic relationship with someone you've never actually met but began talking to online with little/no intention to meet in person, then no, I don't think it's healthy. You really don't know who the other person is—they could be anyone." ES, age 20, California
- "I think online dating can be a good thing, but it isn't something I would venture into unless I had exhausted all of my other options first. I believe that it is a good way to expand your dating pool, but it is always important to be wary of imposters and predators." KK, age 19, Kentucky
- "Online is very risky. The Internet gives people the opportunity to meet people from all over the world; however, the people you meet online may have dishonest intentions." KG, age 19, Texas

have decided to stick together, to support each other in good times and bad. Usually people in committed relationships have common interests, enjoy being together, and share some level of intimacy. People in committed relationships are often attracted to each other, respect each other, and share some of the same values and beliefs. Good communication is necessary to maintain closeness, respect, and trust in a committed relationship. It is especially important to have clear communication about the nature and level of commitment in a relationship.

Committed romantic relationships include exclusive (monogamous) relationships, polyamorous relationships, open and closed relationships, going steady, engagement, marriage, and civil partnerships. Often (but not always) people expect committed relationships to be monogamous. **Monogamy** means having an exclusive relationship with one person.

Polyamory means many (*poly*) lovers (*amor*). A polyamorous relationship may involve one person with two or more partners (who are not in a relationship with each other) or several (more than two) people who are in a relationship together. In the first case, Sue is in a polyamorous relationship: she has two boyfriends (Bob and Andre), but Bob and Andre are not having a romantic relationship with each other. An example of the second case would be Sue, Bob, and Andre all having a romantic relationship together.

Polyamorous relationships can be open or closed. A **closed relationship** is exclusive: it means that the people in the relationship are committed to each other and not romantically involved with anyone outside the relationship. People in an **open relationship** are committed to each other, but they are not exclusive. They may also have intimate relationships with people outside the relationship. To some people, open relationships mean being emotionally intimate and exclusive with their primary partner and having outside sexual relationships. To other people, open relationships mean having an exclusive monogamous sexual relationship with one partner and having outside emotionally intimate (nonsexual) relationships. It's a good idea to clarify what someone expects from an open relationship before committing to be in one. Good communication is needed to make any relationship work; this is especially true of open relationships.

Serious relationships have different levels of commitment. A teen or young adult usually refers to the person he or she is in a committed relationship with as a boyfriend or girlfriend. A marriage or civil partnership is a formal long-term relationship in which people agree to share their resources and establish a household together. Marriage may involve cultural, religious, and legal rituals and contracts. In some states, long-term committed relationships are only legally recognized between a man and a woman; other states allow same-sex marriages. People who share resources and live together in a long-term committed relationship without being married are considered civil partners. People who formally decide to enter into marriage in the future are engaged. Engagement can be a way to signify and formalize a deeper commitment to a relationship and a way to transition from serious dating to marriage or civil partnership.

Falling in Love

There are different types of love: love between parents and children, love between brothers and sisters, love between friends, and romantic love. Each type of love feels different and is shown differently. Romantic love usually develops in adolescence or later. When teens develop and mature, they may start feeling sexual **attraction** to people their own age. Romantic love may help an individual feel very close to someone, important, understood, or secure. Love can provide a feeling of belonging to another or fitting in. Sometimes sexual attraction and romantic feelings are the same, but not always. Some teens want the sense of closeness, belonging, and security that may accompany romance without feeling sexual attraction. Love consists of three qualities: attraction, closeness, and commitment. Some of these qualities are more important to some people—and in some types of relationships—than other qualities.

Attraction is the physical or sexual interest or desire that one person feels for another. Attraction may be a desire to be physically close to someone, a desire to be sexual with that person, or both. In some families, cultures, and religions, it is considered inappropriate for young unmarried people to have sexual relationships. But this doesn't mean that the feelings of attraction aren't there. It is a normal, natural part of being a teenager to feel physical and sexual attraction for other people. It is not necessary to act on feelings of attraction; sometimes it's enough to feel the feelings and hold off on the sexual relationship.

Closeness is an intimate bond that one person feels with another. Closeness involves trusting another person enough to share one's deepest thoughts and feelings. It may mean wanting to spend time with that person. Closeness reflects feelings of being understood, supported, cared for, and accepted by another person. If closeness is reciprocated, it means that one is willing to support, care for, and accept the other person as well.

Commitment involves a promise to stick by someone. It involves a sense of loyalty and trust, a belief that another person will be there through good times and bad.

A love that has closeness without attraction is what someone may feel for a best friend or favorite sibling. Physical or sexual attraction without closeness is a crush or infatuation—when one person is physically attracted but doesn't really know someone well enough to feel close.

Attraction and closeness together make the beginnings of a love relationship. These feelings can be very intense, especially when falling in love for the first time. How can people tell if they are really in love or if it's just a passing fling? If the closeness in the relationship deepens to the point where both individuals see themselves as a couple, they may want to make a commitment. Being in a committed love relationship usually means having hopes of continuing to be together for some time.

During adolescence, romantic relationships may be shorter because teens are growing and changing so fast. Teens are discovering their interests and developing their identities—a sense of self. This may change as people discover who they are: what types of friends and activities they like, how they see themselves in relation to others, and developing a sense of their own **sexual identity**. What a teen wants out of a romantic relationship will change as the teen's interests and identity change. As teens get older and their identities become more established, they will probably have longer—and more stable—romantic relationships.

When feelings of attraction and sexual interest are new, everything seems exciting and intense; these feelings may be confused with love. True love involves an emotional closeness that develops over time. When the initial infatuation wears off and a deep sense of closeness and attachment remains, then one can be more certain of love. Closeness in a relationship develops when both people take turns, learning to give and receive. People listen to and support each other in close relationships. Supportive caring relationships allow people to be themselves and to reveal their true feelings. Sharing thoughts, feelings, interests, fears, dreams, and worries can bring people closer together.

Dealing with Breakups

Sometimes the passion and attraction felt early in a relationship develops into a close, healthy, long-term relationship. Other times, people lose the sense of closeness or the relationship encounters other difficulties. Sometimes each member of a couple wants different things; sometimes there are miscommunications or a loss of trust and commitment. People might just outgrow the relationship. This can happen if one person grows and changes and the other person doesn't.

A breakup can be very painful, especially the first time. It can feel devastating, like the end of the world. The pain may feel so raw that one feels that the pain will never go away. After breaking up the first time, someone may believe that he will never love anyone again or that no one will ever love him as much as his ex did. A breakup may bring feelings of anger, confusion, guilt, jealousy, grief, or low self-esteem. People almost always feel a sense of loss after a breakup. There is no denying how painful and intense breakups feel. But the reality is that people do eventually get over a breakup and move on.

How can someone move on after something as devastating as a breakup? It can help to share feelings with a trusted friend or family member. Someone who has gone through a breakup can empathize—since they have been through it, they know what it feels like. It's okay to cry after a breakup. Sometimes letting the feelings out can help. Other things that can help include taking good care of yourself, keeping busy, engaging in favorite activities, and giving yourself time to heal and recover. If you feel guilt or low self-esteem, it can help to remember your positive attributes. Remind yourself of your good qualities rather than dwelling on your faults.

People need support after a breakup. If a friend or family member has recently gone through a breakup, it can help to be available to talk or offer to do things together. It may help to get out and do things. Sometimes people drop favorite activities when they're caught up in an intense romantic relationship. After a breakup may be a good time to resume favorite activities and reestablish neglected friendships.

What's Not a Good Idea after a Breakup?

Some people feel so bad after a breakup they turn to alcohol or other drugs to try to feel better. Some people feel angry or guilty and hurt themselves. Others try immediately jumping into another relationship. These are all ways that someone may attempt to avoid the pain of the breakup or change how bad they feel about themselves. These are rarely successful solutions. Immediately jumping into another relationship—on the rebound—doesn't allow one time to heal after a breakup. Rebound relationships don't usually turn out well either. Drinking, using drugs, or hurting yourself or others may change the way you feel in the moment. However, these feelings are only temporary and usually have negative consequences. If the pain and sadness following a breakup are very deep and last a long time or if you need to mask the pain with drugs, alcohol, or self-harming behaviors, it may help to talk to a counselor or therapist.

Sexual Relationships

Feeling sexual attraction to another person doesn't mean it's a good idea to have sex with that person right away (if at all). The first thing for a teen to consider is whether he or she is ready to have sex. Sex can be a special intimate experience. It can also lead to misunderstandings, hurt feelings, embarrassment, or pregnancy. Sometimes sex can bring people closer together, but it can also ruin a good friendship.

After people have gotten to know each other, they may decide that they want to have a more intimate sexual relationship. An intimate relationship will be healthier if people have taken the time to get to know each other and if they really care about each other, have mutual respect, and consider the possible consequences of having sex.

It's important to consider the risks as well as the benefits of having an intimate sexual relationship. For example, it's crucial to think about safe sex—preventing pregnancy and not spreading (or picking up) any sexually transmitted diseases (STDs). These issues will be discussed later in this chapter in the section on sexual behavior. STDs are also discussed in chapter 3 of this volume.

Ready for a Sexual Relationship?

People mature at different rates and ages. Usually girls start maturing physically—they start puberty—before boys. But everyone develops at his or her own pace. Just as some people mature physically early and others when they're older, people mature socially and emotionally at different rates. Teens should pay attention to how they feel and not jump into a sexual relationship just because other people their age are doing it. A decision to have sex should not be made because of feeling pressured by peers. Some people may think that having sex will make them fit in or be liked by others. This is probably not a good reason to have sex. A decision to have sex should only be made with full knowledge of the consequences, including safe sex and birth control. Such a decision should only be made by someone who is mature enough to

TABLE 3.2.1 **AM I READY FOR SEX?**

- Am I doing this because *I* want to?
- Do I know my partner well enough?
- Do I feel comfortable enough with my partner to have sex?
- Am I comfortable enough with my partner to have sex sober?
- Do I know enough about sex?
- Is it legal?
- When I'm older, will I be glad that I had sex now?
- Do I know how to have sex safely?
- Is my partner willing to practice safe sex?
- Can I talk to my partner about this easily?
- Do we *both* want to do this?
- Does sex fit with my personal beliefs and my partner's?
- How does sex fit in with my personal and family's religious or cultural values?

Source: Adapted from AVERT (2011a).

fully consent, knows what he or she is doing, and is fully willing to enter into a sexual relationship with another consenting person. Table 3.2.1 lists questions that teens can ask themselves to help figure out if they're ready to have sex.

Even if you decide that you are ready to have sex in general, that's not the same as deciding to have sex in a specific situation. It can be helpful to think about different situations in which you would be willing—or unwilling—to have sex. It's good to think about these situations during a quiet time when you are alone and not being distracted or influenced by other people (such as family members or friends). You can ask yourself, for example, how you feel about kissing on the first date, how far you are willing to go the first time you have a sexual experience, and how well you feel you should get to know someone before having sex. Other questions to ask yourself include whether you consider oral sex to be the same as having sex and under what conditions intercourse would be acceptable. You should also think about what you would do if one of you wanted to have sex and the other didn't.

People have different ideas about what behaviors or activities count as sex. When asked questions about whether certain activities count as sex, opinions vary depending on whether the act is being performed *by* a male or a female, whether the act is being performed *on* a male or a female, and whether the question (about whether the behavior qualifies as sex) is being answered by a male or female. There are also different answers depending on whether both, neither, or only one person (in the hypothetical scenario) has an orgasm. When thinking about whether certain behaviors count as sex, it makes sense to consider more than just whether one or both of the people have an orgasm. For example, it's a good idea to consider the risk of spreading or contracting an STD or of getting pregnant. Table 3.2.2 summarizes how college students responded when asked whether certain behaviors count as sex.

Virginity and Abstinence

Why does it matter whether someone believes that one behavior counts as sex and another doesn't? Sometimes people think that behaviors that don't affect their virginity don't really count as sex. Or as long as someone remains a **virgin**, anything goes. What is virginity, and how is it different than **abstinence**? A virgin is usually considered to be someone who has not had sex before. Some people think that virginity only refers to a girl or woman who has never had vaginal intercourse.

The **hymen**—a thin membrane partly covering the vaginal opening—is usually torn after vaginal intercourse, so some people consider an intact

TABLE 3.2.2 **WHAT COUNTS AS SEX?**

When asked whether certain behaviors qualify as sex, 223 college students responded as follows:

	Percentage of college students who said this was sex	
	If neither partner has orgasm	***If both partners have orgasm***
Vaginal intercourse	90	100
Oral sex on a man	34	54*
Oral sex on a woman	36	41*
Anal sex	89	96

*Only the person receiving the oral sex has an orgasm.
Source: Bogart, Cecil, Wagstaff, Pinkerton, and Abramson (2000).

(untorn) hymen to be proof of virginity. However, the hymen can be torn in ways other than sexual intercourse, so having an intact hymen does not prove that someone has never had sexual intercourse. But some girls reason that as long as they don't have vaginal intercourse—meaning that their hymens may still be intact—they are still virgins. This may contribute to the idea that other types of sex—for example, oral or anal sex—don't really count. Does virginity just apply to girls, or does it also apply to boys? A boy who has never had sexual intercourse may be teased because he is a virgin. A girl may be teased if she is not a virgin or if other people believe she isn't.

Abstinence means not having (abstaining from) sex. Abstinence usually indicates a voluntary or deliberate choice or decision to not have sex. Someone who may have already had sex before (no longer a virgin) may decide to be abstinent. Someone else may still be a virgin and decide to abstain (not have sex) until they are older or until they're married.

Religious, moral, and family beliefs and values play a big role in beliefs about virginity, abstinence, and sexual behavior in teens. For example, some religions state that no one should have sex outside of marriage. This means no type of sex before being married. Others believe that some types of sexual activities are okay (for example, kissing and touching) but that sexual intercourse before marriage is wrong. When someone is deciding whether to have sex or not, religious, cultural, family, and other factors may affect her or his decision.

 WHAT PEOPLE ARE SAYING **TEEN OPINIONS ON VIRGINITY AND ORAL SEX**

Do you think that if someone has only had oral sex they're still a virgin?

- "I don't think they are because I see virginity as more of a mental state rather than a physical one." KK, age 19, Kentucky
- "Yes, I believe that anyone who has not had vaginal intercourse is a virgin." KK, age 18, Louisiana
- "Not really. You and your partner have decided to have a sexual relationship, and the term 'virgin' is really an archaic differentiation between the women and girls of a tribal group, which has only persisted into the modern age through religion's insistence that it still means something." ES, age 20, California

Do you think oral sex counts as sex in the same way as intercourse?

- "I do not, because by definition they are different." KK, age 18, Louisiana
- "No. Because there's no way for conception to happen. Unless you really screw up." PW, age 16, Virginia
- "Not mentally. But in terms of safety and trust, yes. The rest is for you to decide." GBH, age 17, California
- "Yes, because the physical and emotional implications are generally the same." KK, age 19, Kentucky

Deciding whether to have sex is a personal decision. Other people—parents, teachers, siblings, friends—may have opinions about whether an individual should or should not have sex. But the final decision is up to the individual. If someone has sex before he or she is really ready, it could be a bad experience. If one partner wants to have sex and the other doesn't, that can be an unpleasant experience. It's better to ask someone—rather than assuming—if he or she really wants to have sex.

Deciding Not to Have Sex

Some teens may not feel ready to have sex until they are older or until they are in a long-term committed relationship. Some may not want to worry about pregnancy or STDs. Others may have religious or moral reasons or may be reluctant because of personal or family beliefs. And

? Did You Know?

- In a 2005 survey, 47 percent of U.S. high school students reported having had sexual intercourse.
- Most teens (75 percent) have their first sexual encounter within a dating relationship.
- More than three-fifths of teens who are sexually active eventually have sex outside of traditional dating relationships. Casual sexual partners include strangers, friends, ex-boyfriends, or ex-girlfriends.
- In one 2006 survey of 1,316 high school students, about 33 percent reported having had sexual intercourse. Of those who reported being sexually active, 61 percent reported having sex outside a dating relationship.

Source: Liace, Nunez, and Luckner (2011).

some may just not be interested in having sex. If it seems like everyone else at school is talking about having sex, some teens may feel pressured to have sex—even if they're not sexually attracted to anyone—just so they can feel like they fit in.

Even someone who is in a relationship and feels sexually attracted to her or his partner may decide to slow down or wait to have sex. One person might feel a sense of emotional closeness and feel ready to make a commitment, while the other person wants something different out of the relationship. It's a good idea to be honest about feelings and expectations with each other; otherwise, people can have misunderstandings and hurt feelings. Good relationships take work, and communication isn't always easy. But healthy relationships should feel good for both people in the relationship. Having sex before one partner is ready can cause guilt and hurt feelings and will most likely damage the relationship.

Individuals may decide to hold off on having sex—to remain abstinent—for many reasons. They may want to get to know their partner better before having sex or focus on other things (school or sports) without distractions. They may decide to be abstinent because of religious, cultural, or family beliefs. If you have a gut feeling that you're not ready to have sex or that you should wait, you should listen to that gut feeling. People can always decide later to go ahead and have sex, but they can't ever turn the clock back.

WHAT PEOPLE ARE SAYING **TEEN OPINIONS ON TELLING SOMEONE YOU DON'T WANT TO HAVE SEX**

What's a good way to tell someone that you care about her or him but don't want to have sex with that person?

- "You do just that. If they care about you enough they will understand." KK, age 18, Louisiana
- "You say that you're not ready. You shouldn't have to just because they want to." BM, age 21, California
- "That you respect your body and you prefer to show your affection in different ways then having sexual contact." JW, age 16, Texas
- "Tell them you've made a promise to yourself to abstain until you know you're ready." KK, age 19, Kentucky
- "Sharing your reasons behind not wanting to have sex with them is helpful." KG, age 19, Texas
- "It will differ depending on the relationship you have with that person, but generally just telling them simply and honestly that you do care for them but won't sleep with them is the best way." ES, age 20, California

Is Sex Legal? Is It Appropriate?

Some sexual relationships may be appropriate, and others may not be. It is never appropriate for an adult to have sex with a child. The legal **age of consent**—the age at which a person can consent to have sex—varies by state. In some states, it is **illegal** for any **minor** to consent to sex. Other states may have ages of consent less than 18 years. Some U.S. states have **age-gap provisions,** meaning that it is illegal for one person to have sex with another person who is much younger. For example, in some states it would be illegal for anyone over 18 to have sex with a person under 18 but not illegal for a 14-year-old to have sex with a 16-year-old. For teens who are considering having a sexual relationship, it is important to be aware of their state laws. Anyone who has sex with a person under the legal age of consent may be charged with **statutory rape.** This means that even if a minor agrees to have sex with an adult or older teenager, the older person can be charged with rape. Statutory rape has harsher penalties—including longer prison sentences—than other types of sexual assault.

TABLE 3.2.3 **AGE OF CONSENT BY U.S. STATE**

State	Age	State	Age
Alabama	16	Montana	16
Alaska	16	Nebraska	17
Arizona	18	Nevada	16
Arkansas*	14/16	New Hampshire	16
California	18	New Jersey	16
Colorado*	15/17	New Mexico	17
Connecticut	16	New York	17
D.C.	16	North Carolina*	16
Delaware*	16/18	North Dakota	18
Florida*	16/18	Ohio	16
Georgia	16	Oklahoma	16
Hawaii	16	Oregon	18
Idaho	18	Pennsylvania	16
Illinois	17	Rhode Island	16
Indiana*	14/16	South Carolina	16
Iowa*	14/16	South Dakota	16
Kansas	16	Tennessee	18
Kentucky	16	Texas*	17
Louisiana*	17	Utah*	16/18
Maine	16	Vermont	16
Maryland	16	Virginia	18
Massachusetts	16	Washington*	16/18
Michigan	16	West Virginia	16
Minnesota	16	Wisconsin	18
Mississippi	16	Wyoming*	16/18
Missouri	17		

Note: If more than one age is listed, the law within that state varies by region or circumstances. In some cases age of consent is lower when partners are similar ages.

* In some U.S. states a lower age applies when the age gap between partners is small or when the older partner is below a certain age (usually 18 or 21).

Source: AVERT (2011b).

It is inappropriate to have sex with a close family member. For example, it is not appropriate for a parent, grandparent, aunt, or uncle to have sex with a child. It is also inappropriate for brothers and sisters to have sex. This is known as **incest** (sex between close relatives), and it is usually considered a type of sexual abuse. Most cultures have **taboos** on incestuous relationships, and incest is illegal in some communities or states. A taboo is something that is considered immoral or violates cultural or religious values and norms.

One likely reason for the incest taboo is that when close blood relatives have a child, the child may be more likely to have congenital birth defects. If two related people, for example a brother and sister, are both carriers of a defective gene (a gene leading to a birth defect), their child would have a greater chance of being born with that birth defect. Incest may also be a taboo because it can be especially harmful to be betrayed and used for sex by a trusted family member—someone you depend upon for survival.

Sexual Behavior

The teen years are a time of rapid change: bodies are maturing and developing, and so is one's sense of identity. A person changes from a child with certain friends, preferences, and roles within the family to a more independent teen who may have new preferences in music or clothes, hang out with different groups of friends, and start to feel differently about himself or herself. Along with the physical changes of puberty come hormonal changes, feelings of sexual attraction to others, and new feelings about oneself as a sexual being.

Sometimes all of these changes happen so quickly that it can be confusing. At other times, teens feel that things are moving too slowly, and they can't wait to finish growing up. It's important to remember that change happens at different rates for different people. Generally speaking, girls tend to physically mature (reach puberty) earlier than boys. However, many factors affect the rate of maturity, including family, genes, hormones, nutrition, other environmental factors, and individual differences. Someone who looks physically mature may not feel much sexual attraction or have any interest in sex. Another teen may start experiencing feelings of sexual attraction while still appearing physically immature.

Since everyone develops at different rates, a teen might not feel like dating or getting intimate with anyone, even if all of her or his friends are talking about sex and dating. The teen years are a time to discover oneself and gradually develop a sense of one's own sexual identity.

Sex versus Sexuality

Sexuality is the quality or state of being sexual or the expression of sexual interest. The term "sex" can refer to one's biological sex (male or female) or to sexual activities. Sexual activities are an expression of someone's sexuality. However, sexuality does not necessarily involve sexual activity. Sexuality can be expressed in one's sense of oneself as a sexual person, whom one is attracted to, and how one presents oneself to others as a sexual person. This may be reflected in how someone dresses or with jewelry, hairstyles, makeup, or body art (e.g., piercings, tattoos). **Sexual expression** includes sexual desire and sexual behavior.

Sexual Orientation

Sexual identity includes self-concepts related to gender—masculinity, femininity, and **androgyny**—and gender roles. Androgyny is the quality of being or feeling neither specifically masculine nor feminine. Sexual identity also includes feelings about one's sexual orientation—the sex of the person one is attracted to. There is a range of sexual orientations, including **heterosexual**, **homosexual**, and **bisexual**. "Hetero" is the Greek prefix for "other," "homo" is the prefix for "same," and "bi" is the prefix meaning "two." Heterosexual means that one is romantically and physically attracted to people of the opposite sex, such as when boys are attracted to girls. Homosexual means that one is attracted to people of the same sex (such as when girls are attracted to each other). Bisexual (also known as bi) means that one is attracted both to people of the same sex and people of the opposite sex. A bisexual girl might have a girlfriend and then later have a boyfriend. Someone who is heterosexual may be referred to as straight. One who is not heterosexual is known as gay. "Gay" and "queer" are terms that may also be used derogatorily—to bully or tease someone who may or may not actually be homosexual. A homosexual man is referred to as gay; a homosexual woman is a lesbian.

Part of developing one's identity is becoming aware of sexual attraction—to people of the opposite sex, the same sex, or both. One may find that one is attracted only to boys, only to girls, or to both boys and girls at different times. People may have sexual fantasies during adolescence. It is common for teens to have sexual thoughts and feelings about both boys and girls during this time of emerging sexuality. Fantasizing about or sexually experimenting with someone of the same sex does not necessarily mean that a person is gay, straight, or bi.

Media portrayals of gay people may affect how one feels about one's sexual orientation. Sometimes TV shows and movies will portray stereotypes of gay people. Stereotypes may lead a teen to think that all gay men are effeminate (having feminine qualities not typical of men). One stereotype portrays gay men as people with lisps who dress flamboyantly and have occupations such as florists, hairstylists, or interior decorators. Another stereotype portrays heterosexual men as tough manly men who get into fights and never show their feelings. Stereotypes are not reality: the reality is that there are some lesbians who are very feminine and some heterosexual women who are tomboys. People are not gay or straight depending on their occupations. There are homosexual, heterosexual, and bisexual soldiers, police officers, firefighters, doctors, lawyers, chefs, florists, and teachers. It is not possible to tell by someone's appearance, job, or preferences whether he or she is gay or straight.

Families, religions, cultures, or the media may convey attitudes that are homophobic. **Homophobia** is fear of or discrimination against homosexuals. Family members may be more or less accepting and understanding of sexual orientation. Some people believe that homosexuality is a choice or a lifestyle. These people may not understand about different sexual orientations. If one's parents or peers are homophobic, they may react poorly to a teen who comes out—reveals his or her sexual orientation—as gay. Peers may be more or less accepting of **LGBT** (lesbian, gay, bisexual, transgender) individuals. If people at school or at home make jokes or use derogatory terms about gay people, it can be intimidating to even think about the possibility of being attracted to someone of the same sex or to admit being attracted to both boys and girls.

A teen who is gay (or isn't sure) and does not feel safe coming out to family or friends at school may feel pressured to date people of the opposite sex just to show he or she is not gay. This can be uncomfortable and awkward—both for the gay or questioning teen and for his or her date. It can be confusing and distressing to act like one type of person while feeling like a different person inside. It can cause conflict to feel as if one must pretend to be a certain way one place (such as at home) and act like a different person elsewhere (such as at school or with friends). A teen who is attracted to people of the same sex may be afraid that other people may find out or somehow notice the attraction. This might involve anxiety about changing clothes in the school locker room, playing on a sports team, or doing activities with peers.

A gay teen who has not come out or a teen who isn't sure about his or her sexual orientation (questioning) may feel better by talking to a close friend who is not judgmental. It may help to explore the issue with a school counselor or a trusted teacher who has expressed support of LGBT individuals. Resources listed later in the chapter include books and Internet support for LGBT issues. Sexual orientation and gender identity are discussed further in chapter 1 of this volume.

Sexual Activity

Even if one feels an overwhelming attraction or desire to have sex, sometimes it makes sense to take a step back and think about the possible consequences. But it also may make sense to wait awhile before engaging in sex. Feelings of attraction may be intense, but they can also pass quickly. One may decide to wait to see if the feelings of attraction persist or may decide to have sex after considering issues such as pregnancy prevention, safe sex, and whether one is really ready to engage in sex. This section discusses issues related to sexual activity, including **masturbation** (sex with oneself), respecting boundaries in sexual relationships, communicating about safe sex, and sexual desire.

Masturbation

Masturbation means touching oneself to give oneself sexual pleasure. It may be some combination of touching one's genitals and engaging in sexual or erotic fantasies. Masturbation may result in orgasm. Most people masturbate, although people don't talk about it much. This is partly because masturbation is such a private activity. It is generally done by oneself in private or may be shared in the context of sex with an intimate partner.

The idea of masturbation may be embarrassing for some people. It may also be difficult to talk about because some cultures, religions, or families have taboos against masturbation. A taboo is something that is forbidden or discouraged according to social customs, conventions, or morality. Because of taboos, some people may feel that they should not ever masturbate. Other people may be okay with the activity of masturbation, but taboos prevent them from talking about it.

Whether people talk about it or not, masturbation is a natural part of growing up. Most young children explore their bodies, including their genitals, and the sensations caused by different types of touching. Parents usually teach young children what type of self-touching is acceptable in public and what should remain private. However, some kids are given the message that it is never okay to touch oneself in an intimate or sexual way. This may contribute to a teen feeling ashamed for touching himself or herself or for experiencing pleasure during masturbation or sex.

Masturbation is a healthy sexual practice. It is an important part of developing a sexual identity, of learning what types of touching are pleasurable and exploring one's identity through sexual and erotic fantasies. Masturbation can be a good way to relieve stress and tension and reduce feelings of anxiety, depression, and some types of pain. For example, it may ease the pain of menstrual cramps (Planned Parenthood 2011). Masturbation is also the safest form of sex—it cannot result in pregnancy or an STD.

Being in a romantic or intimate relationship does not mean that one has to refrain from masturbating. People in committed relationships may masturbate as much or more often than people who aren't in relationships. Masturbation is not a sign that someone is not getting enough sex or not enjoying the sex within a relationship. It also doesn't mean that a

Fact or Myth?

Masturbation

Myth	*Fact*
Too much masturbation can make people crazy or blind, damage their sex organs, or make them grow hair on their palms.	Masturbation is not emotionally or physically harmful. It can help relieve stress and tension. Masturbation will not stunt someone's growth.
Children don't masturbate before puberty.	It is normal and healthy for children—even young children—to explore their bodies and discover what types of sensations are pleasurable.
Girls don't masturbate.	Some social and cultural conventions say that it is okay for boys to masturbate and express themselves sexually but that this is not okay for girls. The truth is that girls and women do masturbate, and there is no reason they shouldn't.
A girl shouldn't masturbate during her period.	If someone wants to masturbate during her period, there's no reason she shouldn't. In fact, some girls find that it helps reduce menstrual cramps.

Source: Planned Parenthood (2011).

sexual partner doesn't find one attractive. Some people may use masturbation as a way to warm up or get themselves in the mood for sex with a partner. Other people masturbate to learn more about their bodies and what gives them pleasure. Some couples may enjoy watching each other masturbate. Masturbating together (mutual masturbation) is a way to be intimate with someone without worrying about pregnancy or infections.

Is there such a thing as too much masturbation? Only if it gets in the way of daily activities, such as going to school or work or getting together with friends. Masturbating a lot will not reduce a man's fertility. A man has less volume of semen directly after ejaculation, but his long-term fertility will not be affected by masturbation.

Even if someone makes every effort to keep masturbation private, it's possible that someone can be caught masturbating. For example, a parent or sibling may barge into a teen's bedroom while he or she is masturbating. In that situation, it might be a good idea to talk to family members about respecting one's privacy. If one shares a room with someone—for example, a brother or sister—it might make sense to work out a privacy signal, especially if there are no locks on the doors. An example might be asking the roommate to not enter if the door is shut. It might be embarrassing to talk about why one is requesting privacy (especially to a parent). One needn't explain that one is masturbating; just express a desire for privacy.

Respecting Boundaries around Sexual Behavior

A **boundary** is a line or division between one thing and another. For example, the shoreline is the boundary between the land and the sea. Sometimes boundaries are very clear, like the boundary between dark black and stark white. Other times boundaries are not so clear, such as when black and white start fading into shades of gray. Boundaries may be particularly unclear in relationships, especially intimate or sexual relationships. Boundaries may involve behavior other than sex. For example, one person may want to spend all of her or his time with a partner, while the partner may want to also spend time with other people. One person may expect the partner to share all of her or his thoughts and feelings about everything, while the partner may desire more privacy (keeping some things to himself or herself).

There are different levels of sexual behavior and different activities. Consenting to one type of behavior does not mean that one automatically consents to other behaviors. For example, one person may feel comfortable holding hands in public and kissing in private but not comfortable kissing in public. Another person may consent to oral sex but not to sexual intercourse. It is important to be able to communicate with a partner if one feels uncomfortable. Any time one person says that he or she feels uncomfortable, the other person should stop. If one person says "no," expresses discomfort with sexual behavior, or asks the other person to stop, it is important to stop the behavior or activity right away. Not stopping when someone asks to stop is considered sexual assault.

When it comes to sex, it can be especially difficult to know where the boundaries are. It may feel embarrassing to ask someone what he or she wants, to let someone know that one is uncomfortable, or to ask the other person to stop. Consensual sex means that it is okay to stop at any time, to say that the activity is uncomfortable or unwanted, and to refuse to participate in any activity. It is always okay to ask the other person to stop, even if things seem to have gone past the point of no return. It's better to speak up (and risk embarrassment) than to engage in sexual behavior that is uncomfortable or unwanted for either partner.

Communicating about Safe Sex

It can seem awkward to talk about safe sex. You may feel vulnerable or be afraid of being laughed at, teased, or rejected for speaking openly about such a sensitive topic (Gowen 2003). You might be concerned that talking about safe sex may ruin a romantic moment or mood. However, it is better to talk about this with a partner than to leave things to chance. It is better to discuss safe sex, because not planning ahead can lead to unwanted behavior and consequences such as pregnancy or STDs.

One of the elements of a healthy relationship is good communication. Communicating up front about safe sex may improve the chances for an ongoing healthy relationship. Talking about safe sex may also ensure that both partners in the relationship share common values about health and safety and have in mind their own and each other's well-being. After all, if people want to have sex but don't want to take precautions, what does that say about how they feel about a partner's health? What kind of message does it send about the kinds of risks they take with their own health?

The best time to think about safe sex is before finding yourself in a sexual encounter, before things get too involved; it can be difficult to ask your partner to pause when passions are aroused. People may be able to reason more clearly before finding themselves in a moment where passions and desires may overcome their common sense. Safe sex practices include abstaining from or limiting sexual activities, using a condom for all sexual activities, both partners being tested for STDs, maintaining monogamy within a sexual relationship (only having sex with one other person), and discussing birth control and pregnancy.

TABLE 3.2.4 **DEALING WITH OBJECTIONS TO USING CONDOMS**

Objection	Response
"It's uncomfortable."	Suggest a different brand or size. "Wearing a condom takes some getting used to."
"Condoms put me out of the mood."	"Unsafe sex puts me out of the mood—permanently."
"If you really love me, you'd trust me."	"Because I love you so much, I want to be sure we're both safe and we protect each other."
"Do you think you'd catch something from me?"	"Sometimes people don't know when they have an infection. It's better to be safe."
"I won't enjoy sex if I use a condom."	"I won't enjoy sex unless it's safe."
"I don't know how to put it on."	"Here, let me show you."

Source: Adapted from Hirsch (2009a).

Talking about Condoms

Since condoms are one of the best protections against pregnancy and STDs, it is a good idea to know how to use a condom. It is also important to know how to talk to one's sexual partner about using condoms. Before talking with someone about condoms, it's a good idea to be familiar with them. Know what they look like and how to use them. That way, if one partner is unfamiliar with condom use, the other partner can demonstrate how to use one. It's best to talk about condom use before having sex. This will allow time to discuss any objections or challenges. A couple can experiment with different types of condoms to find a brand that works best for both of them. A person should be clear that he or she will not have sex without a condom. Table 3.2.4 discusses some ideas for responding to objections about condom use.

Talking about STDs

Even more than talking about birth control, it can be difficult to talk about STDs. This can be awkward for several reasons. First, one's partner may not seem like someone who would have an STD. People like to believe that they know their partners well, trust people they want to be intimate with, and would never have sex with someone who is carrying a disease. The reality is that you can't tell by looking at others whether they have an STD. An STD is not a reflection of someone's character, nor does it mean that someone is promiscuous (having multiple sex partners). Someone can contract an STD from just one sexual experience. Someone who has no symptoms and doesn't feel sick can transmit an STD.

Before having a conversation with a partner about STDs, it helps to have information about STDs, such as knowing what types of STDs can be transmitted by which sexual behaviors. For example, some people think that the only way to contract an STD is through vaginal intercourse. However, STDs such as HIV, genital herpes, syphilis, gonorrhea, and hepatitis can also be spread through oral or anal sex. It is also useful to know where tests are available for STDs (for example, a clinic or doctor's office) and how much it will cost.

You may be reluctant to discuss STDs with a partner for fear that your partner will assume that bringing up the topic means that you have an STD. Other obstacles may include shyness, embarrassment, or fear of rejection. Your best bet is to bring up the topic and discuss it in a

WHAT PEOPLE ARE SAYING **TEEN OPINIONS ON TALKING ABOUT SAFE SEX**

What's a good way to talk to a partner about having safe sex?

- "Bring it up. Don't leave it to the last minute. Talk about it beforehand." PW, age 16, Virginia
- "It can be awkward, but in the long run it's good for the relationship. You have to be honest." BM, age 21, California
- "I think the decision to have safe sex should be made early in the relationship, before a couple becomes sexually active. Some of the challenges include possible awkward situations if the couple is too young." KK, age 19, Kentucky
- "Sit down and talk about it first. Before having sex." GBH, age 17, California
- "I'd imagine the best way is 'condom or no fun.' The challenge being they don't want to use the condom. (I don't care what anyone says. If you're not using the condom, you're not being safe.)" HH, age 20, California
- "You should talk to them before anything intimate is happening. . . . If you are not comfortable enough talking about sex, you should not be comfortable enough to have sex with them." KK, age 18, Louisiana

matter-of-fact nonjudgmental way. Paying attention to how a partner reacts, listening to his or her point of view, and discussing the topic in a calm way are all good approaches. A partner who responds to the topic by really listening, trying to understand, and respecting your wishes gives some positive indications about the relationship. A partner who reacts by shutting down, acting defensive, or making fun of the other partner may indicate a lack of respect and a troubled relationship (Hirsch 2009b).

Communication Strategies

It can be easier to talk about safe sex in certain situations. It's usually less embarrassing (for both partners) to discuss it when the couple is alone. Timing is also important. Waiting too long to discuss this topic may put a damper on the mood. It may be difficult to make a rational decision in the heat of the moment. A good time to talk about safe sex is probably when the couple is alone, not having (or about to have) sex, and both people are in a reasonably good mood. It's probably not a great idea to bring up the topic in the middle of a heated argument, in a crowd of friends, in class, when either person is sad or upset, or when either partner is drunk or high (Gowen 2003).

Knowing when and where is not enough; one also needs to know how to communicate about safe sex. One should use clear, direct language to communicate about safe sex. Most people are not mind readers. Subtle gestures—such as arching one's eyebrow in the general direction of a condom packet—may not get the message across. Neither will shyly pulling a condom packet out of your pocket and waving it vaguely in the direction of your partner do the trick. It may seem difficult and awkward to make eye contact and speak directly to a partner about birth control,

TABLE 3.2.5 **COMMUNICATING ABOUT SAFE SEX**

- Don't back down: Safe sex is not negotiable.
- If the partner doesn't seem to hear, hold up a hand and repeat the message firmly, in a strong voice.
- Suggest that both partners take time to think it over.
- Explain that practicing safe sex is a way of showing respect for each other.
- If the person still insists on unsafe sex, get up and leave or call someone for help.

Source: Adapted from Gowen (2003).

STDs, and what sexual behaviors one is willing to engage in. However, with practice, this important communication gets easier.

Sometimes, even though one partner communicates clearly about safe sex, the other partner doesn't agree or doesn't seem to hear the message. Maybe one person is pressuring the other to engage in sexual behaviors that are uncomfortable or unwanted. Maybe one partner doesn't want to bother with safe sex practices. Or maybe a partner doesn't see the need for safe sex practices. This could occur for a variety of reasons. Maybe a person does not believe that he or she is at risk of contracting

? Did You Know?

- Of high school students who were sexually active, 61 percent surveyed in 2009 reported using a condom during their last sexual intercourse. This is down slightly from 63 percent in 2005 (Centers for Disease Control and Prevention 2010).

A study from the Guttmacher Institute (Kost, Henshaw, and Carlin 2010) found that:

- In 2006, about 7 percent of American girls ages 15–19 became pregnant.
- In 2005, the states with the highest teen birth rates were New Mexico, Nevada, Arizona, Texas, and Mississippi. The states with the lowest teen birth rates were New Hampshire, Vermont, Massachusetts, Connecticut, and New Jersey.

A 2003 Kaiser Family Foundation survey of young people found that:

- While 75 percent of sexually active adolescents engage in oral sex, 20 percent are unaware that STDs can be transmitted through oral sex.
- 20 percent of young people believe that they would simply "know" if someone else had an STD even if they were not tested.
- One-sixth of teens believe that an STD can only be transmitted when obvious symptoms are present.
- Half of sexually active young people say that they have been tested for STDs and HIV. However, 30 percent mistakenly believe that this screening is a standard part of a routine physical.

Sources: Centers for Disease Control and Prevention (2010); Kaiser Family Foundation et al. (2003); Kost, Henshaw, and Carlin (2010).

or spreading an STD or thinks that certain sexual practices do not carry a risk of pregnancy or STDs. Or maybe the person thinks "it can never happen to me" or "to us." If one person is pressuring another person, is not respecting boundaries regarding desired sexual behaviors, or is not willing to practice safe sex, it is important for the person whose boundaries are being violated to stand up for herself or himself. Table 3.2.5 has some tips for communicating about safe sex. Safe sex is discussed further in chapter 3 of this volume.

Sexual Desire and Asexuality

Sexual abstinence means abstaining from (not having) sex. **Asexual** may describe a person who is not sexually active or someone who is not sexually attracted to other people. Some adults who are not sexually attracted to other people describe their sexual orientation as asexual (or they describe themselves as not having any sexual orientation). However, **libido** (sexual drive) varies greatly in teens. Most teens who do not engage in sexual activities because of little or no sex drive or attraction would probably consider themselves abstinent rather than asexual. Because of differences in rates of maturity and hormone levels, it is typical for some teens to have a great deal of sex drive and for other teens to have very little or none. Sex drive also varies because of individual differences.

Sex at Parties

One type of casual sex—sexual experiences outside of a dating relationship—includes **sex parties,** parties set up for the purpose of people having casual sex. The usual social rules and expectations that relate to dating relationships do not apply at sex parties. For example, with partners at sex parties, there is no expectation of commitment to a relationship. A teenager may have sexual encounters with one or more other teens at a sex party. Sexual behaviors at parties sometimes include vaginal intercourse but more often include other sexual activities, including oral sex.

Among teens who were interviewed (Toscano 2006), most said that alcohol is usually consumed at sex parties. People do not report being coerced or pressured into sexual activity but say that alcohol is used to help teens relax and participate. Teenagers who had attended sex parties described the sexual experiences as different from a usual dating relationship. In a typical dating relationship, there is an expectation of commitment. At sex parties, there is no sense of social obligation; the purpose of the party may be sexual experimentation, or it may be just to have sexual encounters without a sense of obligation. The sex party was used as a place to hook up with no ongoing emotional attachments. People interviewed said that a sex party was usually within someone's peer group. Because teens know most of the other people at the party, they feel safer. Those who had participated described the sex party as a way to get instant gratification. Dating relationships were described as being more committed and lasting longer but also requiring more delay in sexual gratification because of social rules. Most teens described the sex at parties as consensual, without being pressured or coerced. However, some teens experienced a sense of regret or **remorse** after the party. Those who said that they felt regret indicated that alcohol played a role in their decision to have sex and that they might not have agreed to have sex if they hadn't been drinking (Toscano 2006).

Pornography

Pornography (porn) refers to anything that is intended to create sexual excitement or arousal. Pornography may include magazines featuring photos of nude people or sexually explicit pictures or descriptions, erotic literature, or X-rated movies. Pornography may appear in printed forms, on videos or DVDs, or on the Internet. It is illegal for minors to purchase this material. It is also illegal to distribute material containing pornographic or sexually explicit images or other material of children. Even though it's illegal for minors to purchase pornographic material, it is common for teens to have seen pornographic material or at least advertisements for it.

There are different types of porn. Some types of porn could be beneficial. For example, sexually explicit images could help a teen fantasize about what he or she might or might not enjoy during sex and can be safe visual aids during masturbation. However, other types of porn—especially if it contains violent images (such as of rape, forced sex, or bondage)—may be unhealthy. Some studies have shown an association between exposure to violent sexual images and more violence in people's real lives and relationships (Gowen 2003).

Too much use of pornography may interfere with a teen's desire to engage in an actual real-life romantic relationship. Because of the way people are portrayed in porn—everyone is good looking, with perfect bodies, and they always want to have sex—teens may develop unrealistic expectations about actual sexual relationships. In the real world, people don't always have perfect bodies, don't always want to have sex, and have to deal with the messy realities of life, such as discussions of safe sex and pregnancy prevention (Gowen 2003). Pornography may depict a distorted view of sex and relationships, including portraying relationships

 WHAT PEOPLE ARE SAYING **TEEN OPINIONS ON PORNOGRAPHY**

Do you think viewing porn—in magazines, in movies, or online—affects sexual relationships?

- "I think it has a tendency to hold sex to unreasonable standards in people's minds. It can also become an addiction that will damage a relationship emotionally." KK, age 19, Kentucky
- "Yes. I think it can make the person you are in a relationship with feel uncomfortable, and a person viewing porn is probably being dishonest about it to the person they are in a relationship with." KG, age 19, Texas
- "I think it has the potential to give some people unrealistic expectations in a partner, but not everyone. For someone it might be a healthy outlet when they don't have a sexual partner; for someone else it might become an addiction to the point where they have difficulty maintaining a sexual relationship with another human." ES, age 20, California

that are casual (only sexual) and that lack intimacy, love, affection, and commitment.

Studies show that teen boys tend to seek out and use pornography more than girls do (Bleakley, Hennessy, and Fishbein 2011). A study of Swedish teens ages 14 to 20 found that teens used pornography as a source of information and sexual stimulation. Porn use also affected how teens felt about themselves. Teens tended to be critical of their own body images and sexual performance based on unrealistic images portrayed in porn (Lofgren-Mårtenson and Månsson 2010). Girls are more likely to disapprove or dislike pornography, describing it as disgusting, demeaning, or off-putting. This relationship between gender and approval of pornography has been found in sexually open societies, such as in Sweden, as well as in studies in Israel and the United States (e.g., Lofgren-Mårtenson and Månsson 2010; Mesch 2009)

Some pornography is violent, showing forced sex or rape. There is controversy about the possible harmful or beneficial effects of violent pornography and sexual media. People who think that pornography is harmful claim that it contributes to trivialization of the sex act, minimization of the impact of sexual violence, and acceptance of abusive attitudes, especially toward women. On the other hand, those who believe that it can be beneficial say that violent pornography provides a harmless outlet, promotes tolerant attitudes toward sex, and is an expression of free speech in a free society. So who is right: Is violent pornography beneficial or harmful? Research shows that frequent viewing of violent porn may be associated with support for the rape myth in which rape victims are shown as responsible for their own sexual assault (Mesch 2009). Boys are more often perpetrators of sexual harassment and violence, and girls are more often the victims; however, either can be a perpetrator or a victim. In fact, it is not unusual for the same person to be a perpetrator of sexual violence in one situation and a victim in another (Bonino et al. 2006).

Since boys also tend to use porn more than girls do—and especially to view violent pornography—can one say that teen use of violent pornography is linked to perpetrating sexual violence? A 2006 study of 804 Italian high school students (ages 15–19) explored just that question. The study found a strong association between a high level of porn use, increased likelihood to perpetrate sexual harassment or forced sex, and attitudes of greater tolerance toward unwanted sexual behavior. Boys were more likely than girls to sexually harass peers (both boys and girls). Findings suggested that girls—who use less pornography than boys do—were more sensitive to porn and were more likely to be victims of sexual violence than boys. As to type of media, pornographic magazines and comics were most likely to contribute to a teen perpetrating sexual violence. For girls, viewing pornographic films and videos was linked to a greater risk of being a victim of sexual violence (Bonino et al. 2006). These findings tend to support the perspective that viewing violent pornography can be harmful.

Some teens may get accustomed to viewing pornography to the point where it occupies much of their time and energy. The teen may no longer find the idea of actual sex with another human being as exciting as the sex portrayed in porn. This behavior can become problematic if the teen neglects friendships, personal interactions, real intimacy, and responsibilities such as schoolwork. It is also a problem if the teen can no longer experience pleasure without pornography or if the teen's porn use gets in the way of a personal intimate relationship. Some teens discuss their experiences with pornography in the video *Teens Hooked on Porn* (2007), listed in the resources section at the end of this chapter.

People may get in trouble for viewing porn at inappropriate times and places. For example, most schools and workplaces have policies against using school or work computers to view pornography. A person who violates these policies at school may have her or his computer or Internet privileges revoked. Someone who views porn at work may be reprimanded or fired. School and workplace networks may have software that tracks what Internet sites individual network users visit.

Relationship Issues

Healthy Relationships

Healthy relationships are based on mutual trust, respect, consideration, and communication. The term "mutual" means that something goes both ways: If Sam respects Jill but Jill doesn't respect Sam, then there is only one-way respect. If Sam and Jill both respect each other, then that respect is mutual. The same goes for trust and communication. In the healthiest relationships, each individual trusts the other, and each person makes an effort to communicate clearly with the other person.

Relationships are shaped by family background, religion, culture, individual differences, and many other factors. These factors also influence what trust, respect, consideration, and communication mean to different people. Here are some questions to help explore what these concepts may mean within a relationship:

- *Trust:* Does one partner in a relationship trust the other to be honest? Allow their partner to have friends outside the relationship? Get jealous? Jealousy is a natural emotion. However, it's important to notice how people react if they get jealous. Do they talk about their feelings, or do they pressure their partner to not have other friendships or check up on the partner all the time?
- *Mutual respect:* Does one partner feel that he or she has to act, dress, or talk a certain way for the other partner to like her or him or feel that the partner likes her or him for who the person is naturally? Mutual respect means that each partner values the other and understands and respects the other person's boundaries.
- *Consideration:* Is one person caring to the other? Does each person treat the other well? Care about the other's feelings? Consideration means listening if one person says that he or she is uncomfortable doing something and making some adjustments and compromises so that both people are happy. Consideration also involves give and take, such as taking turns choosing what activities to do together. Consideration also involves each person being supportive of the other.
- *Communication:* Healthy communication involves being able to express feelings and ask questions. It doesn't mean automatically knowing what another person is thinking (mind reading). Sometimes communication is easy, and sometimes it takes a lot of work. Sometimes people say things that hurt another's feelings. The important thing is being able to communicate openly

> and honestly about feelings and misunderstandings, apologize if necessary, and move on. There needs to be enough trust in a relationship so that one person feels that it is safe to be honest with the other. Unspoken expectations (assumptions) can cause a lot of stress and misunderstanding in a relationship. It can be helpful to state expectations or ask questions if you are unsure of what the other person's expectations or feelings are. This can help avoid miscommunication.

In addition to mutual respect, trust, consideration, and communication, healthy relationships involve each person having a separate identity. In healthy relationships, people don't have to spend all their time together or share all the same interests. It is healthy to have some separate interests, activities, and friends as well as to have common interests and spend time together. Healthy relationships involve balancing what is shared with the other person and what is separate or individual.

Unhealthy Relationships

If a healthy relationship is one based on mutual trust, respect, consideration, and communication, then an unhealthy relationship is one without these qualities. Specifically, an unhealthy relationship may involve mean, abusive, or disrespectful behavior or lots of arguments. This could be a home in which parents or other family members are mean, fight a lot, or hurt each other.

Difficult Relationships

Relationships can be difficult if there are communication problems or if one or more members of the relationship have low self-esteem or are insecure. Mental health problems or substance use can contribute to an unhealthy relationship. Very intense relationships can be difficult and may not last long. Teenagers are still in the process of establishing their identities, of figuring out who they are. Two teenagers who are learning about themselves, growing, and changing rapidly may not stay together very long. They may start out liking the same things but soon end up wanting very different things. Sometimes it makes sense to end a relationship that isn't working anymore. It's better to deal with the temporary grief of a breakup than to drag on a relationship that isn't healthy for either partner.

If two people are having relationship problems and really want to make the relationship work, counseling may help them learn to communicate more effectively or resolve their differences. However, staying in an unhealthy relationship without taking any steps to make it work is not good for either person. Self-esteem and relationships are also discussed in chapter 1, "Environment and Mental Health," in volume 5.

Abusive Relationships

A dating, friendship, or family relationship in which there is abuse is an unhealthy relationship. Someone who comes from a home or community in which domestic violence or abuse is common may think that abusive behaviors are normal or that these behaviors are acceptable. Abuse is never okay!

Types of Abuse

Abuse can be emotional, physical, or sexual. It can include verbal abuse, bullying, or **hate crimes**. Hate crimes are acts of violence against someone because of her or his race, ethnicity, gender, religion, or sexual orientation. Abuse can happen in families, in intimate or dating relationships, or in friendships. Domestic violence is when someone is physically abusing a family member. Witnessing domestic violence in the family can be traumatic for children, teens, and other family members. Abuse happens in all kinds of families and communities.

Physical Abuse

Physical abuse includes hitting, punching, kicking, or any type of physical violence, fighting, or aggression. Physical abuse may be pulling someone's hair, pinching, choking, burning, beating, throwing, shaking, biting, or physically hurting someone in any manner that causes pain or injury or leaves marks. Physical abuse has the most obvious effects. Sometimes these effects can be seen, such as a broken bone or bruises. The effects of physical abuse aren't always visible, but physical abuse still leaves emotional scars.

Emotional Abuse

Emotional abuse may include teasing, bullying, name calling, put-downs, or humiliation. Intimidation, threats, and betrayal are types of emotional abuse, as is being overly controlling, possessive, or jealous. Yelling, being dismissive, or being overly critical can be types of emotional abuse. Emotional abuse can be difficult to recognize because it doesn't leave a visible scar. But emotional abuse hurts, and the effects can last long after the abuse ends.

Neglect

Neglect is a type of abuse that occurs when someone's basic needs aren't being met, such as if a parent doesn't provide children with food, shelter, clothing, medical care, or supervision. Emotional neglect is when a parent or guardian doesn't provide a child with emotional support or any attention (such as consistently and deliberately ignoring the child or teen). Emotional neglect is not when basic needs are unmet because of things beyond the parent's control, such as homelessness or unemployment. It is not emotional neglect when a teen doesn't get everything that he or she wants (such as a new car or cell phone). Emotional neglect refers to not getting basic needs like love, attention, food, and shelter.

Sexual Abuse

Any sexual contact between an adult and a minor is considered sexual abuse. Incest is when someone sexually abuses a family member. Sexual abuse may mean being forced to have sex. It can also mean being pressured or coerced into any type of sexual activity that is unwanted or uncomfortable. Any sex that is not consensual—meaning that both people are voluntarily, willingly, and knowingly engaging in sexual activity—is sexual abuse. Rape is a form of sexual abuse. Anyone can be sexually abused—men, women, boys, or girls. No one should be forced or pressured into any type of sexual activity that is uncomfortable or unwanted.

What Causes Abuse?

Growing up in an abusive or violent family or community may lead someone to believe that abuse is the right way to treat others. Some people may consider certain behaviors appropriate ways to discipline a child; other people would consider this abuse. People who have never learned to manage their feelings may abuse others. This can be especially true if someone doesn't know how to handle feelings of anger or how to manage stress. Someone who doesn't have good **coping mechanisms**—ways to manage stress—and doesn't know where to turn for help might behave in abusive or hurtful ways when stressed. Situations that may exacerbate stress, such as unemployment or marriage difficulties, could make abuse worse. Alcohol and other drug use can impair judgment and make it difficult for people to manage their feelings and control their anger. Some types of mental health disorders, especially if not treated, can make people more likely to act aggressively or lack

TABLE 3.2.6 **TEEN DATING VIOLENCE**

Percentage of high school students surveyed who reported experiencing violence in a romantic relationship in the 18 months preceding the survey:

	Opposite-sex Relationships (%)	**Same-sex Relationships (%)**
Physical violence	12	11
Psychological violence	29	21

Source: Jouriles, Platt, and McDonald (2009).

self-control. Stress, coping, and anger management are discussed in chapter 2, volume 5.

There is help for abusers. With appropriate treatment, abusive people can learn to manage their feelings and take responsibility for their behavior. For example, people can get help managing their anger. People with mental health disorders can get treatment. And people who are abusive when they use alcohol or other drugs can get help to stop using substances. When abuse occurs in families, family members may all need different types of treatment and support to learn healthier ways of interacting and to heal from the abuse. People who get help to break the cycle of abuse have a better chance of having healthier nonabusive relationships in the future.

Warning Signs of Abuse

Some people may not realize that they are in an abusive relationship. This may be because they grew up in a home where there was abuse, so they think that this behavior is normal or acceptable or cannot be changed. Someone may be used to living in abusive situations and may not realize that things can be different. Someone may think that hitting, humiliating, or putting someone down is a normal way to show love and caring. It can also be confusing if a partner or family member is nice, loving, and caring sometimes and abusive other times. It can be difficult to recognize or admit that someone whom one loves and cares about is being abusive.

A boyfriend, girlfriend, or family member using insults or mean language or putting someone down is a warning sign of abuse. Other signs of abuse include hitting, slapping, or forcing someone into any sexual activity. Some warning signs that may indicate that a relationship is abusive or is becoming abusive include a person who:

- Gets jealous if the partner wants to spend time with other friends
- Doesn't want the partner to have any separate activities
- Wants the partner to give up favorite activities
- Criticizes the way the partner dresses or looks
- Tells the partner that no one else will ever want to be with/date her or him
- Gets angry if the partner doesn't drop everything to be with her or him
- Tries to force the partner into unwanted sex

Someone is exhibiting warning signs of abuse if he or she tries to control a partner, makes the partner feel bad about herself or himself, isolates the partner from friends or family, or tries to harm the partner physically or sexually. Possessiveness, controlling behavior, isolating someone, put-downs, physical violence, and sexual coercion are all types of abuse.

When both partners in a relationship don't respect each other, it may be a sign that the relationship is unhealthy. Other red flags of possible abuse include unwanted sexual advances or feeling obligated to participate in

? Did You Know?

In the United States in 2011:

- 10% of teen boys and girls were victims of physical violence by a dating or romantic partner.
- 20–30% of teens were victims of psychological, verbal, or emotional abuse.
- Teens are more likely than adults to become victims of intimate partner violence.
- Males are less likely than females to report dating abuse or violence.

According to Teen Research Unlimited (2006):

- 15% of teens who have been in a relationship report having been hit, slapped, or pushed by their boyfriend or girlfriend.
- 30% of teens who have been in a relationship have worried about their physical safety in a relationship.

Sources: Ayers and Davis (2011); Teen Research Unlimited, Liz Claiborne Inc. (2006).

sexual acts that make either person uncomfortable. If one person pressures another to do something by saying "if you really loved me, you would . . . ," this is a sign of possible abuse. Any time one person tries to control another through manipulation, coercion, threats, or pressure, warning flags should go up. When one person tries to control another, this means that the person cares more about himself or herself and what he or she wants than about the other person.

Cycle of Abuse

It may be tempting to make excuses for someone who is being abusive, especially if that person has had a rough life. One may feel sorry for someone who is abusive or think that being nice to that person will change the abusive behavior. Unfortunately, being understanding and nice won't cure someone of abusive behavior.

Some people who are abused think that if they were nicer, more understanding, or a better partner or lover, the abuse wouldn't happen. A victim may blame himself or herself because the abuse is happening. Abuse is never the fault of the victim (the person being abused). No one deserves to be abused!

Sometimes an abuser will feel remorseful after the abuse. Remorse is a feeling of guilt or shame for one's behavior. The abuser may apologize to the victim for being abusive, give the victim gifts to make up, and swear that it will never happen again. However, abuse often happens over and over in a pattern or cycle.

The cycle of abuse starts with a build-up of tension followed by a violent incident or explosion—the abuse. The abuse is followed by reconciliation. Reconciliation is when the abuser apologizes to the victim, gives gifts to make up, and promises that it will never happen again. Reconciliation may be followed by a period of relative calm, when things seem practically normal. The calm time is when the victim focuses on the abuser's good qualities, remembering what attracted him or her to the abuser in the first place. During this calm time, the victim may believe that the abusive behavior was just a one-time thing, that it may have been her or his own fault, and that it will never happen again. The calm period is followed by another period of tensions building, and the cycle starts all over again. Figure 3.2.1 shows the cycle of abuse.

Effects of Abuse

Someone who has been in an abusive relationship—whether the abuse is physical, emotional, or sexual—may be at increased risk of experiencing

Cycle of Abuse

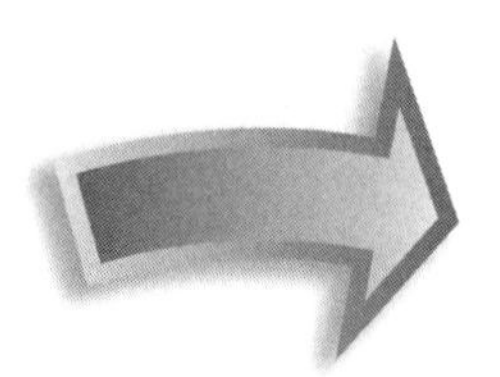

4. Calm
- Honeymoon period
- Abuser and victim 'forget' the abuse ever happened, and believe the relationship is 'normal' again

1. Tensions Build
- Tension increases, communication breaks down
- Victim becomes fearful and tries to smooth things over with abuser

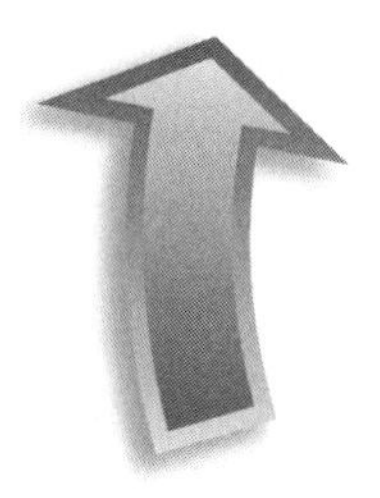

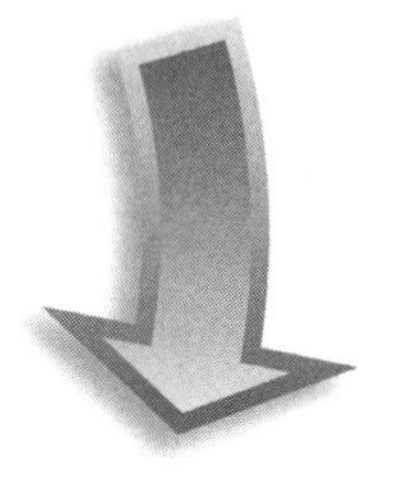

3. Reconciliation
- Abuser apologizes, offers excuses, or blames the victim
- Abuser may deny that abuse occurred, or may say it wasn't as bad as the victim believes
- Abuser may give make-up gifts or promise that it will never happen again

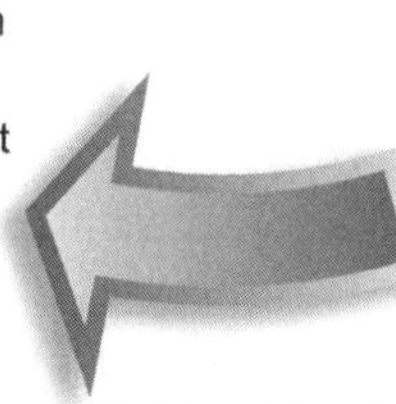

2. Abuse
- Violent incident, explosion
- Verbal, emotional, physical, or sexual abuse
- Arguments, anger, blaming, threats, intimidation

FIGURE 3.2.1 **CYCLE OF ABUSE.**
(Yvette Malamud Ozer, 2012)

mental health symptoms or distress. Symptoms following abuse could manifest as depression, anxiety, or stress.

It can be confusing and traumatic if abuse involves keeping secrets—not talking about the abuse outside the relationship or family. Friction, arguments, or misunderstandings can happen in any relationship. It is not unusual for teens to get into arguments with parents or other family members. Sometimes people get mad and yell. Parents may discipline and punish children in ways that seem unfair, such as privileges being taken away or children being grounded. Teens in a romantic relationship may get into arguments and get mad at each other. All these things can feel bad, but they aren't necessarily abuse. If punishments, yelling, and arguments go on for a long time, are very intense, are deliberately hurtful, or escalate to physical violence, then abuse may be occurring.

Being abused affects all aspects of someone's life. Effects of abuse may vary depending on the type of abuse, how severe the abuse is, and how long it goes on. Abuse can especially affect someone's self-esteem: how one feels about oneself, one's self-confidence and self-respect. Abuse can make someone feel afraid, jittery, jumpy, and insecure. Abuse may contribute to stress, difficulties concentrating, learning difficulties, and problems with eating or sleeping. Someone who is being abused may feel sad, angry, or frightened or may just not care anymore.

Abuse can make someone afraid to be around other people or afraid to be alone. Someone who has been abused may have difficulty trusting other people or making or keeping friends and may have trouble with relationships. Teens who have been abused have an increased risk of depression and sometimes turn to alcohol or other drugs to feel better. Some people who have been abused try to feel better by hurting themselves—for example, cutting themselves or attempting suicide. Self-injurious behavior and suicide are discussed further in chapter 3, volume 5.

Someone who has been abused may feel angry, confused, lonely, numb, upset, guilty, embarrassed, or ashamed. This is especially true if the abuser is manipulative or blames the victim. It can be difficult to report abuse if a victim doesn't want to get someone he or she loves in trouble. A victim might be afraid of the consequences of reporting abuse, such as

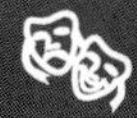

Fact or Myth?

Abusers in intimate relationships are usually males.

Myth:

- Males and females tend to be abusers in intimate relationships at equal rates.
- However, the majority of physical abuse resulting in injuries is usually perpetrated by male abusers on female victims.
- Female abusers are more likely to inflict emotional or verbal abuse on their victims.
- Because of social and cultural gender expectations, males are more reluctant to report being abused by a female.

Source: Ayers and Davis (2011).

child protective services intervening, having a parent arrested, or being removed from an abusive home. A teenager may be afraid to report an abusive boyfriend or girlfriend because of the fear of peers and teachers finding out about the abuse. Because of the feelings and fears that go along with abuse, much abuse does not get reported.

Because abuse is accompanied by such intense and confusing feelings, symptoms, and consequences, painful feelings can last for a long time after the abuse stops. Sometimes working with a therapist or counselor can help victims heal from the effects of abuse.

Getting Help If You Are Being Abused

It is not healthy to stay in an abusive relationship, and it is important to get out of the abusive situation as soon as possible. A victim may need help to get out of the relationship, stay safe, and heal from the abuse. A friend or trusted adult may be able to help a victim get to a safe place. If a victim is afraid of being hurt, he or she can call the police or 9-1-1 for help. If someone has been physically attacked or raped, it may be necessary to see a doctor or go to an emergency room for medical care.

People who have been abused may feel isolated from friends and family. This may be an aspect of the abuse and may be related to feelings of guilt or shame. People who are trying to get out of an abusive relationship should avoid isolating themselves. It is usually safer to be around trusted friends and family. It may be difficult to ask for help; this is especially difficult if the person being abused still loves the abuser or feels guilty about leaving. Asking for help takes a lot of courage and may be the first step to getting out of an abusive situation.

Helping a Friend Who Is Being Abused

Signs of abuse may include broken bones, bruises, secrecy, isolating from friends or family, avoiding school or social events, expressing or showing excessive feelings of guilt or shame, or making excuses that don't make sense. A friend may be reluctant to talk about being abused. This may be because he or she is afraid of getting the abuser in trouble, being hurt more by the abuser, or being pressured into ending the relationship.

Victims of abuse may feel guilty or ashamed, that they don't deserve to be treated better, or that the abuse is their fault. A friend who is being abused needs patience, understanding, caring, and someone who will listen. It's important to listen without being judgmental and to let abuse victims know that the abuse is not their fault and that they deserve better.

Where to Find Help

Abuse victims should be encouraged to tell a parent, counselor, or other trusted adult about the abuse so they can get help. There may be resources for help at school, including trusted teachers, school counselors, school psychologists, or school nurses. A teen might also turn to doctors, nurses, therapists, other health care professionals, or religious or spiritual leaders for help. The resources section at the end of this chapter lists hotlines, teen help lines, youth centers, and shelters where teens who are being abused can find help.

How to Stop Being Abusive

So far there has been a lot of focus on victims of abuse. What about the abuser? With enough motivation and some outside help, it is possible for a person who is abusive to change. People may be abusive for many reasons, including coming from abusive homes or families, difficulty with communication skills or anger management, difficulty managing feelings, fear of being alone, or not knowing what healthy relationships are like. Table 3.2.7 has tips for anyone who is thinking about changing his or her abusive behavior.

Rape

Rape is a form of sexual violence involving forced or coerced sex and may involve physical force, violence, or manipulation or coercion to have sex. Any type of forced sex—sex without consent—is rape. Sexual assault is the same thing as rape.

Girls and women are raped more often, but boys and men may also be victims of rape. Rape is an aggressive and violent act; it has nothing to do with love. Rape is about power, dominance, and control. Even though some of the behaviors are similar to those that occur in consensual sex, rape is not sex. No one asks to be raped, and no one deserves to be sexually assaulted. Even someone who is wearing **provocative** clothing or is flirting is not asking for or consenting to sex. Rape is always the rapist's fault; it is never the victim's fault.

Rape is illegal. Anyone who has sex with a person under the legal age of consent may be charged with statutory rape. Laws about what age is considered too young to consent vary by state. Statutory rape may be committed by a stranger or by someone known to the victim (an acquaintance or family member).

TABLE 3.2.7 **TIPS FOR ABUSIVE TEENS**

- *Take responsibility for your behavior.* Even if your boyfriend or girlfriend sometimes does things that make you angry, no one deserves to be controlled or abused.
- *Change for yourself.* Getting help to stop abusing will help you in your current and future relationships.
- *Find a friend you can be honest with.* Talk about your concerns and your plans to change; ask your friend to hold you accountable if he or she sees you being abusive.
- *Take a break.* Try spending some time away from your girlfriend or boyfriend.
- *Walk away from an argument before it escalates.* Make a decision to walk away before things get out of hand.
- *Look at the people around you.* If possible, spend less time with family or friends who are abusive in their relationships. Pay attention to how you feel when you witness others being abused.
- *Be patient with yourself.* Admitting that you have a problem and that you want to change is a big step. Be patient; things don't change overnight.
- *Look for a class or counseling locally.* Contact loveisrespect.org, the National Teen Dating Abuse Helpline. A peer advocate can help you locate local help and talk to you about your concern.

Source: Adapted from Love Is Respect (2011).

Acquaintance or Date Rape

Sometimes a stranger sexually attacks someone, but often the attacker is someone the victim knows. Acquaintance (or date) rape occurs when nonconsensual sex happens between two people who know each other—whether they've been friends for a long time or are going out on a date for the first time.

Forced sex between people who are dating is known as date rape. Spousal rape is when forced sex happens between married people. Familial rape is forced sex with a family member, a type of incest. Acquaintance rape could be committed by a neighbor, someone at school, or someone in the community who is known by the victim. All of these are types of acquaintance rape.

Gang rape is when two or more people sexually assault an individual, either at the same time or sequentially (one after the other). The attackers

? **Did You Know?**

- 75% of American adolescents who have been sexually assaulted were victimized by someone they knew well.
- 13% of American teen sexual assaults were reported to police, 6 percent to child protective services, 5 percent to school authorities, and 1 percent to other authorities.
- 86% of sexual assaults against American adolescents went unreported.
- In 2007, teens ages 12 to 19 experienced nearly 1.6 million violent crimes, including 57,511 reported sexual assaults and rapes.

Source: National Center for Victims of Crime (2011).

may be acquaintances of the victim or may be strangers. Gang rape can be particularly traumatic, because in addition to the person actively attacking the victim, other people are witnessing the event. In fact, there may be people in the room watching who are not participating in the attack, but they are not trying to help the victim either. This can be devastating and humiliating and can reinforce a sense of helplessness and worthlessness in the victim.

Consent

Consent is when both people want to have sex and agree about what types of sexual behavior they want to have. If one person is not sure whether he or she wants to have sex, it is not okay for the other person to assume consent and go ahead. If one person says "maybe" or "no" to a request for sex, then consent has not occurred. "No" never means "yes" when it comes to sexual consent. "No" does not mean that it is okay to keep asking and pressuring someone until he or she agrees to have sex.

Both parties have to be able to truly consent. Someone who is drunk on alcohol or under the influence of other drugs cannot legally consent. A person who is asleep or passed out cannot consent. Someone who is mentally or emotionally challenged may not be able to consent. A child can never legally consent to sex.

A person can say no to sex at any time, even after initially consenting. Just because someone has already consented to sex doesn't mean that anything goes. Someone may agree to one type of sexual activity (for example, kissing or oral sex) but may not consent to other types of sex.

Alcohol, Drugs, and Rape

Use of alcohol or other drugs can play a part in sexual assault. Being under the influence makes a person more vulnerable to sexual assault. Alcohol and other drugs can loosen inhibitions and impair judgment. Someone who is under the influence of substances may find themselves in an unsafe situation. Being under the influence makes it difficult to judge the dangerousness of a situation, what someone's intentions are, and how to stay safe.

Some people get more aggressive after drinking or using drugs. People who are drunk or high may act in ways that they wouldn't normally act, including being more sexually aggressive. Someone may not feel drunk but may show less common sense than he or she normally would.

Date rape drugs may be used as part of sexual assaults. Drugs such as rohypnol (also known as roofies), GHB (gamma-hydroxybutyrate), and ketamine (also known as Special K) may be mixed into a drink without someone's knowledge. Rohypnol and GHB are colorless and odorless, so someone might not be aware that the drug is in her or his drink. Date rape drugs can cause someone to black out and forget what happened. People who have been given date rape drugs say that they felt paralyzed, had blurred vision, or couldn't remember what happened. Effects of drugs can be intensified when mixed with alcohol. If a friend at a party feels more intoxicated (fuzzy, woozy, or sleepy) than one would expect, he or she may have been drugged. If someone is having trouble remembering things or feels as if he or she may pass out, the safest thing may be to find a trusted friend and leave the party. It may be necessary to take someone to the hospital to ensure that person's safety, especially if he or she may have been given date rape drugs.

Preventing Sexual Assault

People can take precautions to avoid sexual assault, such as going on dates with groups of friends rather than just as a couple. This is a good idea when dating someone you don't know very well. Another safety precaution is going to a party with a good friend rather than alone.

Some people may think it's funny to spike drinks at parties with drugs or alcohol, that it will make the party more fun. Other people add drugs or alcohol to someone's drink so they can take advantage of that person, including sexually assaulting the person. Going to a party with a good friend gives you more of a chance to keep an eye on each other's drinks. It's not a good idea to leave a drink unattended at a party. It's safer to drink something that comes out of an unopened bottle or can so that you know exactly what you are drinking. Friends who go to a party together can arrange to check on each other every hour, especially if there is drinking at the party. It's a good idea to let a friend or family member know where you are going and when you plan to return.

Meet in a public place when dating a new person—someone you don't know very well. Avoid meeting alone or in isolated places until after you get to know someone better. Don't be alone with someone you feel uncomfortable or unsafe around. Think about how intimate you want to be with someone when dating someone new. It's easier to communicate and establish boundaries before things get uncomfortable.

Some commonsense precautions include avoiding isolated secluded places, especially at night, and walking with someone (rather than alone) after dark. If it is necessary to walk alone or at night, be alert, sober, and aware of your surroundings. Self-defense courses, including some martial arts, can help you feel more confident and learn physical techniques that you can use to get away from an attacker. If you find yourself in a dangerous situation, you can yell "fire" or "police" or run toward a well-lighted public place.

Dealing with a Rape

No matter how many precautions one takes, rape still can happen. Remember that rape is never the victim's fault. Someone who has been raped should go someplace where he or she feels safe or should call a trusted friend or family member who can help get him or her somewhere safe. In dangerous situations, it may be necessary to call the police or dial 9-1-1. If someone is injured, he or she should go straight to an emergency room.

At the hospital, the victim's injuries will be assessed and treated. He or she will be examined, and evidence such as photographs and fluid samples will be taken. The victim's clothing may be collected as evidence. It is important to preserve this material as evidence to aid in prosecution of a rapist.

A friend who has been sexually assaulted may feel embarrassed, ashamed, or afraid to talk about it. The best way to support victims of sexual assault is to listen, believe in them, and be patient. If the abuse is still going on—for example, if a family member is molesting them or they are in an abusive dating situation—encourage them to get help. This is especially important if they are in an unsafe situation.

If someone has been raped and does not immediately report it, he or she can still get help. Some places to find support include trusted family members, school counselors or school psychologists, trusted teachers or clergypersons, child protective services, or a crisis center or rape hotline. Several resources are listed at the end of this chapter.

Reporting Sexual Assault

Someone who wants to report a sexual assault should go to a hospital or emergency room. It's important not to change clothes, wash up, bathe, or take a shower in order to preserve any evidence of a rape. Sometimes evidence collected after a rape can be used to prosecute a rapist. Write down anything remembered from the assault, including descriptions of the attacker, the location, any possible witnesses, and any vehicles involved.

Doctors or hospital personnel conduct a special exam after someone has been sexually assaulted. This may be difficult or embarrassing and may seem frightening to someone who has recently been assaulted. These exams may involve photographing injuries, collecting material by combing the victim's hair and checking under the victim's fingernails, and taking swabs from the victim's mouth, vagina, or rectum. Clothing may also be brushed, photographed, or taken. This exam may provide evidence that can be used to prosecute a rapist.

Local rape crisis centers, if available, have information about victim's rights, local resources, or tips for preventing or recovering from sexual assault. Many are also listed at the end of this chapter.

Sexual Harassment

Sexual harassment is any unwanted sexual behavior and can be considered a type of bullying. A harasser may be a teen or an adult. Both the person being sexually harassed and the harasser may be male or female, and they can be the same or opposite gender. Boys can sexually harass other boys, and girls can harass each other. Teasing someone about sexual orientation, touching in an unwanted sexual way, or making fun of someone's body characteristics are all forms of sexual harassment. Examples of sexual harassment include:

- *Physical contact:* Pinching or touching someone's breast, buttocks, or other body part without permission.
- *Assault:* Kissing or hugging someone intimately when that person doesn't want that type of contact. Pulling off someone's clothing.
- *Intimidation:* Cornering or blocking someone in a sexual way.

- *Sexual comments:* Calling someone a whore or a slut or making derogatory (unkind) comments about someone's sexual orientation or gender identity. Making comments about someone's physical characteristics, such as breast size or the appearance of someone's genitals. Spreading sexual rumors about someone, including on the Internet, on social networking sites, or through text messages or e-mails.
- *Obscene or sexual gestures:* Making sexual gestures toward or about someone.
- ***Sexual innuendo*** (implied or suggestive behavior): Can include words, gestures, or images that imply or suggest sexual behavior about somebody.

? Did You Know?

- 81% of students will experience some form of sexual harassment during their school lives.
- 27% of students experience sexual harassment often.
- 85% of students report that students harass other students at their schools.
- Almost 40% of students report that teachers and other school staff sexually harass students in their schools.
- 9% of youth Internet users surveyed said that they had been harassed online in 2005, up from 6% in 2000.
- 86% of LGBT youths have been verbally harassed at school because of their sexual orientation.
- 44% of LGBT students have been physically harassed (e.g., pushed or shoved) and 22% had been physically assaulted because of their sexual orientation.
- 61% of LGBT students who were harassed or assaulted at school did not report the incident to school officials, 33% because they doubted that anything would be done and 25% because they feared that reporting would make the situation worse.

Sources: AAUW Educational Foundation Sexual Harassment Task Force (2004); National Center for Victims of Crime (2011).

- *Sexual drawings or photographs:* Making sexual drawings or posting or passing around a provocative or sexual photograph of someone, including on the Internet.
- *Sexual propositions:* Asking or pressuring someone to have sex after that person has said "no."
- *Unwanted communication:* Repeated phone calls, texts, e-mails, or letters. Stalking someone.

Flirting or Sexual Harassment?

Flirting is common between teens, and it isn't always unhealthy. However, it's never acceptable for an adult to flirt with a teen. Sometimes it's hard to know when the line is being crossed between flirting and sexual harassment. Table 3.2.8 shows some examples of differences between flirting and sexual harassment.

Someone may not appreciate being flirted with if he or she seems uncomfortable, uninterested in flirting back, afraid, or embarrassed. If someone does not flirt back, does not laugh at a sexual joke, or starts avoiding someone who is flirting, then that person does not want to flirt. Continuing to flirt after receiving any of these signals would be considered harassment.

A victim of sexual harassment might feel scared, embarrassed, depressed, helpless, or hopeless. Someone who is sexually harassed may feel physical symptoms of stress such as headaches, stomachaches, or

TABLE 3.2.8 **FLIRTING OR SEXUAL HARASSMENT?**

Flirting	Sexual Harassment
• Welcome attention	• Unwelcome attention
• Goes both ways	• One-sided
• Makes someone feel: ○ attractive or flattered ○ in control ○ good about herself or himself	• Makes someone feel: ○ ugly or put down ○ out of control ○ bad or dirty

Source: Adapted from New York City Alliance against Sexual Assault (2010).

difficulty sleeping (New York City Alliance against Sexual Assault 2010). Being sexually harassed may affect someone's academic performance.

When Is Sexual Harassment Illegal?

Sexual harassment is illegal and may also violate school rules or workplace polices. Sexual harassment of students is illegal. A federal law, Title IX of the Education Amendments of 1972 (U.S.C. §§1681–1688 [1972]), prohibits sexual harassment in all education programs and activities that receive any federal funds. Title IX applies to harassment that occurs at school or at school-related activities, such as extracurricular sports and field trips. Title IX applies to a student being harassed by an adult or by another student (Office for Civil Rights, U.S. Department of Education 2008). In the workplace, sexual harassment violates Title VII of the Civil Rights Act of 1964 (P.L. No. 88-352, 78 Stat. 241 [1964]).

Dealing with Sexual Harassment

What Can a Victim of Sexual Harassment Do?

Depending on where it occurs, who is doing it, and what type of harassment it is, there are different steps that a victim can take. If sexual harassment takes place at school, it should be reported to a principal, school counselor, trusted teacher, or parent. Being aware of workplace and community policies and rules is a starting place to knowing how to report sexual harassment. An adult sexually harassing a teen should always be reported. Other steps to deal with sexual harassment include the following:

- Ask the person who is harassing to stop. Be specific about what behavior is unwelcome or uncomfortable.
- Don't ignore the harassment, and don't be afraid to speak up.
- Keep a journal of the harassment. Write down what, where, and when it happened; the name of the perpetrator; and whether there were any witnesses. Making a note of how the harassment made the victim feel, any steps that were taken to stop the harassment, and how the harasser responded are all useful information in case a victim decides to file a complaint or press charges.
- Be persistent about finding someone who will listen and is willing to help.

- Victims of sexual harassment should not blame themselves. (Fogarty 2008; New York City Alliance against Sexual Assault 2010)

How Can Someone Help a Victim of Sexual Harassment?

A witness to sexual harassment can help in several ways:

- Do not participate in the harassment.
- Step in and try to intervene, unless it is not safe to do so.
- Report the incident.
- Suggest to the victim that he or she talk to an adult or report the harassment.

Resources

Websites, Help Lines, and Hotlines

AVERT: AVERTing HIV and AIDS

An international organization working to avert HIV and AIDS: http://www.avert.org/aids-hiv-charity-avert.htm

Am I Ready for Sex? http://www.avert.org/ready-sex.htm

Boston Alliance for Gay and Lesbian Youth

A youth-led social support organization committed to social justice and advocating for programs, policies, and services for the LGBTQ youth community: http://www.bagly.org/

Boys Town International

Nationwide programs to help children and families in need: http://www.boystown.org/national-hotline

24/7 National Hotline (Spanish-speaking counselors and translation services in 140 languages available): 1-800-448-3000

TDD: 1-800-448-1833

Break the Cycle

An organization that addresses teen dating abuse: http://www.breakthecycle.org/

Child Help

Child abuse hotline that includes crisis intervention, information, literature, and referrals to emergency, social service, and support resources: http://www.childhelp.org/pages/hotline

National Child Abuse Hotline: 1-800-4-A-CHILD

Coalition for Positive Sexuality (CPS)
A site for teens who are sexually active or thinking about having a sexual relationship; information about decision making, contraception, STDs, and pregnancy: http://www.positive.org/

COLAGE
A national movement of children, youths, and adults with one or more LGBT parents; building community and working toward social justice through youth empowerment, leadership development, education, and advocacy: http://www.colage.org/about/

Covenant House
For runaways and homeless youths: http://www.covenanthouse.org/

Teens who are on the street, need a place to stay, are struggling with drugs, or having thoughts of suicide, call: 800-999-9999

Gender Equity Resource Center
LGBT resources; definition of terms: http://geneq.berkeley.edu/lgbt_resources_definiton_of_terms#asexual

GLSEN (Gay, Lesbian, & Straight Education Network)
Safe Space programs for schools; free downloadable Safe Space posters and stickers. Resources for LGBT students, allies, and families; support to create a school GSA (gay-straight alliance): http://www.glsen.org/

Go Ask Alice! (Columbia University)
Information about alcohol and other drugs, fitness and nutrition, emotional health, general health, sexuality, sexual health, and relationships: http://www.goaskalice.columbia.edu/

Healthy Relationships (Jewish Women International)
Resources and information about self-esteem and healthy relationships: http://www.jwi.org/Page.aspx?pid=320

I Wanna Know! American Sexual Health Association (ASHA)
Information about sexual health, relationships, LGBT, pregnancy, and parenthood: www.iwannaknow.org

Love Is Not Abuse
Information, resources, and quiz to test knowledge about teen dating violence: http://loveisnotabuse.com/

Love Is Respect
Online home of the National Dating Abuse Helpline, a community with support, resources, and information on dating abuse: http://www.loveisrespect.org/

National Dating Abuse Helpline
1-866-331-9474

TTY: 1-866-331-8453

National Domestic Violence Hotline
http://www.thehotline.org/

1-800-799-SAFE

Our Family Coalition
Promotes the rights and well-being of LGBT families with children through education, advocacy, social networking, and grassroots community organizing: http://www.ourfamily.org/

Pandora's Project
Support and resources for survivors of rape and sexual abuse: http://www.pandys.org/index.html

PFLAG (Parents, Families, and Friends of Lesbians and Gays)
Resource for families and friends of LGBT individuals: http://community.pflag.org/

Planned Parenthood Info for Teens
Information for teens about the human body, sex, relationships, pregnancy, and LGBTQ: http://www.plannedparenthood.org/info-for-teens/our-bodies-33795.htm

Rape, Abuse & Incest National Network (RAINN)
National hotline and information about sexual assault: http://www.rainn.org

1-800-656-HOPE

Safer Sex
Everything you wanted to know about safer sex: http://safersex.org/

Sex, Etc.
Sex education by teens and for teens but overseen in part by the Center for Psychology at Rutgers University and in service for 30 years: http://www.sexetc.org/topic/emotional_health

Sex Info SF
A sexual health text-messaging program for youths in San Francisco:
http://www.isis-inc.org/sexinfo.php
http://www.sextextsf.org/

Sexuality Information and Education Council of the United States (SIECUS)
A nonprofit with access to accurate information on sex and sexual health:
http://www.siecus.org/

TeensHealth
Website with information in English and Spanish for teens about the body, the mind, physical and emotional health, relationships, drugs and alcohol, sexuality, and many other topics from the Nemours Foundation, which provides children's health information and care: http://teenshealth.org/teen/

Teen Source
Sexual health for youths to encourage informed decision making:
http://www.teensource.org/

Teens in Charge (Chinese Community Health Resource Center)
Health topics in English, Chinese, and simplified Chinese, including dating and relationships, diseases, emotional and sexual health, addiction and substance misuse, nutrition and fitness, and general health: http://www.teensincharge.org/en/health-topics

The Trevor Project
Suicide prevention and resources for LGBT youths, including 24-hour crisis intervention phone line and suicide prevention resources:
http://www.thetrevorproject.org/
866-4-U-TREVOR (1-866-488-7386)

We Are Talking: Teen Health (Palo Alto Medical Foundation)
Health information for teens: http://www.pamf.org/teen/

Youth Resource
Information on sexual health for LGBT and questioning youths:
http://www.amplifyyourvoice.org/youthresource

Videos

Glazier, Lynn. 2009. *Wired for Sex, Lies and Power Trips.* New York: Women Make Movies. http://www.wmm.com/filmcatalog/pages/

c777.shtml. E-mail orders@wmm.com to place an order. *An inside look at the culture of sexual harassment and bullying widespread among many teens today; examines the price that adolescents, especially girls, pay to be cool, hip and popular.*

Teens Hooked on Porn. 2007. Films for the Humanities & Sciences, PO Box 2053, Princeton, NJ, 08543-2053, 800-257-5126, 609-671-0266. Distributor e-mail: custserv@films.com. *Follows stories of teenage porn addicts and discusses the role that the Internet has played in escalating teen exposure to pornography. The teen boys in the video tell their own stories, some admitting and some not admitting to having a problem.*

Further Reading

Basso, Michael. 2003. *The Underground Guide to Teenage Sexuality.* 2nd ed. Minneapolis: Fairview.

Beam, Cris. 2011. *I Am J.* New York: Little, Brown. *A thoughtfully researched and written novel about a transgender teen.*

Corinna, Heather. 2007. *S.E.X.: The All-You-Need-to-Know Progressive Sexuality Guide to Get You through High School and College.* New York: Marlowe.

Eugenides, Jeffrey. 2002. *Middlesex: A Novel.* New York: Picador. *An excellent novel about an intersex individual who starts life as a girl and begins developing male characteristics at age 14.*

Fine, Cordelia. 2010. *Delusions of Gender: How Our Minds, Society, and Neurosexism Create Difference.* New York: Norton.

Gowen, L. Kris. 2003. *Making Sexual Decisions: The Ultimate Teen Guide.* Lanham, MA: Scarecrow.

Haney, John Mark. 2006. "Teenagers and Pornography Addiction: Treating the Silent Epidemic." *Vistas: Compelling Perspectives on Counseling*, edited by Garry R. Walz, Jeanne C. Bleuer, and Richard K. Yep, 49–52. Alexandria, VA: American Counseling Association. http://counselingoutfitters.com/vistas/vistas06/vistas06.10.pdf.

Hasler, Nikol. 2010. *Sex: A Book for Teens; An Uncensored Guide to Your Body, Sex, and Safety.* San Francisco: Zest Books.

López, Ralph I. 2002. *The Teen Health Book: A Parent's Guide to Adolescent Health and Well-Being.* New York: Norton.

Norman-Eady, Sandra, Christopher Reinhart, and Peter Martino. 2003. "Statutory Rape Laws by State." *OLR Research Report.* http://www.cga.ct.gov/2003/olrdata/jud/rpt/2003-R-0376.htm.

Pascoe, C. J. 2007. *Dude, You're a Fag: Masculinity and Sexuality in High School.* Berkeley: University of California Press.

Rye, B. J., and Maureen T. B. Drysdale. 2009. *Taking Sides: Clashing Views in Adolescence.* New York: McGraw-Hill/Dushkin.

Smith, Joanne, Meghan Huppuch, Mandy Van Deven, and Girls for Gender Equity. 2011. *Hey, Shorty! A Guide to Combating Sexual Harassment and Violence in Schools and on the Streets.* New York: Feminist Press at CUNY.

Taverner, William, and Ryan McKee. 2011. *Taking Sides: Clashing Views in Human Sexuality.* New York: McGraw-Hill/Dushkin.

Teen Research Unlimited, Liz Claiborne Inc. *A Teen's Handbook: What You Need to Know about Dating Violence.* http://loveisnotabuse.com/c/document_library/get_file?uuid=33617cde-3a17-46a8-afc8-f4d383b5e623&groupId=10123.

Weston, Carol. 2004. *Girltalk: All the Stuff Your Sister Never Told You.* 4th ed. New York: Harper Perennial.

References

AAUW Educational Foundation Sexual Harassment Task Force. 2004. *Harassment-free Hallways: How to Stop Sexual Harassment in School.* Washington, DC: American Association of University Women. http://www.aauw.org/learn/research/upload/completeguide.pdf.

AVERT. 2011a. "Am I Ready for Sex?" http://www.avert.org/ready-sex.htm.

AVERT. 2011b. "Worldwide Ages of Consent." http://www.avert.org/age-of-consent.htm.

Ayers, Jim, and Susan Davis. 2011. "Adolescent Dating and Intimate Relationship Violence: Issues and Implications for School Psychologists." *School Psychology Forum: Research into Practice* 5(1): 1–12.

Bleakley, Amy, Michael Hennessy, and Martin Fishbein. 2011. "A Model of Adolescents' Seeking of Sexual Content in Their Media Choices." *Journal of Sex Research* 48(4): 309–315. doi:10.1080/00224499.2010.497985.

Bogart, Laura M., Heather Cecil, David A. Wagstaff, Steven D. Pinkerton, and Paul R. Abramson. 2000. "Is It Sex? College Students' Interpretations of Sexual Behavior Terminology." *Journal of Sex Research* 37(2): 108–116. doi:10.1080/00224490009552027.

Bonino, Silvia, Silvia Ciairano, Emanuela Rabaglietti, and Elena Cattelino. 2006. "Use of Pornography and Self-Reported Engagement in Sexual Violence among Adolescents." *European Journal of Developmental Psychology* 3(3): 265–288. doi:10.1080/17405620600562359.

Centers for Disease Control and Prevention. 2010. "National Youth Risk Behavior Survey (YRBS): Trends in the Prevalence of Sexual Behaviors, 1991–2009." http://www.cdc.gov/HealthyYouth/yrbs/pdf/us_sexual_trend_yrbs.pdf.

Fogarty, Kate 2008. "Teens and Sexual Harassment." University of Florida, IFAS Extension. http://www.education.com/reference/article/Ref_Teens_Sexual/.

Gowen, Kris L. 2003. *Making Sexual Decisions: The Ultimate Teen Guide.* Lanham, MA: Scarecrow.

Hirsch, Larissa 2009a. "Talking to Your Partner about Condoms." TeensHealth from Nemours. September. http://kidshealth.org/teen/sexual_health/guys/talk_about_condoms.html#.

Hirsch, Larissa 2009b. "Talking to Your Partner about STDs." TeensHealth from Nemours. September. http://kidshealth.org/teen/sexual_health/stds/the_talk.html.

Jouriles, Ernest M., Cora Platt, and Renee McDonald. 2009. "Violence in Adolescent Dating Relationships." *Prevention Researcher* 16(1): 3–7.

Kaiser Family Foundation, Tina Hoff, Liberty Greene, and Julia Davis. 2003. *National Survey of Adolescents and Young Adults: Sexual Health Knowledge, Attitudes, and Experiences.* Pub. No. 3218. Menlo Park, CA: Henry J. Kaiser Family Foundation. http://www.kff.org/youthhivstds/upload/National-Survey-of-Adolescents-and-Young-Adults.pdf.

Kost, Kathryn, Stanley Henshaw, and Liz Carlin. 2010. "U.S. Teenage Pregnancy, Births, and Abortions: National and State Trends and Trends by Race and Ethnicity." Guttmacher Institute. January. l http://www.guttmacher.org/pubs/USTPtrends.pdf.

Liace, Lisa K., Jessica B. Nunez, and Amy E. Luckner. 2011. "Casual Sex in Adolescence: Outcomes and Implications for Practice." *NASP Communiqué* 39(6): 1, 26–27. http://www.nasponline.org/publications/cq/39/6/casual-sex-in-adolescence.aspx.

Lofgren-Mårtenson, Lotta, and Sven-Axel Månsson. 2010. "Lust, Love, and Life: A Qualitative Study of Swedish Adolescents' Perceptions and Experiences with Pornography." *Journal of Sex Research* 47(6): 568–579. doi:10.1080/00224490903151374.

Love Is Respect. 2011. "Help for an Abusive Teen." National Dating Abuse Helpline. http://www.loveisrespect.org/get-help/help-for-an-abusive-teen/.

Mesch, Gustavo S. 2009. "Social Bonds and Internet Pornographic Exposure among Adolescents." *Journal of Adolescence* 32(3): 601–618. doi:10.1016/j.adolescence.2008.06.004.

National Center for Victims of Crime. 2011. "Teen Victims." http://www.ncvc.org/ncvc/main.aspx?dbName=DocumentViewer&DocumentID=38721.

New York City Alliance against Sexual Assault. 2010. "Sexual Harassment Information for Teens." Factsheets. http://www.svfreenyc.org/survivors_factsheet_60.html.

Office for Civil Rights, U.S. Department of Education. 2008. *Sexual Harassment: It's Not Academic.* September. http://www2.ed.gov/about/offices/list/ocr/docs/ocrshpam.html.

Planned Parenthood. 2011. "Myths and Facts about Masturbation." http://www.plannedparenthood.org/info-for-teens/sex-masturbation/myths-facts-about-masturbation-33824.htm.

Teen Research Unlimited, Liz Claiborne Inc. 2006. "Topline Findings: Teen Relationship Abuse Survey." March. http://loveisnotabuse.com/c/document_library/get_file?p_l_id=45693&folderId=72612&name=DLFE-205.pdf.

Toscano, Sharyl Eve. 2006. "Sex Parties: Female Teen Sexual Experimentation." *Journal of School Nursing* 22(5): 285–289. doi:10.1177/10598405060220050701.

Glossary

abstinence: Not having (abstaining from) some behavior, such as sex (sexual abstinence) or drug or alcohol use.

age-gap provisions: State laws specifying that it is illegal for one person to have sex with another person who is much younger.

age of consent: The age at which a person can legally consent to have sex.

androgyny: The quality of being or feeling neither specifically masculine nor feminine.

asexual: A person who is not sexually active or is not sexually attracted to other people.

attraction: The physical or sexual interest or desire that one person feels for another.

bisexual (bi): A person who is attracted both to people of the same sex and people of the opposite sex.

boundary: A line or division between one thing and another.

closed relationship: An exclusive, usually monogamous, relationship; contrast with open relationship.

closeness: An intimate bond that one person feels with another.

commitment: In a relationship, a sense of loyalty and trust; a promise or agreement to stick by the other person.

coping mechanism: A way to manage stress.

domestic violence: When someone is physically abusing another family member.

hate crime: act of violence against someone because of race, ethnicity, gender, religion, or sexual orientation.

heterosexual: One who is romantically and physically attracted to people of the opposite sex.

homophobia: Fear or hatred of or discrimination against homosexuals.

homosexual: One who is romantically and physically attracted to people of the same sex.

hymen: A thin membrane partly covering the vaginal opening.

illegal: Against the law.

incest: Having sex with a family member or close blood relative.

LGBT (lesbian, gay, bisexual, transgender): An initialism that refers to members of sexual orientation or gender identity minorities.

libido: Sex drive.

masturbation: Touching oneself to give oneself sexual pleasure.

minor: A person under the legal age, usually 18 years of age. This age varies by state for different things such as voting, drinking, and consenting to sex.

monogamy: Having an exclusive relationship with one person.

mutual: Sharing; each person in a couple having the same feelings for the other person; something that goes both ways; reciprocity or give and take in a relationship.

neglect: A type of abuse that occurs when someone's basic needs aren't being met.

open relationship: A relationship that is committed but not exclusive; contrast with closed relationship.

polyamory: Having more than one lover or relationships with more than one person; contrast with monogamy.

pornography: Anything intended to create sexual excitement or arousal.

provocative: Something that excites, provokes, or stimulates.

remorse: A feeling of guilt or shame for one's behavior.

sex: A person's biological sex (male or female) or sexual activities.

sex parties: Parties set up for the purpose of people having casual sex.

sexual abstinence: Abstaining from, or not having, sex.

sexual expression: Sexual desire and sexual behavior.

sexual harassment: Any unwanted sexual behavior.

sexual identity: Self-concepts related to gender—masculinity, femininity, and androgyny—and gender roles.

sexual innuendo: Words, gestures, or images that are sexually suggestive or imply sexual behavior.

sexual orientation: The sex of the person one is attracted to; see bisexual, homosexual, and heterosexual.

sexuality: The quality or state of being sexual or the expression of sexual interest.

statutory rape: Illegal act of having sex with a person under the legal age of consent.

taboo: Something that is forbidden or discouraged according to social customs, conventions, or morality.

virgin: Someone who has not had sex; sometimes refers to someone who has never had sexual intercourse.

CHAPTER 3

Safe Sex

Sexuality is a central part of many people's self-concept as well as their romantic and reproductive goals for the future. Certain social norms and gender roles pertain to sexual expression in males and females. The role of being a spouse, sweetheart, or parent may contain aspects of sexuality. Generally, people consider sexual activity a very positive experience—one that is exciting and fun—as well as a way to express love and affection. Sexual experience may be a topic of pride or embarrassment to people, especially teens. Peer pressure may play a role in how teens regard their sexual knowledge and experience.

Many teens are faced with a decision about whether or not to begin having sex. Teens' own feelings and values, influences from parents and family, religious teachings and beliefs, and the opinions of friends and other peers may affect this decision. Trust, feelings, and attraction to the potential sexual partner are also considerations. Sexual appetite is an aspect of human nature; our species reproduces and survives because humans naturally want to have sex. Hormones emerging during puberty may bring very strong urges and curiosity about sex. Although the body feels ready for sex and reproduction, a teen's mind and emotions may not be mature enough to deal with all the consequences of a sex life (Lyness 2010). When people decide to have sex, they are responsible for protecting themselves and their partners from **sexually transmitted diseases** (**STDs**) and pregnancy. **Safe sex** includes sexual practices that prevent pregnancy and the spread of illness.

Abstinence

Abstinence in this case refers to refraining from having sex. Sexual abstinence is the most reliable way to prevent pregnancy and to avoid STDs. STDs are also known as **sexually transmitted infections** (**STIs**) and venereal disease (VD). Someone who has had sex may decide to abstain from sex in the future. Someone who has never had sex may decide to refrain from sex for a continued period of time. Abstinence is 100 percent effective at preventing pregnancy because there is no opportunity for sperm to fertilize an egg (Planned Parenthood 2011a).

Because sexual intercourse is the most common way that STDs are spread, abstinence also offers some protection from STDs. Abstinence only completely prevents STDs when there is no contact with another person's genitals. STDs can be spread through **oral sex** and skin-to-skin contact as well as anal or vaginal sex. **Consistent abstinence** means that a person refrains from sexual activity all the time (Hirsch 2009a). Abstinence may be difficult to maintain at times due to one's own natural sexual desires and pressures from others. Breaking abstinence should not be done impulsively. People should begin having sex only if they are prepared to protect themselves from pregnancy and STDs or to face the consequences of pregnancy. It is best to delay decisions about abstinence until the issues can be considered calmly and carefully. These decisions

---

WHAT PEOPLE ARE SAYING **TEEN OPINIONS ON ABSTINENCE**

Do you think sexual abstinence is a good idea?

- "It is a good idea because you may not be ready for sexual activity." NK, age 15, Louisiana
- "I think abstinence is a good idea. Sex can sometimes lead to consequences such as pregnancy or STDs that require responsibilities that would be hard for a teen to handle." KG, age 19, Texas
- "I think with waiting often comes maturity—as we age (physically, mentally, sexually) we learn about ourselves and what we are capable of. If being abstinent until we reach maturity is the way to actually consider all consequences and risks of sexual activity, then yes, I think it is a good idea. But the age of maturity might not be 18 for everyone; it could be 16, it could be 25." ES, age 20, California
- "It's not necessarily a good or bad idea. For me it's not something I would really do. Waiting until I'm 18 makes sense but not until I'm married." PW, age 16, Virginia
- "I absolutely believe this is a good idea. Sex can provide a complexity to relationships that younger people may not be able to handle. The physical consequences are also better understood as an adult." KK, age 19, Kentucky

---

should not be made in situations when people are charged with sexual desire and emotions.

A **virgin** is a person who has never had sex. The term usually means that a person has never had sexual intercourse; some people consider a virgin as someone who has no sexual experience at all. Much thought may go into deciding when to begin having sex and lose one's virginity. Having sex for the first time only happens once in each person's life. Many want the event to be special and expect to feel happy, loved, and safe during their first sexual experience. People who are molested, raped, or forced to have sex suffer many injustices, including being robbed of having choices about their first sexual experience. For everyone, choosing the right time, place, and person for oneself—and waiting for all that to work out—can be difficult. Virginity and abstinence are also discussed in chapter 2 of this volume.

Being pressured by others to have sex can make it difficult to wait. Boyfriends and girlfriends may be ready for sex at different points in the relationship or in their own lives. A virgin may feel conflicted, wanting to stick by what's best for him or her but also wanting to make a partner happy. In something as important as beginning one's sex life, what is best for oneself must be the deciding factor, not what other people want (Lyness 2010).

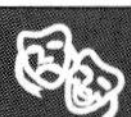

Fact or Myth?

Most teens have had sexual intercourse.

Myth:

- A 2009 survey of over 16,000 U.S. high school students found that only 46 percent of students surveyed reported that they had ever had sexual intercourse.
- Among students who reported that they had sexual intercourse, rates were highest among 12th-graders (62.3 percent), followed by 11th-graders (53.0 percent) and 10th-graders (40.9 percent). Among 9th-graders, 31.6 percent reported having had sexual intercourse.
- Fewer than 6 percent of students nationwide reported having had sexual intercourse before the age of 13.

Source: Centers for Disease Control and Prevention (2010g); Planned Parenthood (2011p).

People who push for sex before their partner is ready are probably thinking only of their own needs. They are not showing respect for the other person's right to make independent decisions. Someone who would end a relationship because another person will not have sex may not be the right choice for a relationship (Lyness 2010). Sex should be something very wonderful to share with another person, an expression of feeling and regard for the other person. Truly caring boyfriends or girlfriends do not ask partners to do something they do not want to do.

Contraception

Contraception (**birth control**) is the prevention of pregnancy using artificial or natural methods. Artificial methods of birth control include **condoms** (and other **barriers**) or birth control pills, while natural methods involve abstaining from sex or avoiding sex during **fertile** periods. There are many methods of contraception; each has advantages and drawbacks. When deciding which method is best, one should consider the method's level of reliability, convenience, disease prevention, and safety given one's health history. Health care practitioners may prescribe or dispense some methods of birth control; they can be consulted for advice about any of

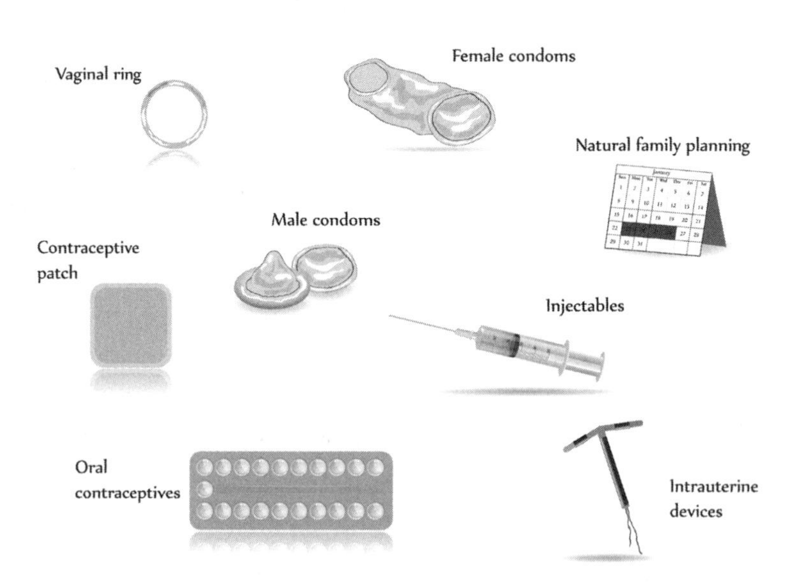

Contraceptive methods. *(Shutterstock.com)*

the methods described in this chapter. Abortion (the termination of a pregnancy) is discussed in chapter 4 of this volume.

Natural Birth Control Methods

Some people look for methods to prevent pregnancy that do not involve barriers (such as condoms) or medications (birth control pills). The most well-known natural birth control method may be **withdrawal**, also called pulling out or **coitus interruptus** (*coitus*, Latin for "sexual intercourse," and *interruptus*, meaning "to interrupt"). Withdrawal means pulling the penis out of the vagina before sperm comes (ejaculation). Sperm is deposited somewhere outside the vagina. Another practice that some people use to prevent pregnancy is **outercourse**—sex activities that do not involve vaginal sex (or any penetration). **Fertility awareness–based birth control** involves monitoring ovulation cycles to decide when to have sex. This method is also called natural family planning or the **rhythm method** (using the rhythm of one's menstrual cycle to prevent pregnancy). Breastfeeding may also reduce a woman's chances of becoming pregnant.

Withdrawal

Several factors make withdrawal a risky method of birth control. Some experts state that the **preejaculate** can carry enough sperm to cause a pregnancy. Preejaculate (also known as preseminal fluid or Cowper's fluid) is a clear fluid that comes out of the penis before ejaculation. Pregnancy may also occur if sperm is spilled on the **vulva** (vaginal area). Withdrawal requires women to trust that partners know when to pull out. The man needs to have enough control to pull out before ejaculating. The withdrawal method is especially ineffective for teens and sexually inexperienced men. It is very difficult for men with limited experience to be sure they will know when to pull out. The method will not work for men who have **premature ejaculations** (Planned Parenthood 2011t). Premature ejaculation is ejaculation before it is intended—during early stages of sexual excitement or soon after inserting the penis in the vagina. Around 4 percent of women using the withdrawal method will become pregnant each year if the method is done correctly. If it is not done correctly, 27 percent of women using withdrawal will become pregnant each year (Planned Parenthood 2011t).

There are no side effects to withdrawal except the pregnancies that occur because of mistakes in pulling out and ineffectiveness of the method. Withdrawal does not protect either partner from STDs unless a condom is used. Some couples also use a condom to reduce the risk of STDs and pregnancies from withdrawal mistakes (Planned Parenthood 2011t).

Outercourse

Outercourse is a method of pregnancy prevention that may involve many sexual activities. It does not include sexual intercourse. Because semen does not contact the vagina, this method is a very effective way to prevent pregnancy except for small chances of pregnancy if semen is spilled on the vulva (Planned Parenthood 2011q). Outercourse also reduces risks of contracting **human immunodeficiency virus (HIV)** and some STDs except when bodily fluids are exchanged in oral or **anal sex**. HIV is a virus that may lead to AIDS (acquired immunodeficiency syndrome). **Herpes** and some other STDs may be passed through skin-to-skin contact and may not be prevented during outercourse. Latex or plastic barriers can reduce the risk of transmission of herpes and other STDs (Planned Parenthood 2011q).

Teens may find several advantages to outercourse as a method of preventing pregnancy. Both boys and girls can be sexually satisfied without pressure to proceed to sexual intercourse. Outercourse may allow teens to learn about sexual responses and each other's bodies and how to satisfy themselves and their partners. Some activities included in outercourse are kissing various parts of the body, body-to-body rubbing, and using sex toys. Other sex acts may include manual stimulation of the partner's genitals or masturbation while holding or watching each other.

Oral and anal sex may be considered outercourse. Oral sex involves using one's mouth on a partner's genitals. Anal sex includes exploring the buttocks, anus, and rectum of a partner with hands, mouth, sex toys, or genitals. These sex acts cannot cause pregnancy but may spread STDs. STDs may be prevented by using barriers in oral sex. A dental dam (a thin square piece of rubber placed over the vulva) or plastic wrap can be used over the genital area or anus while oral sex is performed. Condoms can be used to protect men and women from STDs during oral and anal sex.

Outercourse has no negative side effects but does have some drawbacks. Sperm may accidently come into contact with the vagina, resulting in pregnancy (Planned Parenthood 2011q). Some people may find it difficult to resist the urge to have intercourse, especially when aroused by other sex acts during outercourse. They may not be prepared at the time to prevent pregnancy and STDs.

Fertility Awareness–Based Birth Control

Fertility awareness–based birth control involves being aware of the woman's menstrual cycle and the days when a woman is most fertile—most able to become pregnant. The most fertile time is usually the five days before ovulation, the day of ovulation, and one or two days after ovulation. Several methods of predicting ovulation may be used; descriptions are available at the Women's Health website and other sources, listed in the resources section at the end of the chapter.

The **calendar method** is one way to calculate the day of ovulation. First track the length of the menstrual cycle—the number of days between the first day of one period and the first day of the next period—for several months. Then subtract 18 from the shortest number of days and use that number to count from day 1 of the next period. That date is the first day in the cycle that the woman is fertile.

For example, Louisa keeps track of the number of days between her menstrual periods in September (30), October (29), November (30), December (28), January (31), February (28), March (29), and April (30). She uses information from at least eight cycles. The smallest number of days is 28; subtracting 18 from 28 leaves 10. Louisa starts her next period on May 7. Counting 10 days from May 7, Louisa will be fertile starting May 17.

Fertility awareness–based birth control is not effective for women with irregular periods (ovulation dates may not be predictable), nor is it effective without careful records about the cycle. Both partners must agree to abstain on fertile days. Among couples who correctly and carefully use fertility awareness–based methods, 9 percent will still become pregnant each year (Planned Parenthood 2011m).

Breastfeeding

Breastfeeding offers a natural method to decrease pregnancy risk. When a woman feeds her baby only breast milk, her body does not make the hormone that causes ovulation. Without ovulation, fertilization cannot take place. Mothers must breastfeed their baby at least every four hours by day and every six hours at night for breastfeeding to remain effective as birth control. Among women who follow this schedule, 1 percent will become pregnant each year (Planned Parenthood 2011h). Birth control effects of breastfeeding may last up to six months after birth, provided the mother has not menstruated. Breastfeeding is not an effective method for birth control if parents decide to give the baby formula or other foods.

Sex during the Menstrual Period

Some women believe that they will not become pregnant from sex during their menstrual periods. In fact, a woman may become pregnant when she has vaginal bleeding. The bleeding may occur from ovulation rather than menstruation. During ovulation, chances of becoming pregnant are usually very high. Ovulation may also occur near the end of a menstrual period or a few days after the period. During the period, sperm from sex may still be alive in a women's reproductive tract. In this case as well, a pregnancy may occur (Hirsch 2009c). Additionally, having **unprotected sex** at any time may expose either partner to an STD. Girls and women should always remove a tampon before having sex because the penis may push a tampon deeper into the vagina, making it difficult to remove (Hirsch 2009d).

Artificial Methods of Birth Control

Contraceptive Medications

Contraceptive medications contain female hormones (estrogen and progesterone) that change women's natural hormonal cycles. These medications are prescribed by health care practitioners. It is crucial that those who use artificial methods of birth control talk to a professional health care practitioner to prevent the possibility of harmful side effects for some existing conditions, such as heart disease. Hormone shots and implants require practitioners to administer the medication. Birth control pills are daily dosages of estrogen and progesterone or estrogen alone. With extra amounts of hormones in the system, ovulation does not occur and there is no ovum (egg) to become fertilized (Planned Parenthood 2011e). Birth control shots are given every three months. Progesterone is released into the body, preventing ovulation (Planned Parenthood 2011f).

A **birth control implant** (etonogestrel, brand name Implanon) is a small rod about the size of a matchstick. A health care provider inserts it under the skin on a woman's upper arm. Implanon prevents pregnancy for up to three years by releasing progesterone into the body to prevent ovulation (Planned Parenthood 2011c). A **birth control patch** releases estrogen and progesterone. A small plastic patch with medication is worn on the skin for one week. The patch is replaced with a new patch for two more weeks, and then the woman has no patch for one week (Planned Parenthood 2011d). A **birth control ring** is a small flexible ring placed by a woman in her vagina to prevent pregnancy. The ring releases hormones (estrogen and progesterone) that prevent ovulation (Planned Parenthood 2011s). The ring is inserted monthly, left in place for three weeks, and then discarded. A new ring is inserted one week later.

The **morning-after pill** (**emergency contraception**) is a pill that may be used up to five days after unprotected sex to prevent pregnancy. Emergency contraception may be used if people have not used birth control correctly and are concerned about the risk of pregnancy. The morning-after pill contains hormones that prevent ovulation. It prevents pregnancy; it does not end a pregnancy. The morning-after pill is for use in emergencies and is not recommended for regular birth control use (Planned Parenthood 2011o).

TABLE 3.3.1 **BIRTH CONTROL (BC) MEDICATIONS**

Talk with your doctor or professional health provider before using these medications, as they can have some harmful side effects in people with certain health conditions.

Effectiveness	Advantages	Drawbacks (Side Effects or Contraindications)	Costs
BC Pills			
91–99%	• Simple, safe, convenient • Reduces menstrual cramps • Some protection against PID	• Breast tenderness, nausea, vomiting • Some bleeding between periods	• $15–50/ month
BC Patch			
91–99%	• Safe, effective, convenient • No prescription required • Periods lighter, shorter, more regular	• Breast tenderness, nausea, vomiting • Some bleeding between periods	• $15–70/ month
BC Shot			
94–99%	• Safe, effective, convenient • No prescription required • No daily pill to remember • Lasts three months	• Irregular bleeding • Change in sex drive; depression • Change in appetite; weight gain • Headache, nausea, sore breasts • Hair loss/increase on face/body • After discontinuing, can take a long time to get pregnant	• $15–70/ injection

(*continued*)

TABLE 3.3.1 **BIRTH CONTROL (BC) MEDICATIONS** (*Continued*)

Effectiveness	Advantages	Drawbacks (Side Effects or Contraindications)	Costs
BC Ring			
91–99%	• Safe, effective, convenient • No prescription required • Lighter, shorter, more regular periods • Can use continuously, eliminating monthly periods	• Breast tenderness, nausea, vomiting • Some bleeding between periods • Change in sexual desire	• $15–70/ month
Implantable Contraception			
99%	• Safe, effective, convenient • Usable while breastfeeding • Suitable for women who can't take estrogen • Ability to become pregnant returns quickly after discontinuing	• Must be inserted by health care professional • Irregular bleeding, change in sex drive, headache, nausea, sore breasts • Pain at insertion site • Some medications reduce effectiveness of contraceptive	• $400–800 up front but lasts up to three years
Morning-After Pill (Emergency Contraceptives)			
89%*	• Can be used to prevent pregnancy up to five days after unprotected sex • Safe, effective • Available at health centers, drugstores	• Nausea, vomiting, breast tenderness • Irregular bleeding • Dizziness, headaches	• $10–70

*When started within 72 hours after unprotected sex. Less effective as time passes.
Source: Planned Parenthood (2011b, 2011j).

The birth control methods described in this section do not provide any protection from STDs. Condoms must be used with these methods to ensure prevention against diseases. Many people decide to use medications for birth control for the best chance of preventing pregnancy plus a condom to reduce the spread of STDs.

Intrauterine Device

An **intrauterine device (IUD)** is a small plastic device shaped like a "T." A health care practitioner places the IUD into the uterus to prevent pregnancy. An IUD affects the way sperm move and prevents them from joining with an egg. One brand of IUD also releases hormones that prevent ovulation. The IUD has a string that extends about two inches into the vagina. Pulling this string might loosen the IUD and destroy effectiveness. The health care practitioner may use the string to remove the IUD when indicated, but no one else should try to remove an IUD. IUDs with hormones may remain effective for 5 years, and those without hormones may last as long as 10–12 years (Wheaton 2011). IUDs offer no protection against STDs.

Barrier Birth Control

Barrier birth control refers to methods that place a barrier—an obstacle or hindrance—in the path of sperm as they move toward the egg. Pregnancy is avoided by preventing the union of sperm and egg. A condom, also called a rubber or a safe, is a thin plastic or latex sleeve-like object worn to cover the penis. Condoms are the most common barrier method used to prevent pregnancy and STDs (Planned Parenthood 2011k). The condom collects the ejaculate (semen, cum) in its tip; pregnancy is prevented because sperm are not released into the vagina. Condoms prevent STDs by covering and protecting the penis from contact with bodily fluids. The condom protects the partner from STDs by keeping semen from contacting partner's tissues (vaginal, anal, or oral). A **female condom** is a thin plastic pouch placed inside a woman's vagina. It may be used for anal sex when placed in the anus. The female condom has a ring at the closed end that is placed near the cervix to hold it in place. The ring at the open end stays outside the vaginal opening during intercourse.

A **diaphragm** is a flexible latex cup placed inside the vagina to cover the cervix and prevent pregnancy. This keeps sperm from entering the cervix and uterus. Pregnancy prevention is most effective when **spermicide** is spread in and around the cup before placement in the vagina (Planned Parenthood 2011l). Spermicide is a cream or jelly containing chemicals that stop sperm from moving, decreasing the chances of sperm getting around the barrier.

? Did You Know?

When to Put on a Condom

- Put condom on *before* the penis touches the vulva.
- Only use each condom once and then dispose of it; use a fresh condom for each erection.

How to Put on a Condom

- Check the expiration date to be sure the condom is still good.
- Open the condom package with hands, not teeth; be careful not to tear. Dispose of damaged condoms (torn, brittle, sticky, or stiff).
- Use two drops of lubricant inside the rolled condom. With latex condoms, use only water-based lubricants (AstroGlide or K-Y Jelly).
- Pull back foreskin.
- Place rolled condom over the tip of the hard penis, leaving a half-inch space at tip (a space for semen to collect).
- With one hand, pinch air out of condom tip.
- With the other hand, unroll the condom over the penis.
- Roll the condom down to the base of penis. Smooth out any air bubbles.
- Lubricate the outside of the condom.
- After ejaculation, remove the condom before the penis softens. Keep semen inside the condom and discard the condom in a plastic bag.

See the resources section for more information about condom use.

Source: Planned Parenthood (2011n).

A **cervical cap** is a silicone cup that is placed over the cervix to prevent pregnancy. Like the diaphragm, it is most effective when used with spermicide. The cervical cap serves as an obstacle to sperm moving toward the egg, and spermicide stops the sperm from moving (Planned Parenthood 2011i). Neither the diaphragm nor the cervical cap provides any protection from STDs. A condom is still needed to prevent the spread of STDs.

A **birth control sponge** is a round piece of soft plastic foam containing spermicide that is placed deep into the vagina. The sponge has a two-inch diameter and is equipped with a nylon loop, used to remove the

TABLE 3.3.2 **BARRIER METHODS FOR BIRTH CONTROL**

Effectiveness	Advantages	Drawbacks (Side Effects or Contraindications)	Cost
Diaphragm			
88–94%	• Safe, immediately effective, convenient • Lasts up to two years • No effect on female hormones • Can insert ahead of time • Usable while breastfeeding • Usually not felt by either partner	• Some have difficulty inserting • May be pushed out of place • Must insert with each act of intercourse • May need refitting • Urinary tract infections, vaginal irritation	• $15–75
Condom			
82–98%	• Prevents pregnancy and STDs • Inexpensive, easy to get, lightweight, disposable • No prescription required • May relieve premature ejaculation • Usable with other birth control methods, decreasing risk of pregnancy and STDs	• May dull sensations • Must interrupt sex to put on; some people may lose sexual excitement or be frustrated • Use plastic condom if either partner has latex allergy	• About $1 each

(*continued*)

TABLE 3.3.2 **BARRIER METHODS FOR BIRTH CONTROL** (*Continued*)

Effectiveness	Advantages	Drawbacks (Side Effects or Contraindications)	Cost
Female Condom			
79–95%	• Prevents pregnancy and STDs • Usable for vaginal or anal intercourse • Safe, effective, convenient, easy to get • No effect on female hormones • Usable with water- and oil-based lubricants • Usable by people with latex allergies • Stays in place even if erection is not maintained	• May irritate vagina, vulva, or anus • May slip or reduce sensation during intercourse • Can be noisy	• About $4 each
BC Sponge			
76–91%	• Safe, convenient, easy to use • Can carry in pocket, purse • Usually cannot be felt by either partner • No effect on female hormones • Can insert ahead of time • Usable while breastfeeding	• May have difficulty inserting or removing • Vaginal irritation • Sex may be messy or dry	• $9–15 for package of three

(*continued*)

TABLE 3.3.2 **BARRIER METHODS FOR BIRTH CONTROL** (*Continued*)

Effectiveness	Advantages	Drawbacks (Side Effects or Contraindications)	Cost
Cervical Cap			
71–86%	• Safe, effective, convenient • Lasts up to two years • Can carry in pocket, purse • Usually not felt by either partner • Immediately effective and reversible • Usable while breastfeeding • No effect on female hormones	• Cannot use during menstruation • Difficult to insert for some • May be pushed out of place • Must insert for each act of intercourse • May need larger cap after pregnancy	• $60–75
Spermicide			
71–85%	• Can carry in pocket, purse • Can be inserted by either partner • No effect on female hormones • Easy to get • No prescription required • Usable while breastfeeding	• May be messy • May cause irritation • Less effective if good barrier is not formed over cervix	• About $8/ package

Source: Planned Parenthood (2011b).

sponge. The sponge prevents pregnancy by covering the cervix and creating a barrier to sperm. The sponge releases spermicide, making sperm less able to move (Planned Parenthood 2011g).

Spermicide may be used alone to prevent pregnancy. Spermicide is available in several forms, including foams, creams, gels, and **suppositories**. The spermicide is inserted deep in the vagina to cover the cervix, often using an applicator-type stick. Used properly, spermicides cover the cervix and provide a barrier to sperm, and chemicals in spermicides stop sperm movement.

Sterilization

Sterilization is surgery that changes the reproductive system so that the body is no longer fertile, preventing pregnancy. After female sterilization, women are unable to conceive or carry a pregnancy to term. Male sterilization prevents men from getting women pregnant. Sterilization is intended to be permanent.

Women may have a **tubal ligation,** a procedure that removes small segments of each fallopian tube to prevent the union of sperm and ovum (egg). **Hysterectomy** (surgical removal of the uterus) and **oophorectomy** (surgical removal of the ovaries) are sometimes performed for health reasons. Sterilization surgeries usually result in the woman being unable to become pregnant.

Men may have a **vasectomy,** which surgically blocks or closes the tubes that carry sperm from the testes. Because sperm are prevented from getting into the semen, men are no longer able to make a woman pregnant. A vasectomy does not interfere with the ability to have sex, reach a climax, and ejaculate.

Sterilization surgeries are almost 100 percent effective, but vasectomy is not immediately effective. Sperm may take about three months to be totally eliminated from the man's reproductive system. After procedures to block or cut the fallopian tubes, 3 to 5 of every 1,000 women may still become pregnant (Planned Parenthood 2011s).

One disadvantage of sterilization surgery is a permanent loss of the ability to reproduce. Surgeries may attempt to reverse a tubal ligation or a vasectomy by reattaching the ends of the severed tubes. These surgeries are very expensive, and **fertility** may not be restored. Because sterilization is permanent, it must be carefully considered and should be discussed with one's partner. Counseling is recommended before deciding to have sterilization.

Some teens and young adults may believe that they will never want to reproduce or be parents. If they change their minds as they grow older,

TABLE 3.3.3 **EFFECTIVENESS OF BIRTH CONTROL METHODS**

Birth Control Method	Percentage of Couples Who Will Get Pregnant This Year Using This Method	Effectiveness in Pregnancy Prevention	Protects against STDs?
Abstinence (consistent)	None	Completely	Yes
Birth control patch	8	Effective	No
Birth control pill	8	Effective	No
Birth control ring	8	Effective	No
Female condom	21	Less effective	Yes
Male condom	15	Moderate	Yes
Birth control shot	3	Effective	No
Diaphragm	16	Moderate	No
Emergency contraception (morning-after pill)	1 to 2	Very	No
IUD	<1	Very	No
Fertility awareness	25	Less effective	No
Withdrawal (pulling out)	29	Less effective	No
No birth control	27	Less effective	No

Source: Hirsch (2009b); Planned Parenthood (2011a).

they will be relieved that they did not have sterilization surgery. The laws regarding sterilization and the age at which a person can give consent for the procedure vary across states and other countries. Some sterilization laws came about after questionable practices of sterilizing to limit growth of certain populations (**eugenics**). Sterilization has been forced upon people with intellectual disabilities, prisoners, people convicted of sexual crimes, and certain ethnic groups to limit reproduction among these people.

After comparing birth control methods in terms of cost, availability, effectiveness, benefits, and drawbacks, one can make an informed choice of method. While people are single, they may use one or two methods to prevent STDs and pregnancy. These same people may later use a method that only protects from pregnancy if they are in a monogamous relationship with both partners testing negative for STDs. If people decide that they want to have children, they may make another change in birth control methods.

Safe Sex

Safe sex refers to sexual practices that decrease risks for contracting an STD or infecting a partner with an STD. Many people use the term "**safer sex**" as a more accurate way to describe the methods used for protected sex, because the risks are still present but at a lesser degree. **Unsafe sex**, in contrast, refers to unprotected sex. STDs are caused by organisms that may live on the vagina, penis, skin, mouth, or anus. Many of these diseases are transmitted to other people by contact with a sore on the genitals or mouth. Others are present without any visible sores. STDs are most commonly transmitted during vaginal intercourse but may also spread through anal or oral sex or skin-to-skin contact. STDs can lead to later problems with getting pregnant, that is, **infertility**; illnesses to babies born of mothers with active STDs (for example, **chlamydia**); or other serious illnesses or conditions, some of which can lead to death (such as from AIDS). These issues are discussed below.

Oral sex is often considered a safer way to have sex because it cannot result in pregnancy. However, oral sex may result in contracting an STD. Body fluids received in the mouth and throat can transmit HIV/AIDS, **genital herpes**, **syphilis**, **gonorrhea**, and hepatitis (Downs 2010). Oral sex has been found to increase the risk for throat cancer, because **human papillomavirus (HPV)** infections can be transmitted through oral sex. Researchers have found that HPV is the probable cause of some throat and tonsil cancers. The risk of cancer caused by HPV is higher in people who have had oral sex with more than six partners. This illness occurs in both men and women (Downs 2010).

Using a condom or dental dam for oral sex greatly reduces the chances of contracting an STD. However, a 2004 survey of single adults found that 91 percent never used any protection during oral sex (Downs 2010). Oral sex is popular among teens, in part because of a belief that it is safe. In a 2005 survey, most ninth-graders said that they believed that oral sex would not put them at risk for health problems. Teens gave five primary reasons to explain why teens participate in oral sex. Reasons included seeking pleasure, improving relationships, gaining popularity, curiosity, and oral sex being less risky than vaginal sex. Boys in the survey said that seeking pleasure was the top reason, while girls said that improving a relationship was the most important reason for having oral sex. Girls were more likely to report feeling guilty about having oral sex and believed that a relationship had been damaged by oral sex. Boys were more positive in their feelings, saying that having oral sex brought social and emotional benefits (Downs 2010).

Measures for Safer Sex

Because people sometimes make jokes or gossip when they hear that someone has an STD, someone may be embarrassed by having one himself or herself. Someone who contracts an STD may have judged others, thinking that it would never happen to himself or herself. People with STDs may have negative feelings toward themselves and believe that others will look down on them or find them undesirable. They may regret having placed themselves in a situation where they contracted a disease. Distress about having an STD may make it difficult to talk to people about the condition.

It is important to talk with one's potential sexual partner about STDs before having sex. This conversation may be embarrassing and may not seem very romantic, but caring for personal safety is important. It could be seen as romantic to make sure sex is not risky for your partner. A person with an STD who needs to inform a potential partner may fear that the news will end the relationship. People who reject others or end relationships because they do not want to use condoms or other precautions are not showing respect for their partner or themselves. The discomfort of talking about STDs is a good deal less than the discomfort of having an STD. Talking about it before sex is easier than regretting giving an STD to someone else.

Telling a new sexual partner that one has an STD is best done in a straightforward manner, with respect for oneself for having the courage to do the right thing and speak up (Hirsch 2009f). It may be helpful to listen to your partner's response and allow time before pressing for a decision about having sex. Inviting questions allows the other person to learn more about the condition and what protection is needed to prevent spreading the disease.

A discussion about STDs should include information about each person's sexual health history and each partner's intentions to practice safe sex. Each partner needs to ensure that the other agrees to use safer sex practices, such as wearing a condom. Hearing other people say that they are disease-free does not ensure that they do not have an STD. Some people do not know that they have an illness, while others may not believe that the condition is important or contagious. Some may not be truthful, fearing rejection. Having tests for STDs is a much better way to be confident about sexual health status.

It is recommended that both partners be tested for STDs and HIV before proceeding to have sex. Getting tested, perhaps together, should be a part of the discussion about safe sex. (See the "Tests for STDs and HIV" section at the end of the chapter for how to find testing locations.) If tests for STDs come back positive (meaning the person has an STD), the infected person needs to notify any sexual partners—past or present—that they may be infected, should be tested, and may need treatment. This is important even if safe sex measures were used; safe sex practices are not always 100 percent effective.

STDs may develop into serious or even life-threatening infections. STDs may damage reproductive organs, leading to infertility. Not letting someone know that he or she might be infected is very unfair. Some states have laws against having sex without informing partners of one's HIV status. In any state, a person who knowingly endangers another's well-being and does not warn the person that he or she may be in danger can face legal action (lawsuit). Laws vary by state, including whether it is illegal to infect someone intentionally (on purpose) versus recklessly (through carelessness). Reckless endangerment could mean not taking adequate precautions to prevent transmission of HIV or an STD. AVERT (2011) summarizes different state and international laws as well as prosecutions for transmission of HIV. Many public health clinics offer a service to inform past sex partners about possibly having been exposed to an STD, without mentioning the name of the person who has the STD. The InSPOT website (listed in the resources section at the end of this chapter) allows people to anonymously notify current or former sexual partners that they may have been exposed to an STD.

A positive STD test result may seem to indicate that one's partner has been having sex with someone else. However, some STDs may be present for a long period of time and could have been contracted before the current relationship began. Talking to a health care practitioner or reviewing the facts about transmission of an illness may increase understanding about the STD and the probable behaviors of the infected person. If the facts do point to a partner being unfaithful—having sex with someone else—the partner should be asked to provide information about how and where he or she may have contracted the disease. Your partner's other sex partners may have an impact on your own health.

If someone has been unfaithful (for example, to a girlfriend) and developed an STD, it is important for him to tell his girlfriend about it because of the health dangers involved. Being honest and responsible—about the decision to have sex outside the relationship—may help the conversation go better. People who learn that a partner has been unfaithful are usually very angry, hurt, and upset; they may need time to deal with the information. Sometimes talking about safe sex and STDs and dealing with any related problems may reveal sensitivity and consideration in one's partner. Going through the process of protecting each other and valuing a safe and healthy relationship may bring a couple closer together.

Another important conversation in safe sex practice addresses the use of condoms. Using condoms is the best protection against STDs. However, some people have objections to using condoms (Hirsch 2009e). For safety's sake, these objections need to be addressed without giving up on this important protection. Some men complain that condoms are not comfortable. Making sure that they have the right size and know how to properly wear the condom may help.

People may feel that insisting on using a condom indicates a lack of trust in one's partner, but being willing to ensure each other's safety is a way to increase trust. Some people say that a condom diminishes pleasure in sexual activity—not feeling safe is also a deterrent to enjoying sex. People may complain that stopping to use a condom spoils a spontaneous or romantic moment. When putting on a condom becomes a part of the romance or sexual fun, it is no longer seen as an interruption. Talking about safe sex and use of condoms is discussed further in chapter 2 of this volume.

Practicing safe sex requires calm and consistent decision making. Drinking alcohol or using other drugs may interfere with being aware of one's behavior and decisions. Staying sober in situations where sex may be involved is very important to prevent careless behavior that may result in getting an STD or becoming pregnant. At the time it may seem fun to be drunk and abandon caution, but it will not be fun later to have an illness or to deal with an unwanted pregnancy. When people are impaired by substance use, they may not have the attention or coordination needed to apply condoms properly or to use birth control methods correctly (U.S. National Library of Medicine and National Institutes of Health 2010).

A teen who stands up for his or her beliefs and decisions about having safe sex should be proud of these convictions. It may not be easy to do the right thing, but doing the right thing usually brings rewards. By sticking with intentions to prevent pregnancy and STDs, teens may avoid regrets and problems. If a mistake is made or a person has sex without taking precautions, the incident should be addressed, and the safe sex practices should begin again.

Legal Issues Pertaining to Sexual Activity

Laws about sexual activity and about consent to receive medical care have an effect on people's safety decisions. If there is a state law against a 19-year-old having sex with a 16-year-old, that fact should influence the older person to not have sex with the younger person. Even if the younger person is willing to have sex or is insistent upon sex, the older participant can be charged with a crime and may go to jail. Laws may also limit the options for getting health care in the case of STDs or obtaining medications for birth control. If teens are not legally allowed to have these services without their parents' consent, some teens may decide not to receive the health care or not to use contraception.

Laws about the Legal Ages for Sexual Participants

Each state in the United States has its own rules about the legal ages at which people can have sex without it being called rape or assault. Legal charges may be brought when a person who is older (usually 18 or over) has sex with someone who is considered too young to make a mature decision about consenting to sex. **Age of consent** refers to the age at which the law states that a person is old enough to decide to have sex. Before that age the sex act may be considered rape, even if the younger partner consents to have sex. This situation is sometimes called **statutory rape**.

States may also have laws about reporting when an older person has sex with a person who is too young to legally give consent. Many states place statutory rape in the category of child abuse. **Mandatory reporting** requires that people who know of an act of child abuse must, by law, report the abuse. All states have laws requiring certain professionals to report child abuse, and many states also have broad statutes requiring any citizen to report child abuse. Mandatory reporting by any citizen who knows of child abuse is the law in 18 states and Puerto Rico (Child Welfare Information Gateway 2010). These reports are made to police or child protection agencies. In a third of U.S. states, the sexual interaction is only considered child abuse when the older person is the minor's parent or caregiver (Glosser, Gardiner, and Fishman 2004). Under these laws, consensual sex between a 15-year-old girl and her 19-year-old boyfriend would be considered illegal but not reportable as child abuse. Other states have mandatory reporting for any known act of sex with a person under the age of consent, regardless of the relationship (Connecticut General Assembly 2003). For further discussion of age of consent and statutory rape, see chapter 2 of this volume.

Laws about Confidentiality of Minors Receiving Medical Care

Parents and guardians are responsible for making decisions about young children. They must give consent before their children receive medical care. As children become more mature, parents and guardians may decide that minors have a right to some privacy and confidentiality with their medical care and decisions. Health care practitioners may recognize this level of maturity and feel ethically obliged to protect an adolescent's privacy to some extent (Neinstein 1987). Confidentiality means that communications are private—between a patient and the patient's health care provider. Except under certain circumstances, confidential information cannot be shared with anyone else without permission.

At any age, people who are a danger to themselves or others must be protected. To protect and get help for these people, health care practitioners may have to break confidentiality. Some illnesses are monitored for public health, and government agencies may mandate the reporting of these problems. Some injuries—for example, those related to child abuse or another crime—must be reported. With these exceptions, many states have laws providing for older minors to seek birth control, abortions, mental health treatment, and treatment for STDs (University of Illinois

TABLE 3.3.4 **MINORS' RIGHT TO CONSENT TO HEALTH CARE**

Some states allow minors to consent to health care services but do not guarantee confidentiality of medical records. The following table shows the types of health care services to which minors are allowed to consent and the number of states (including the District of Columbia) in the United States that allow minor consent.

Type of Health Care Service	**Number of States That Allow Minor Consent**
Contraceptive services	27
Prenatal care/delivery services without parental consent or notification	28
Testing and treatment for STDs, including HIV*	51
Confidential drug or alcohol counseling and treatment	45
Outpatient mental health services	21
Require at least one parent to be involved in a minor's abortion decision	31

*Three states limit this authorization to testing only.

Sources: Boonstra and Nash (2000); Dailard (2003).

at Chicago College of Medicine 2011). These laws have been written to allow teens to get important or life-saving treatment when their parents may not consent.

HIV/AIDS

HIV is a virus that destroys a type of white blood cells called **T cells.** These cells help the body protect itself from disease. HIV can develop into acquired immunodeficiency syndrome (AIDS). HIV is thought to have originated in apes in West Africa. Humans hunted and ate the meat of apes there and came into contact with the infected blood. The disease spread throughout Africa and gradually was brought to other parts of the world by travelers (Centers for Disease Control and Prevention 2010a).

HIV is transmitted (passed) from one person to another through contact with infected blood and other body fluids such as vaginal fluid, semen, preseminal fluid, and breast milk. Sexual contact and IV drug use with contaminated needles are the most common forms of HIV transmission. The most likely way to get HIV is by having anal sex with an infected partner who is not using a condom. Unprotected anal sex is more likely to result in HIV infection than unprotected vaginal sex. The high blood supply in the rectal area and the irritation and tearing of rectal tissues make it easier for HIV to get into the bloodstream. In men who have sex with infected men, the man who receives unprotected anal sex is more at risk for getting HIV than a man who inserts his unprotected penis in the anus of an infected man.

The risk of contact is higher in people who have any type of unprotected sex with several partners or in people who have other STDs. Unprotected oral sex increases the risk for HIV but poses less risk than vaginal or anal sex (Centers for Disease Control and Prevention 2010a). Some people do not know that they have HIV or may conceal their HIV status. It is safest to always use a condom for any type of sexual contact.

Using contaminated needles is a route for getting an HIV infection. People who are accidentally stuck by a contaminated needle or receive infected blood products through transfusions can develop HIV. Tattoos, piercings, or dental treatment done with unclean equipment containing HIV-infected blood can cause an infection. Babies can get HIV from an infected mother, either during pregnancy, through the birth process, or from breastfeeding. Being bitten by an infected person or contaminated blood coming in contact with one's own open wound has rarely resulted in HIV infections (Centers for Disease Control and Prevention 2010a).

There is no cure for HIV infection, and it is a very dangerous disease. Measures to prevent contracting the disease must be taken very seriously.

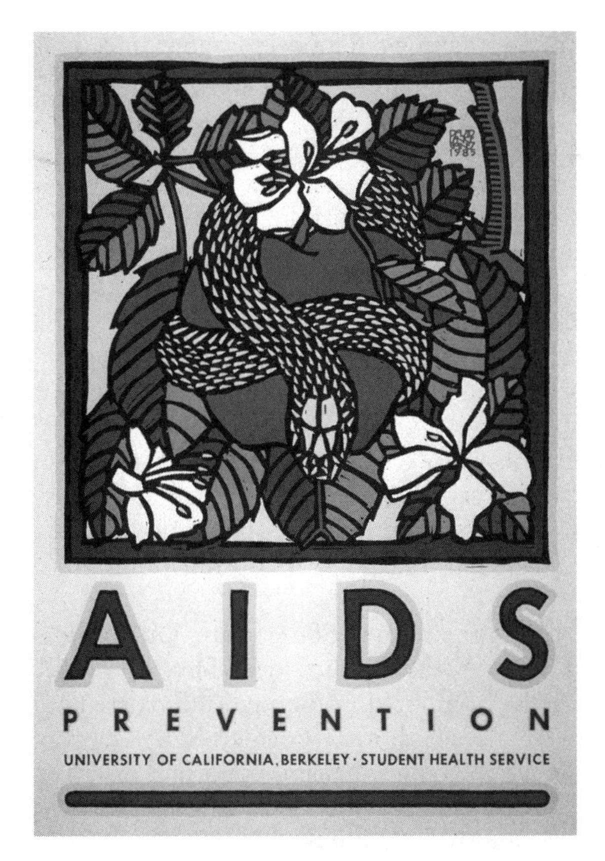

AIDS prevention poster. *(David Lance Goines/LOC)*

Medications can slow the progression of HIV to AIDS and improve the health and quality of life for people with the disease. Current medications do prolong and improve life for those with HIV and AIDS, but the medications have serious side effects. Individuals with HIV or AIDS need to take these medications daily for the remainder of their lives. Most people who develop AIDS will die from the disease.

Early symptoms of HIV infection are mild fever, achiness, headache, and swollen lymph glands. Many people do not have any symptoms. They may feel well and appear healthy for several years. Nevertheless, these people still need treatment to control damage from the virus. Over time, they may notice having more infections, fevers, sore throats, weight loss, and diarrhea.

HIV is diagnosed using blood tests that confirm that the virus is present. If a person is diagnosed with HIV, tests are done to check T cell counts and amounts of the virus and whether the person is responding to medications.

People with HIV have a higher risk for tuberculosis (TB), hepatitis and liver disease, STDs, kidney disease, and urinary tract infections (UTIs).

Salmonella (a bacteria found in contaminated food and water) infections are also more likely to occur. Salmonella infections cause diarrhea, fever, chills, and abdominal pain. People with HIV also have an increased risk of **toxoplasmosis**, a deadly infection related to parasites found in cat feces (Mayo Clinic 2010b).

People with immune systems impaired with HIV or AIDS are more likely to develop cancer. **Kaposi's sarcoma,** a cancer of the blood vessel walls, is a common complication of AIDS. It results in red- or purple-colored **lesions** (sores) on the skin or in the mouth. **Lymphoma** (lymph node cancer) can occur in people with HIV/AIDS. The earliest symptom of lymphoma is swelling of the lymph nodes in the neck, armpits, or groin (Mayo Clinic 2010b).

Dementia (thinking difficulties) may develop in a person with AIDS. AIDS damages brain tissue, which causes problems with memory. A person with AIDS dementia may have social problems, poor concentration, confusion, problems with movement, and loss of coordination (Mayo Clinic 2009b).

HIV medications interfere with the growth of the virus. The medications block proteins needed for the virus to reproduce. They also block HIV from affecting certain cells. Combinations of medications are used and are carefully monitored by the health care provider. Side effects of these medications include weakened bones, nausea, vomiting, diarrhea, and shortness of breath.

Several health measures can improve the course of HIV illness. Eat a healthy diet, and avoid foods that may be contaminated. Raw eggs, meats, seafood, and unpasteurized dairy products can be dangerous. Cook meats thoroughly, and wash fruits and vegetables carefully. Choose pets carefully; cats and reptiles can carry diseases that are deadly for people with HIV. Get immunizations against pneumonia and influenza, as these diseases are more common in people with HIV. People with HIV should not receive vaccines that contain live viruses.

It is usually terrible news to receive a diagnosis of a life-threatening condition. Many emotions may be connected to a diagnosis of HIV. A person who learns of an HIV diagnosis may fear dying from the disease and dread the many hardships that often accompany the disease. AIDS is very debilitating and costly; it may interfere with one's ability to work, and the treatments can be very expensive. People with HIV or AIDS may feel depressed about the consequences of the illness for themselves and for their loved ones. The person may have concerns about other people that he or she may have infected with the virus and may feel angry if he or she contracted HIV from someone who was dishonest about having the illness.

HIV often strikes people when they are in the prime years of life, because risks and activities that can lead to HIV are more common with young people. Having HIV may rob people of opportunities and hopes they had for the future and may cause people to isolate themselves from others. People with HIV who seek intimate or romantic relationships will have to explain their HIV status. Some people with HIV do not want anyone to know their status because they fear being unwanted or treated differently. The family of an HIV-positive individual may be socially isolated because of fears that others have of being infected with the disease.

About 66 percent of men with HIV or AIDS are men who have sex with men. The spread of HIV has been the strongest among this population (Centers for Disease Control and Prevention 2010d). Since the 1980s, the gay community has suffered the deaths of many men from AIDS. Prejudices against homosexual people may be made stronger due to poor understanding about AIDS and the people who have it. Support groups and AIDS awareness groups have educated the public and decreased negative attitudes toward people with AIDS.

Untreated HIV proceeds to AIDS, usually in about 10 years. People with AIDS have severely damaged immune systems, making them very susceptible to infections that would have been minor before AIDS. In the early years of AIDS, the progression from HIV to AIDS was rapid—only a few years. With proper treatment, some people now live for decades before AIDS develops. AIDS is diagnosed when the person's T cell count falls below a certain level or when any serious complications of the disease have developed (Mayo Clinic 2010b).

Prevention of HIV consists of avoiding contact with the virus. Using condoms for all types of sex is essential in preventing the spread of the disease. Knowing the HIV status of sexual partners, limiting the number of sexual partners, and never sharing needles or using unclean needles all help prevent the disease. Being careful about equipment used in tattoos, piercings, and dental procedures reduces the risk of HIV. Some people get tested regularly for HIV. People can ask their sexual partners to be tested. Even if both partners test negative for the virus, it is still advisable to have protected (safer) sex.

Sexually Transmitted Diseases

STDs are illnesses that are spread through sexual contact. Some of these infections are cured rather easily by medications, but others are **chronic** (long lasting) in nature. STDs may be spread easily. It is important to understand methods of transmission and how to best prevent becoming infected or infecting others.

Chlamydia

Chlamydia is a very common bacterial infection of the genital tract. The infection spreads to others through vaginal, anal, and oral sex. Many with the disease do not know they are infected because the bacteria (*Chlamydia trachomatis*) causes very few or no symptoms. Chlamydia affects people of all ages, but the majority of cases are teens (Mayo Clinic 2009a). Because their cervixes are not fully mature, teens and young women are more prone to being infected.

Women may have mild symptoms that could go unnoticed. Slight vaginal discharge and pain with sex may occur. Men may have pain in the testicles and a discharge from the penis. Pain in the lower abdomen and painful urination are other symptoms of chlamydia. The treatment for chlamydia is antibiotics and avoiding sex for two weeks (the time that the infection usually takes to clear). All partners must be treated, or the bacteria will repeatedly pass between them and reinfections will occur.

If untreated, chlamydia can cause permanent damage to the reproductive organs of women. Problems with infertility (inability to become pregnant) may also occur. Women may also develop chronic pelvic pain and **pelvic inflammatory disease (PID)**, described later in this chapter. Men may have **epididymitis**—inflammation of an organ in the scrotum—and inflammation of the prostate gland, which is located in the pelvis. Rectal inflammation may occur if infected through anal sex. Throat inflammation may occur when chlamydia is contracted through oral sex. Eye infections may be caused if hands carry the bacteria to the eye area. Blindness may occur with these eye infections. People with chlamydia have an increased risk for being infected with HIV and for developing other STDs. A baby may be exposed to chlamydia from an infected mother through vaginal birth. The infant may then develop pneumonia and an eye infection that might cause blindness.

Prevention of chlamydia includes regular screening for STDs. Because a person may not note any symptoms with chlamydia, screening may be the only way of finding this "secret" disease and getting treatment before permanent damage takes place. Using a condom and limiting the number of sexual partners may decrease one's chances of contracting an infection. **Douching** should be avoided because it reduces the amount of helpful bacteria in the vaginal area and increases chances of chlamydia developing.

Genital Candidiasis

Genital candidiasis (also called yeast infections) is a fungal infection that occurs in the genital area. *Candida*, a fungal organism, is normally present in small amounts in the body. Hormonal changes, changes in vaginal acidity, and antibiotics may kill bacterial **flora** in the genital tract. Flora are normal helpful organisms that live in the body (for example, in the digestive and genitourinary tracts). This imbalance may allow *Candida* to multiply and cause infections. Diabetes or taking steroid medications may increase risk for *Candida* infections.

Women with candidiasis may experience itching and irritation of the vaginal area and a smelly discharge that looks like cottage cheese. The illness is rare in men, but if infected they may have an itchy rash on the penis. The cause of candidiasis is usually overgrowth of one's own fungal organisms. Sometimes one person may pass the infection to another during sex. Antifungal medications are available in creams or suppositories (tablets) inserted into the vagina. Single-dose treatments or those used for as many as seven days may be used to treat candidiasis. Health care practitioners may also prescribe a one-time oral medication. It is important to be sure that the problem is a fungal infection, because using antifungal medications too often can lead to eventual resistance to medication (Centers for Disease Control and Prevention 2010b).

Genital Herpes

Herpes in general refers to a viral infection. There are various strains of herpes, including **herpes simplex** (the virus that causes cold sores) and **herpes zoster** (the virus that causes shingles and chicken pox). Genital herpes is a viral infection that is caused by a herpes simplex virus type 2 (HSV2). The virus enters a person's body through small breaks in the skin or mucous membranes. Sexual activity is the most common form of transmission (Mayo Clinic 2009c). Genital herpes may also be caused by herpes simplex virus type 1 (HSV1), the cause of cold sores, that may be passed from a cold sore to the genitals during oral sex. Genital herpes is a very common STD, affecting one in six people ages 14–49 in the United States (Centers for Disease Control and Prevention 2010c).

There is no cure for genital herpes. The infection is usually recurring, but symptoms may be lessened by medication. Many people who are infected with the virus do not know that they have it because they have no symptoms. Symptoms are usually the most severe during the first outbreak of the infection, but even the first outbreak may be so mild as to go unnoticed. Symptoms of genital herpes include small red bumps, ulcers, or blisters on the genital or anal area and pain or itching in these areas and on the buttocks or upper thighs. The bumps or blisters may become ulcers that rupture and bleed. The ulcers will eventually develop scabs and heal. When the ulcers are present, urination may be painful.

An initial outbreak may also include flu-like symptoms—fever, headache, and muscle aches. Swelling of the lymph nodes in the groin may also occur (Mayo Clinic 2009c).

Having genital herpes may increase the risk of contracting other STDs and HIV/AIDS. The herpes virus may be passed to a baby during delivery if the mother has an outbreak of genital herpes. Having genital herpes does not rule out safe pregnancy; steps can be taken to safeguard the baby from an infection. Genital herpes infections may lead to urinary retention in women. It can also lead to inflammation of the lining of the rectum, especially in men who have sex with men (Mayo Clinic 2009c).

Recurrences of genital herpes outbreaks may happen several times a year or every year or so. Some people never experience a second outbreak. As time passes, the outbreaks may become less frequent (Mayo Clinic 2009c). Certain factors may trigger an outbreak. Stress, fatigue, illness, and surgery may bring on an outbreak. Menstruation, friction (as with sex), and immune system suppression may also increase the chances of an outbreak. Antiviral medications may decrease the severity of symptoms in genital herpes and may reduce the number of recurrences. These medicines may also decrease the chances of spreading the virus to others. Some health care practitioners advise taking antivirals at the start of an outbreak. Some people are told to take the medication on a regular basis to reduce the chance of outbreaks. Those who have more than five outbreaks a year are more often told to take the medication daily. Learning about the condition and one's own body may help in minimizing the hardships of having genital herpes.

Having an STD that will not go away and may flare up when it is least convenient is challenging. Those with genital herpes may fear being rejected by potential romantic partners who are disturbed by the threat of herpes transmission. Knowing how to protect a sexual partner from the illness may decrease concerns about having sex. An understanding and caring partner will want to work out the details of the relationship in spite of the condition.

Gonorrhea

Gonorrhea is caused by *Neisseria gonorrhoeae*, bacteria that are passed through sexual contact. These bacteria grow easily in warm moist areas such as the cervix, uterus, and vagina in women and in the urethra of men and women. The germs can also grow in the mouth, eyes, and anus. Gonorrhea is spread through sexual contact with the penis, vagina, mouth, or anus.

Symptoms of gonorrhea include a burning sensation when urinating and a whitish or yellow or green discharge from the penis. Some men have painful and swollen testicles with gonorrhea. Many women do not have any symptoms. If they have burning with urination or vaginal discharge, they may dismiss this as a minor passing problem. Even without symptoms, women may be at risk of serious complications from gonorrhea infections. Rectal symptoms may include itching, discharge, and pain with bowel movements. Mouth infections usually do not show symptoms but may cause a sore throat (Centers for Disease Control and Prevention 2011). Gonorrhea is diagnosed by testing a tissue sample from the infected area.

Untreated gonorrhea can lead to PID, discussed later in this chapter. In men, gonorrhea can lead to epididymitis, a painful inflammation of the ducts within the testicles that can lead to infertility. People with gonorrhea are more susceptible to being infected with HIV. Gonorrhea infections in the blood or joints can lead to death.

Antibiotics are the main treatment for gonorrhea. Gonorrhea that does not respond to certain antibiotics is more complicated to treat (Centers for Disease Control and Prevention 2011). Prevention of the disease involves avoiding sexual contact, particularly with infected people. Using a condom for all types of sex can reduce the chances of contacting gonorrhea. If someone is diagnosed with gonorrhea, any recent sexual partners must be notified and tested. Sexual contact should be stopped until after the infection has cleared in both parties. Having gonorrhea does not create immunity; the infection could be contracted again (Centers for Disease Control and Prevention 2011).

Human Papillomavirus (HPV)

HPV is the most common STD in the United States. There are more than 40 types of HPV. Most people infected with HPV are not aware that they have it. HPV is most often passed through genital contact, usually during vaginal or anal sex.

The body is likely to clear itself of HPV within two years after contact, but in some people the virus is present much longer, lying dormant (inactive). HPV can be present even if it has been years since a person had sexual contact with an infected person. Because most people are not aware of the virus, they do not seek treatment or try to prevent spreading the virus.

HPV is associated with serious complications. HPV can make a woman more likely to develop cervical cancer. The HPV cells can make cervical cells abnormal, causing cancer cells to develop. Cervical cancer can become very advanced before it is detected, and it may be very hard to treat. Regular screening tests, such as a pap smear, may detect signs of cervical cancer early enough to prevent the disease. HPV may also be related to cancer of the penis, vagina, anus, and vulva.

HPV is diagnosed through pap tests, tests for the presence of HPV genetic material, or other measures. There is no treatment for HPV, but there are medications and treatments for the diseases that the virus can cause. Procedures or surgeries can remove cancerous or precancerous cells found in genital areas. **Genital warts** may be treated with medications to remove the warts (Centers for Disease Control and Prevention 2010e).

HPV infections may be prevented with a series of vaccinations. Vaccines for women protect against the common HPV types that can cause cervical cancer. HPV vaccine can also be given to boys to prevent genital warts. Vaccinations are recommended for girls ages 11–12 and for older girls who have not already had the vaccination. Using condoms from beginning to end of every sex act can also reduce HPV risk. Limiting the number of sexual partners reduces potential exposure to HPV, as will having sexual partners who have not had many sex partners.

Genital Warts

Genital warts (also called venereal warts or *condylomata acuminata*) are caused by HPV. The virus invades warm, moist genital regions of the body and forms small gray or flesh-colored bumps. The bumps may be few, or they may multiply into large clusters that may have a cauliflower-like appearance. These warts may grow on the vulva, inside the vagina, and on the cervix. In men, they may grow on the penis, scrotum, or anus. Genital warts may also grow in the throat or mouth of a person who has had oral sex with an infected person. The virus is spread through sexual contact with an infected person. Almost two-thirds of people who have sex with someone with genital warts will develop the condition themselves (Mayo Clinic 2010a). The risk for contracting genital warts is increased by having unprotected sex with multiple partners, by having sex at a young age, and for people who have other STDs.

Infected people may experience itching and discomfort in the genital area and may have bleeding during sex. For some people, genital warts cause no symptoms or are too small to be noticed. The infection is still a problem, however, because of the link between HPV and cervical cancer. Genital warts may also cause problems during pregnancy and childbirth. The warts may grow and make urinating difficult, and they decrease the ability of the vaginal walls to stretch during delivery of the baby. The baby may develop warts in the throat and may be at risk for an obstructed airway and breathing difficulties (Mayo Clinic 2010a).

Almost one-third of the cases of genital warts resolve without treatment. If the infection is causing discomfort, creams may be used that will strengthen the immune system to fight the virus. A health care practitioner may apply a solution that destroys the genital warts. This solution must not be applied to internal tissues (inside the body) and is not safe during pregnancy. Surgery may be used for warts that are very large or that may interfere with pregnancy. Freezing the wart (**cryotherapy**), laser treatments, **electrocautery** (electrical current to burn off the wart), and surgically cutting the wart away are methods used to remove warts. Prevention of genital warts includes using a condom, knowing your partner's sexual history, limiting sexual contact, and getting HPV vaccinations.

Pelvic Inflammatory Disease (PID)

PID is an infection—usually bacterial—of the female reproductive organs. STDs are the primary source of these bacteria; getting treated promptly for STDs can prevent PID. **Biopsies** (removal of a small amount of cervical tissue), abortion, miscarriage, and childbirth may also provide opportunities for bacteria to enter the reproductive tract.

Many women do not experience symptoms with PID. The condition may be discovered when the person has pain or difficulty getting pregnant. Some signs of PID are heavy, bad-smelling discharge from the vagina and irregular menstrual periods. Women with PID may also have fever, diarrhea, or vomiting. Women may experience pain in the back, pelvis, or lower abdomen and during urination or sex. PID may lead to infertility and **ectopic pregnancy** (pregnancy in the fallopian tube). Scarring of the reproductive organs may cause long-term pain (chronic pelvic pain) that may continue for months or years (Mayo Clinic 2009d).

Antibiotics are usually prescribed for PID, and pain medications and bed rest may also be recommended. If the infection is very severe or if the woman is pregnant or HIV positive, hospitalization may be required. **Intravenous** antibiotics—injected into the bloodstream through a vein—may be needed. Surgery is sometimes necessary to treat the effects of PID.

PID is best prevented by practicing safe sex and having regular screening for STDs. Using good hygiene and avoiding douching (which removes helpful bacteria) may lower the risk of PID (Mayo Clinic 2009d). Birth control devices inserted into the uterus (intrauterine devices) can increase the risk of PID.

Syphilis

Syphilis is caused by the *Treponema pallidum* bacteria. This infection is spread through sexual contact with syphilis sores on the skin. Syphilis sores are found on the penis, anus, vagina, or rectum. Sores may also form on the lips or mouth. Syphilis is passed through oral, anal, or vaginal sex. It is not spread through contact with toilet seats or in any other fashion except sexual contact.

The first stage of syphilis usually results in a single sore in the genital or anal area. The sore, called a **chancre**, will appear at the spot where the germ entered the body. It is a small firm lesion that is usually painless and may not be recognized as a problem. The second stage involves a rash over areas of the body. Other symptoms may include fever, sore throat, swollen lymph glands, weight loss, and fatigue. Syphilis has been called "the great pretender" because its symptoms can mimic several other diseases. Without treatment, syphilis can progress into a very serious or fatal disease. Later stages of the disease include damage to the organs (brain, eyes, heart, bones, and blood vessels). Syphilis can cause blindness, dementia, coordination problems, paralysis, and numbness. Organ damage may progress to the point of death (Centers for Disease Control and Prevention 2010f).

Syphilis is diagnosed through tests on a tissue sample from the sore or through blood tests. In the earlier stages, a single injection of an antibiotic can end the infection. Antibiotics will cure the infection but cannot undo any damage that the disease has already done. A syphilis infection does not create immunity; the illness can develop again if someone is exposed to an infected person.

Prevention of syphilis includes using a condom for all types of sex. Abstaining from sex is a certain way to avoid this disease. Once syphilis is diagnosed, all sexual partners need to be told of the infection and tested. Sex should be avoided until the infection has cleared (Centers for Disease Control and Prevention 2010f).

Trichomoniasis

Trichomoniasis is an STI caused by **protozoa** (tiny one-celled parasites). The protozoa are passed between people during sexual intercourse. Trichomoniasis may take from 5 to 28 days to develop (Mayo Clinic 2010c). Women may have symptoms of pain with sex and genital redness and itching. Another symptom is a foul-smelling vaginal discharge (white, yellow, gray, or green in color). Some women may have no symptoms, while others will be very irritated by the discharge and itching. Most men do not have symptoms when infected with trichomoniasis, or they may have mild pain with urination. The risks of developing this infection are increased in people who have multiple sexual partners, other STDs, or a previous case of trichomoniasis. Using condoms and limiting the number of sex partners may reduce the risk of contracting trichomoniasis.

Women with trichomoniasis may have an increased risk of contracting HIV. They also may be at risk for premature birth, for having a baby with low birth weight, and for passing the illness along to the baby during a vaginal birth. Trichomoniasis is treated by a large dose of medications that eliminate the organisms. Creams may also be prescribed to reduce discomfort in the genitals. All sexual partners must be treated to avoid reinfection. The illness takes about one week to clear, and unprotected sex should be avoided until the illness is cured (Mayo Clinic 2010c).

Tests for STDs and HIV

Tests for STDs are available at many health care clinics, public health departments, and health care practitioner offices. A local Planned Parenthood health center may have information about STD testing and costs involved and may offer other types of health care and financial

TABLE 3.3.5 **STD TESTING**

STD—Test or Tests Used

- HIV/AIDS—a blood test or a swab test (scraping cells from the inside of the mouth)
- Chlamydia—physical exam, urine test, tests on anal, urethral, or vaginal discharge or cell samples from the cervix, penis, vagina, or anus
- Genital warts—physical exam; warts are viewed with the naked eye or using a colposcope (a special instrument that helps detect very small warts)
- Gonorrhea—urine test; tests on anal, urethral, or vaginal discharge; or cell samples from the cervix, penis, vagina, or anus
- Hepatitis—blood test
- Herpes—blood test, tests on fluid from a herpes sore
- High-risk HPV—test on cervical cell samples (no HPV test for men)
- Pelvic inflammatory disease (affects only women)—pelvic exam, blood test, test of cervical or vaginal discharge, or exam by laparoscopy procedure (this inserts an instrument through a small cut in the navel and examines internal reproductive organs)
- Syphilis—blood test, tests of fluids from syphilis sores
- Trichomoniasis—test of urethral or vaginal discharge (Planned Parenthood 2011j)

assistance (Planned Parenthood 2011r). HIV testing is also available at medical offices and clinics, health departments, and hospitals. Some may offer free or low-cost testing. Sites may conduct HIV tests anonymously and label samples with numbers rather than names. Other testing sites place a report in the medical record about the patient's HIV status. Laws pertaining to HIV testing and results differ among states. Local health departments may have information about local regulations regarding HIV testing (Hirsch 2008a).

Resources

Websites, Help Lines, and Hotlines

Act Against AIDS
Information about HIV and AIDS prevention:
http://www.actagainstaids.org/

AVERT: AVERTing HIV and AIDS
An international organization working to avert HIV and AIDS:
http://www.avert.org/ready-sex.htm

Coalition for Positive Sexuality (CPS)
A site for teens who are sexually active or thinking about having a sexual relationship; information about decision making, contraception, STDs, and pregnancy: http://www.positive.org/

Go Ask Alice! (Columbia University)
Information about alcohol and other drugs, fitness and nutrition, emotional health, general health, sexuality, sexual health, and relationships:
http://www.goaskalice.columbia.edu/

I Wanna Know! American Social Health Association (ASHA)
Information about relationships, sexual health, STIs, pregnancy, parenthood, myths and facts about sexual health, and more:
http://www.iwannaknow.org/

InSPOT, I.S.I.S, Inc.
A way to anonymously notify a current or previous sexual partner that he or she may have been exposed to an STD: http://www.inspot.org/

The Naked Truth (Idaho Department of Health & Welfare)
Sexual health information to prevent the spread of STDs and HIV:
http://www.nakedtruth.idaho.gov/

Planned Parenthood
Birth Control: http://www.plannedparenthood.org/health-topics/birth-control-4211.htm

Fertility Awareness–Based Methods (FAMS): http://www.plannedparenthood.org/health-topics/birth-control/fertility-awareness-4217.htm

How to Put on a Condom (YouTube video: 2.5 minutes): http://www.plannedparenthood.org/health-topics/birth-control/condom-10187.htm

Information for Teens: http://www.plannedparenthood.org/info-for-teens/our-bodies-33795.htm

Safer Sex
Everything you wanted to know about safer sex: http://safersex.org/

Sex, Etc.
Sex education by teens, for teens: http://www.sexetc.org/topic/emotional_health

http://www.sextextsf.org/

Text "sexinfo" to 61827

TeensHealth from Nemours
Information in English and Spanish for teens about the body, the mind, physical and emotional health, relationships, drugs and alcohol, sexuality, and many other topics: http://teenshealth.org/teen/

Teen Source
Sexual health for youths to encourage informed decision making: http://www.teensource.org/

We Are Talking: Teen Health (Palo Alto Medical Foundation)
Health information for teens: http://www.pamf.org/teen/

Women's Health
Information on various aspects of female health. A federal government website managed by the Office on Women's Health at the U.S. Department of Health and Human Services: http://womenshealth.gov/pregnancy/mom-to-be-tools/ovulation-due-date-calc.cfm

Youth Resource
Information on sexual health for LGBT and questioning youths: http://www.amplifyyourvoice.org/youthresource

Further Reading

Basso, Michael. 2003. *The Underground Guide to Teenage Sexuality*. 2nd ed. Minneapolis: Fairview.

Boonstra, Heather, and Elizabeth Nash. 2000. "Minors and the Right to Consent to Health Care." *Guttmacher Report on Public Policy* 3(4): 4–8. http://www.guttmacher.org/pubs/tgr/03/4/gr030404.pdf.

Corinna, Heather. 2007. *S.E.X.: The All-You-Need-to-Know Progressive Sexuality Guide to Get You through High School and College*. New York: Marlowe.

Dailard, Cynthia. 2003. "New Medical Records Privacy Rule: The Interface with Teen Access to Confidential Care." *Guttmacher Report on Public Policy* 6(1): 6–7. http://www.guttmacher.org/pubs/tgr/06/1/gr060106.pdf.

Gowen, L. Kris. 2003. *Making Sexual Decisions: The Ultimate Teen Guide*. Lanham, MA: Scarecrow.

Hasler, Nikol. 2010. *Sex: A Book for Teens; An Uncensored Guide to Your Body, Sex, and Safety*. San Francisco: Zest Books.

Norman-Eady, Sandra, Christopher Reinhart, and Peter Martino. 2003. "Statutory Rape Laws by State." *OLR Research Report*. http://www.cga.ct.gov/2003/olrdata/jud/rpt/2003-R-0376.htm.

References

AVERT. 2011. "Criminal Transmission of HIV." http://www.avert.org/criminal-transmission.htm.

Boonstra, Heather, and Elizabeth Nash. 2000. "Minors and the Right to Consent to Health Care." *Guttmacher Report on Public Policy* 3(4): 4–8. http://www.guttmacher.org/pubs/tgr/03/4/gr030404.pdf.

Centers for Disease Control and Prevention. 2010a. "Basic Information about HIV and AIDS." August 11. http://www.cdc.gov/hiv/topics/basic/index.htm.

Centers for Disease Control and Prevention. 2010b. "Candidiasis." July 6. http://www.cdc.gov/nczved/divisions/dfbmd/diseases/candidiasis/index.html#what.

Centers for Disease Control and Prevention. 2010c. "Genital Herpes." CDC Fact Sheet. July 13. http://www.cdc.gov/std/Herpes/STD Fact-Herpes.htm.

Centers for Disease Control and Prevention. 2010d. "HIV among Gay, Bisexual, and Other Men Who Have Sex with Men (MSM)." September. http://www.cdc.gov/hiv/topics/msm/index.htm.

Centers for Disease Control and Prevention. 2010e. "Human Papillomavirus." September 16. http://www.cdc.gov/hpv/Treatment.html.

Centers for Disease Control and Prevention. 2010f. "Syphilis." CDC Fact Sheet. September 16. http://www.cdc.gov/STD/syphilis/STD-Fact-Syphilis.htm.

Centers for Disease Control and Prevention. 2010g. "Youth Risk Behavior Surveillance, United States, 2009." *Morbidity and Mortality Weekly Report* 59 (June 4). http://www.cdc.gov/mmwr/pdf/ss/ss5905.pdf.

Centers for Disease Control and Prevention. 2011. "Gonorrhea." CDC Fact Sheet. April 5. http://www.cdc.gov/STD/Gonorrhea/STD Fact-gonorrhea.htm#How.

Child Welfare Information Gateway. 2010. "Mandatory Reporters of Child Abuse and Neglect: Summary of State Laws." U.S. Department of Health and Human Services, Administration for Children and Families. April. http://www.childwelfare.gov/systemwide/laws_policies/statutes/manda.cfm.

Connecticut General Assembly. 2003. "Statutory Rape Laws by State." http://www.cga.ct.gov/2003/olrdata/jud/rpt/2003-r-0376.htm.

Dailard, Cynthia. 2003. "New Medical Records Privacy Rule: The Interface with Teen Access to Confidential Care." *Guttmacher Report on Public Policy* 6(1): 6–7. http://www.guttmacher.org/pubs/tgr/06/1/gr060106.pdf.

Downs, Martin F. 2010. "Four Things You Didn't Know about Oral Sex." WebMD. February 18. http://www.webmd.com/sex-relationships/features/4-things-you-didnt-know-about-oral-sex.

Glosser, Asaph, Karen Gardiner, and Mike Fishman. 2004. "Statutory Rape: A Guide to State Laws and Reporting Requirements." Office of the Assistant Secretary for Planning and Evaluation, Department of Health and Human Services. December 15. http://www.hhs.gov/opa/pubs/statutory-rape-state-laws.pdf.

Hirsch, Larissa. 2008a. "HIV Testing Resources." TeensHealth from Nemours. November. http://kidshealth.org/teen/sexual_health/stds/hiv_tests.html?tracking=T_RelatedArticle#.

Hirsch, Larissa. 2009a. "Birth Control: Abstinence." TeensHealth from Nemours. September. http://kidshealth.org/teen/sexual_health/contraception/abstinence.html#.

Hirsch, Larissa. 2009b. "Birth Control Methods: How Well Do They Work?" TeensHealth from Nemours. October. http://kidshealth.org/teen/sexual_health/contraception/bc_chart.html#.

Hirsch, Larissa. 2009c. "Can a Girl Get Pregnant If She Has Sex during Her Period?" TeensHealth from Nemours. November. http://kidshealth.org/teen/expert/sex_health/sex_during_period.html.

Hirsch, Larissa. 2009d. "Can a Girl Have Sex with a Tampon in?" TeensHealth from Nemours. August. http://kidshealth.org/teen/expert/sex_health/remove_tampon.html.

Hirsch, Larissa. 2009e. "Talking to Your Partner about Condoms." TeensHealth from Nemours. September. http://kidshealth.org/teen/sexual_health/girls/talk_about_condoms.html?tracking=T_RelatedArticle#.

Hirsch, Larissa. 2009f. "Telling Your Partner You Have an STD." TeensHealth from Nemours. September. http://kidshealth.org/teen/sexual_health/stds/stds_talk.html?tracking=T_RelatedArticle#cat20017.

Lyness, D'Arcy. 2010. "Virginity: A Very Personal Decision." Teens-Health from Nemours. November. http://kidshealth.org/teen/sexual_health/guys/virginity.html.

Mayo Clinic. 2009a. "Chlamydia." April 29. http://www.mayoclinic.com/health/chlamydia/DS00173.

Mayo Clinic. 2009b. "Dementia Causes." April 17. http://www.mayoclinic.com/health/dementia/DS01131/DSECTION=causes.

Mayo Clinic. 2009c. "Genital Herpes." http://www.mayoclinic.com/health/genital-herpes/DS00179.

Mayo Clinic. 2009d. "Pelvic Inflammatory Disease." May 23. http://www.mayoclinic.com/health/pelvic-inflammatory-disease/DS00402.

Mayo Clinic. 2010a. "Genital Warts." February 9. http://www.mayoclinic.com/health/genital-warts/DS00087.

Mayo Clinic. 2010b. "HIV/AIDS Dementia Causes." April 11. http://www.mayoclinic.com/health/hiv-aids/DS00005.

Mayo Clinic. 2010c. "Trichomoniasis." January 23. http://www.mayoclinic.com/health/trichomoniasis/DS01163.

Neinstein, Lawrence S. 1987. "Consent and Confidentiality Laws for Minors in the Western United States." *Western Journal of Medicine* 147 (August): 218–224. http://www.ncbi.nlm.nih.gov/pmc/articles/PMC1025802/pdf/westjmed00144-0120.pdf.

Planned Parenthood. 2011a. "Abstinence." http://www.plannedparenthood.org/health-topics/birth-control/abstinence-4215.htm.

Planned Parenthood. 2011b. "Birth Control." http://www.plannedparenthood.org/health-topics/birth-control-4211.htm.

Planned Parenthood. 2011c. "Birth Control Implant (Implanon)." http://www.plannedparenthood.org/health-topics/birth-control/birth-control-implant-implanon-4243.htm.

Planned Parenthood. 2011d. "Birth Control Patch (Ortho-Evra)." http://www.plannedparenthood.org/health-topics/birth-control/birth-control-patch-ortho-evra-4240.htm.

Planned Parenthood. 2011e. "Birth Control Pills." http://www.plannedparenthood.org/health-topics/birth-control/birth-control-pill-4228.htm.

Planned Parenthood. 2011f. "Birth Control Shot (Depo-Provera)." http://www.plannedparenthood.org/health-topics/birth-control/birth-control-shot-depo-provera-4242.htm.

Planned Parenthood. 2011g. "Birth Control Sponge (Today Sponge)." http://www.plannedparenthood.org/health-topics/birth-control/birth-control-implant-implanon-4243.htm.

Planned Parenthood. 2011h. "Breastfeeding as Birth Control." http://www.plannedparenthood.org/health-topics/birth-control/birth-control-shot-depo-provera-4242.htm.

Planned Parenthood. 2011i. "Cervical Cap (FemCap)." http://www.plannedparenthood.org/health-topics/birth-control/cervical-cap-20487.htm.

Planned Parenthood. 2011j. "Comparing Effectiveness of Birth Control Methods." http://www.plannedparenthood.org/health-topics/birth-control/birth-control-effectiveness-chart-22710.htm.

Planned Parenthood. 2011k. "Condom." http://www.plannedparenthood.org/health-topics/birth-control/condom-10187.htm.

Planned Parenthood. 2011l. "Diaphragm." http://www.plannedparenthood.org/health-topics/birth-control/diaphragm-4244.htm.

Planned Parenthood. 2011m. "Fertility Awareness–based Methods." http://www.plannedparenthood.org/health-topics/birth-control/fertility-awareness-4217.htm.

Planned Parenthood. 2011n. "How Do I Use Condoms?" http://www.plannedparenthood.org/health-topics/birth-control/condom-10187.htm.

Planned Parenthood. 2011o. "Morning-After Pill (Emergency Contraception)." http://www.plannedparenthood.org/health-topics/emergency-contraception-morning-after-pill-4363.asp.

Planned Parenthood. 2011p. "Myths and Facts about Sex." http://www.plannedparenthood.org/info-for-teens/sex-masturbation/myths-facts-about-sex-33825.htm.

Planned Parenthood. 2011q. "Outercourse." http://www.plannedparenthood.org/health-topics/birth-control/outercourse-4371.htm.

Planned Parenthood. 2011r. "STD Testing." http://www.plannedparenthood.org/health-topics/stds-hiv-safer-sex/std-testing-21695.asp.

Planned Parenthood. 2011s. "Vaginal Birth Control Ring (NuvaRing)." http://www.plannedparenthood.org/health-topics/birth-control/birth-control-vaginal-ring-nuvaring-4241.htm.

Planned Parenthood. 2011t. "Withdrawal (Pull Out Method)." http://www.plannedparenthood.org/health-topics/birth-control/withdrawal-pull-out-method-4218.htm.

University of Illinois at Chicago College of Medicine. 2011. "Topics: Confidentiality and Duty to Report." http://www.uic.edu/depts/mcam/ethics/confidentiality.htm.

U.S. National Library of Medicine and National Institutes of Health. 2010. "Safe Sex." June 5. http://www.nlm.nih.gov/medlineplus/ency/article/001949.htm.

Wheaton, Joy Mara. 2011. "A Woman's Guide to Understanding IUDs." Association of Reproductive Health Professionals. http://www.arhp.org/Publications-and-Resources/Patient-Resources/printed-materials/Understanding-IUDs.

Glossary

abstinence (sexual): The decision to refrain from having sex.

age of consent: The age at which a person can consent to have sex; *see* **statutory rape.**

AIDS: Acquired immunodeficiency syndrome; an immune disease caused by HIV.

anal sex: Sex that includes exploring the buttocks, rectum, and anus of a partner with hands, mouth, sex toys, or genitals.

barrier: An obstacle or hindrance.

barrier birth control: Birth control methods that place a barrier in the path of the sperm as the sperm move toward the egg.

biopsy: Removal of a small amount of tissue for analysis.

birth control: *See* **contraception**.

birth control implant: A small rod (about the size of a matchstick) that is inserted by a health care provider under the skin on a woman's upper arm.

birth control patch: An adhesive birth control patch that releases estrogen and progesterone to prevent ovulation.

birth control ring: A small flexible ring placed by a woman in her vagina to prevent pregnancy.

birth control sponge: A round piece of soft plastic foam containing spermicide; used to prevent pregnancy.

calendar method: Fertility awareness–based birth control method used to help calculate the day of ovulation.

cervical cap: A silicone cup that is placed over the cervix to prevent pregnancy.

chancre: A syphilis sore.

chlamydia: A very common bacterial infection of the genital tract.

chronic: Long-lasting, persistent.

coitus interruptus: The withdrawal method of birth control, or pulling out.

condom: A thin plastic or latex sleeve-like object worn to cover the penis; used to prevent pregnancy and protect against STDs; also called a rubber or a safe.

consistent abstinence: Refraining from sexual activity all the time.

contraception (birth control): The prevention of pregnancy using artificial or natural methods.

cryotherapy: Freezing; used as a treatment for genital warts.

dementia: Thinking difficulties; can develop in a person with AIDS.

diaphragm: A flexible latex cup that is placed inside the vagina to cover the cervix and prevent pregnancy.

douching: Cleansing a body cavity (usually the vagina) with a liquid cleansing solution (douche).

ectopic pregnancy: Pregnancy in the fallopian tube; this type of pregnancy is not viable (cannot come to term) and may be life-threatening.

electrocautery: A treatment using electrical current to burn off genital warts.

emergency contraception (morning-after pill): A pill that may be used up to five days after unprotected sex to prevent pregnancy.

epididymitis: Painful inflammation of the epididymis, ducts within the testicles in the scrotum.

eugenics: A controversial practice involving encouraging breeding among people with positive, desirable qualities while limiting breeding of people with less desirable qualities; has been used in an attempt to eliminate disease or disability and increase the proportion of people with desirable characteristics.

female condom: A thin plastic pouch placed inside a woman's vagina or anus; used to prevent pregnancy and for protection against STDs.

fertile: Likely or able to become pregnant; the time in a woman's monthly cycle when she is most likely to get pregnant.

fertility: Ability to reproduce; to make someone pregnant or to get pregnant.

fertility awareness–based birth control: A method of birth control that uses information about ovulation to make a decision about when to have sex; also known as natural family planning and the rhythm method.

flora: Normal helpful organisms that reside in the body, such as in the gastrointestinal and genitourinary tracts.

genital candidiasis: A fungal infection that occurs in the genital area; also called yeast infections.

genital herpes: A viral infection that is caused by a herpes simplex virus type 2 (HSV2); may also be caused by HSV1, which causes cold sores.

genital warts: An STD caused by HPV; also called venereal warts and *condylomata acuminata.*

gonorrhea: An STD caused by the *Neisseria gonorrhoeae* bacteria; passed through sexual contact.

herpes: A viral infection; *see* **genital herpes**, **herpes simplex**, and **herpes zoster**.

herpes simplex: The virus that causes cold sores; herpes simplex virus type 1 (HSV1).

herpes zoster: The virus that causes shingles and chicken pox.

HIV: Human immunodeficiency virus; a virus that destroys T cells and may lead to AIDS.

HPV: Human papillomavirus.

human immunodeficiency virus (HIV): A virus that destroys T cells and may lead to AIDS.

human papillomavirus (HPV): The most common sexually transmitted disease in the United States, passed from one person to another through genital contact, usually during vaginal or anal sex.

hysterectomy: Surgical removal of the uterus.

infertility: Inability to sexually reproduce; unable to make someone pregnant or to get pregnant.

intrauterine device (IUD): A small plastic device, shaped like a T, that is placed into a woman's uterus to prevent pregnancy.

intravenous: Injected into the bloodstream.

IUD: Intrauterine device.

Kaposi's sarcoma: A cancer of the blood vessel walls; common complication of AIDS.

lesions: Sores.

lymphoma: Cancer in the lymph nodes; can develop in people with AIDS.

mandatory reporting: Requirement for certain professionals or institutions to report suspected cases of abuse or neglect.

morning-after pill: *See* **emergency contraception**.

oophorectomy: Surgical removal of the ovaries.

oral sex: Sex involving using one's mouth on a partner's genitals.

outercourse: Sex activities that do not involve sexual intercourse, penetration, or vaginal sex; used as a method of birth control.

pelvic inflammatory disease (PID): An infection of the female reproductive organs.

PID: Pelvic inflammatory disease.

preejaculate: A clear fluid that comes out of the penis before ejaculation; also known as preseminal fluid and Cowper's fluid.

premature ejaculation: Ejaculation before it is intended during early stages of sexual excitement or soon after insertion of the penis into the vagina.

protozoa: Tiny one-celled parasites; cause of trichomoniasis.

rhythm method: Using the rhythm of a woman's menstrual cycle to prevent pregnancy; also known as natural family planning. *See also* **fertility awareness–based birth control**.

safe sex: Sexual practices that prevent pregnancy and the spread of illness.

safer sex: A more accurate way to describe the methods used for protected sex; the risks are still present but at a lesser degree; compare with safe sex.

salmonella: A bacteria found in contaminated food and water.

sexually transmitted disease (STD): Disease caused by organisms that may live on the vagina, penis, mouth, or skin or in the anus and are transmitted to others through contact with a sore on the genitals or the mouth. Also known as a sexually transmitted infection (STI) or venereal disease (VD).

sexually transmitted infection (STI): *See* **sexually transmitted disease**.

spermicide: A cream or jelly containing chemicals that stop sperm from moving, decreasing the chance of any sperm finding a way around a barrier (such as a diaphragm) and preventing pregnancy.

statutory rape: Illegal act of having sex with a person who is younger than the legal age of consent.

STD: Sexually transmitted disease.

sterilization: A surgery that changes the reproductive system so that the body is no longer fertile. *See also* **hysterectomy**, **oophorectomy**, **tubal ligation**, **vasectomy**.

STI: Sexually transmitted infection; *see* **sexually transmitted disease**.

suppository: A solid medication, often in the shape of a cone or cylinder, usually inserted into the rectum or vagina.

syphilis: An STD caused by the *Treponema pallidum* bacteria and spread through sexual contact with syphilis sores on the skin.

T cells: A type of white blood cells that help the body protect itself from disease; destroyed by HIV.

toxoplasmosis: A deadly infection related to parasites found in cat feces.

trichomoniasis: A sexually transmitted infection caused by protozoa.

tubal ligation: A surgical sterilization procedure that removes a small segment of each fallopian tube to prevent the union of sperm and ovum, preventing pregnancy.

unprotected sex: Sexual practices that do not protect against pregnancy or STDs; also known as unsafe sex; contrast with safe sex and safer sex.

unsafe sex: Sex that is unprotected from pregnancy and STDs; contrast with safe sex and safer sex.

vasectomy: Surgical sterilization procedure that blocks or closes the tubes that carry sperm from the testes, preventing pregnancy.

VD: Venereal disease; *see* **sexually transmitted disease**.

venereal disease: VD; *see* **sexually transmitted disease**.

virgin: Someone who has not had sex; sometimes refers to someone who has never had sexual intercourse.

vulva: Vaginal area.

withdrawal: When the penis is pulled out of the vagina before ejaculation; used as a method of birth control. Also known as pulling out and coitus interruptus.

CHAPTER 4

Pregnancy and Parenting

Pregnancy and the parenting of children are relevant topics for some teens. Some are dealing with pregnancy and children themselves; others may be interested because they look forward to this experience later in their lives. Many teens are involved in caring for children, either for their younger brothers and sisters or through being involved in child care as a job.

In the United States, close to 7 percent of teenage girls became pregnant in 2006 (Wind 2010). Pregnancy and parenting can be a challenge, especially when faced by teens. This chapter discusses some aspects of pregnancy and parenting. Being well informed can help when faced with decisions about pregnancy or parenthood.

Pregnancy

The news of a pregnancy may result in many reactions from an expectant mother or father. Expectant parents may feel a mixture of joy, fear, anger, or sadness at the many changes ahead for everyone involved. Pregnancy—which means that there is a **fetus** (baby) developing in the mother—can be a challenging time. Most pregnancies are the result of **sexual intercourse**. Sexual intercourse occurs when the penis is placed in the vagina. When the male ejaculates, sperm comes out of the penis and can travel through the vagina to an **ovum** (egg) in the female.

Pregnancies may also occur through special medical procedures. **Artificial insemination** is a process using a small tube to insert sperm through a woman's cervix into the uterus. The sperm may then reach an egg to achieve fertilization. **In vitro fertilization** involves combining eggs from a woman and sperm from a man in a laboratory dish to achieve fertilization. The **embryos** created by this procedure are later placed in the mother's uterus.

Conception happens when sperm from the male fertilizes (joins with) the egg of the female. Conception is when the pregnancy begins. The

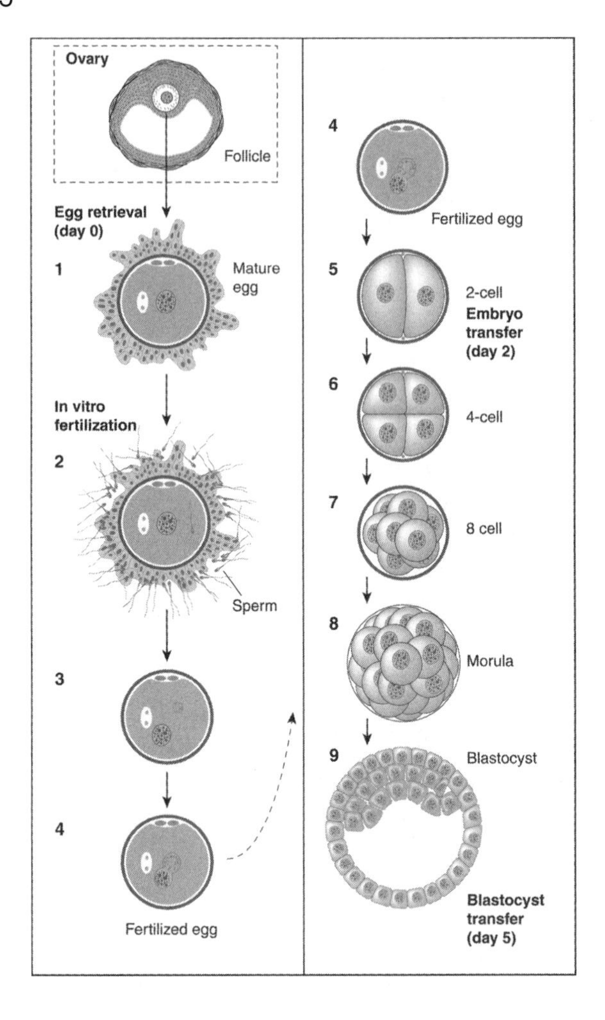

Process of in vitro fertilization. *(Shutterstock.com)*

fertilized egg is called a **zygote;** it develops over time to become a fetus. Conception and pregnancy can occur even if birth control measures are used (see also chapter 3 of this volume). Conception does not occur when a female swallows sperm. Sperm on a female's skin will not cause fertilization unless the sperm is very close to the vagina.

Diagnosing Pregnancy

A missing or late menstrual period may be the first sign of a pregnancy. A woman may have spotty or very light vaginal bleeding and may feel tired, faint, or weak. A woman may notice sore or full breasts, darker nipples,

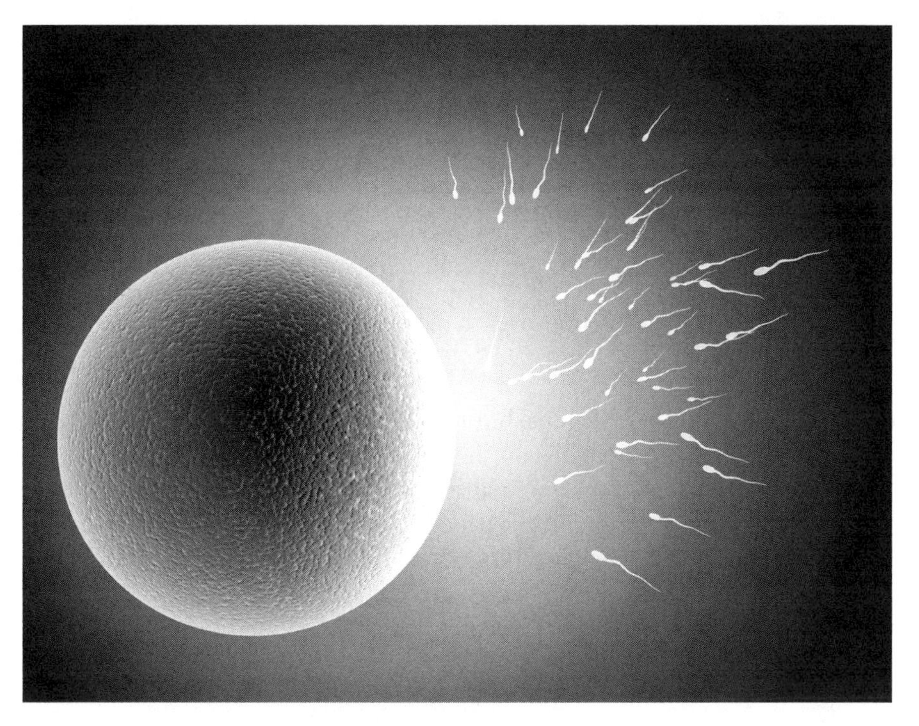

Conception occurs when sperm from the male fertilizes the female's egg (ovum). *(Shutterstock.com)*

and a bloated tummy area. Urinating more often may be another symptom of pregnancy. Other common signs are headaches, slightly elevated body temperature, and feeling moody or stressed. Pregnant women often notice constipation, nausea, or vomiting. They may have new dislikes for some foods or cravings for unusual foods. Later the pregnancy causes a visible increase in the size of the abdomen and may bring lower abdominal pressure or cramps (Wiener 2007).

Pregnant women may worry about which symptoms are normal and which are a problem. Some people give pregnant women advice or tell stories that may be confusing or scary. The truth or wisdom of these comments may vary. During pregnancy, a woman may get used to her changed body and may sometimes know what feels normal for her. When in doubt, contacting a health care professional may be the best way to decide if there is anything to worry about.

Certain symptoms require an immediate call to the health care practitioner. A pregnant woman should call right away if she sees has heavy bleeding, any bleeding with cramps, bloody diarrhea, severe headache, or severe pain in the lower abdomen. Other reasons for making an urgent call to the health practitioner include:

- Being very thirsty and urinating less
- High fever (over 101.5 degrees Fahrenheit)
- Rapid and major swelling around hands and face
- Sudden significant weight gain
- Disturbed vision for more than a few minutes (Murkoff and Mazel 2008)

Some problems are less urgent, but the woman should call the health care practitioner that same day or within 24 hours. Some reasons to call within 24 hours include bloody urine, painful or burning urination, and severe nausea or vomiting, dizzy or faint feelings, frequent diarrhea, fever over 100 degrees, or significant itching over the body (Murkoff and Mazel 2008). More information can be found in Murkoff and Mazel's 2008 book *What to Expect When You're Expecting*, listed under further reading at the end of this chapter.

Pregnancy Tests

Human chorionic gonadotropin (HcG) is present in a woman's blood and urine when she is pregnant. HcG is a hormone that is produced when the fertilized egg implants in the uterus. The egg implants about six days after fertilization. The amount of HcG builds up quickly in the early days of pregnancy. Home pregnancy tests detect the presence of HcG in the female's urine. Other tests measure the level of HcG in the blood; these tests are done in a doctor's office or medical clinic. The blood test can detect a pregnancy as early as 6–8 days after **ovulation.** Ovulation occurs when an egg is released from the ovary, usually 14 days after the beginning of the monthly menstrual cycle. Blood tests that measure the amount of HcG are very accurate; they detect small amounts of the hormone. Those blood tests that check the presence of HcG are only as accurate as a urine test. A positive result on a pregnancy test is usually accurate. A woman can be fairly sure she is pregnant if a pregnancy test shows a positive result (Women's Health Information 2006).

Many home pregnancy tests can be done on the first day of a missed menstrual period. Tests may also be done 19 days after unprotected sex. If a home pregnancy test taken early is negative but the woman still has pregnancy symptoms, the test may have been done too soon. The test should be repeated 3–4 days after the first test. To improve test accuracy, read instructions carefully and follow them exactly. Waiting 10 minutes

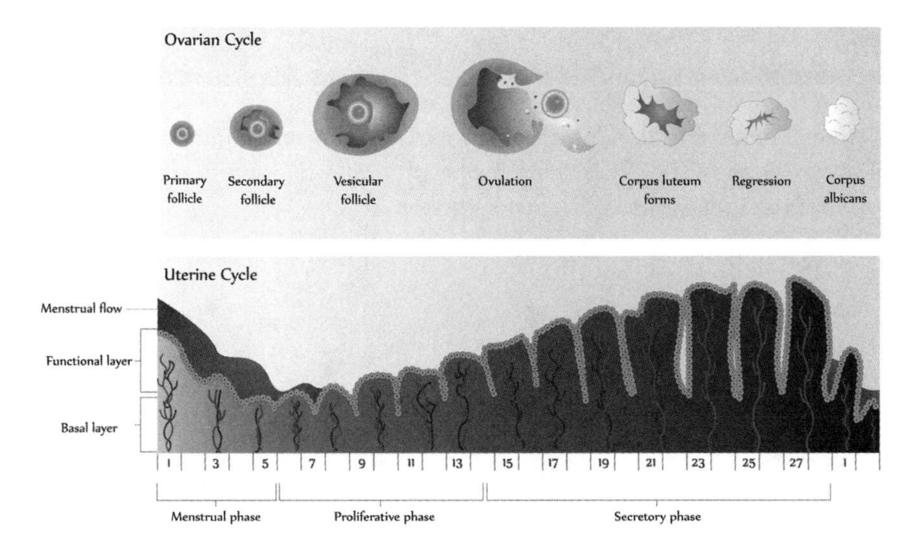

Ovulation cycle. *(Shutterstock.com)*

after taking the test to view the results gives the most dependable results (Women's Health Information 2006). A woman who has a positive home pregnancy test should get medical advice.

The health care practitioner will conduct a physical exam to confirm the pregnancy and check the mother's overall health. Examinations can find any problems that may need to be watched during pregnancy. Knowing the size of the uterus can help determine when the baby is due. Blood tests will likely be conducted.

Other tests that may be done during pregnancy include **ultrasounds**. These tests use high-frequency sound waves to produce pictures of the inside of the body. The sound waves are aimed from outside the body to the uterus and are bounced off internal structures to create an image. Ultrasounds may be done through a smooth object moved across the woman's abdomen or through a smooth small object moved gently within the vagina. The test is conducted by an ultrasound technician. Ultrasounds can be used to learn the size and age of the fetus and to check on the position and growth of the fetus. They may also find problems in the fetus or the pregnancy. Ultrasounds can reveal the presence of multiple fetuses, such as twins or triplets. These tests may also reveal if the fetus is male or female.

Some mothers are advised to have an **amniocentesis** in which a needle is placed into the pregnant uterus. The needle removes a small amount of the fluid from the amniotic sac. The fluid is used for genetic and other diagnostic tests about the fetus. These genetic tests can be used to show the sex of the fetus. This test is used more often in older mothers who

? Did You Know?

- Pregnant women can develop **gestational diabetes.** Hormones present during pregnancy can block the function of insulin and cause high blood sugar in pregnant women. Risk factors are:
  - High blood pressure
  - Glucose in the urine
  - Family history of diabetes
  - Over age 25
  - Overweight
  - History of stillbirth or large babies
- Gestational diabetes may cause blurred vision, fatigue, frequent infections, increased urination, and thirst. The mother and fetus will be monitored carefully. Careful diet and exercise are advised to control blood sugar. Untreated gestational diabetes rarely results in fetal death; mothers and babies do well when the diabetes is controlled. The babies tend to be larger, and a C-section may be necessary. The baby's blood sugar may briefly be low. The baby and mother's blood sugars are likely to be normal soon after delivery (Storck 2010).

may have a higher risk of genetic abnormalities in the fetus. Parents in higher-risk groups are advised to have the test so they can be ready for any problems the baby may have.

During the pregnancy, the mother's blood may be tested for hormone levels. This can help the doctor monitor the progress of the pregnancy. Tests can also be done on the mother's blood to look for problems in the fetus. Other tests include glucose testing to monitor the mother for development of **gestational diabetes**. Group B streptococcus (GBS) is a type of bacteria that can cause infections in the newborn after vaginal delivery. Tests can screen the genital area for GBS. If GBS is found, the woman can be treated with antibiotics to reduce the risk to the infant.

At times, genetic testing will be recommended. These tests can detect some possible genetic problems, including cystic fibrosis, sickle cell disease, hemophilia, and muscular dystrophy (Lucille Packard Foundation for Children's Health 2011).

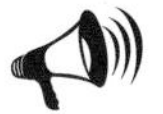 WHAT PEOPLE ARE SAYING **TEEN OPINIONS: WHO SHOULD BE A PARENT?**

Should there be restrictions on who should be a parent?

- "I know people who should simply not be allowed to reproduce because they would be in no way capable of caring for a child. I think it depends a great deal on whether the parent would be raising the child alone or with a partner. If the parents would actually be able to care for the child and function as a healthy family, then I see no reason they should not be allowed to be parents." ES, age 20, California
- "No one should be denied the right of having their own reproductive system. But if someone has a disability, maybe the government should help with the parenting. While I agree that some people shouldn't have a child, it's not the government's job to say no. But they should consider adoption. Maybe there should be counseling to help people decide if they should really have a child." GBH, age 17, California
- "I believe everyone has the natural right to reproduce, but if the child is thought to be in any danger whatsoever, he or she should be removed from that household." KK, age 19, Kentucky
- "Criminals shouldn't be allowed to be parents." MR, age 20, California
- There should be limitations against people who are violent being parents." JH, age 21, California

Responses to Pregnancy

Some parents may not welcome pregnancies in their lives. Parents may not have the finances, maturity, or desire to care for a child. They may feel that they are not suited to be parents or that a baby would be too disruptive to their present lives. Others may fear shame, disappointment, or more serious problems from their families. People may deal with an unwanted pregnancy in different ways, including adoption or **abortion**.

Abortion

If a mother has certain medical problems, carrying the baby to full term may be dangerous. Some parents decide to end a pregnancy when testing shows that the baby is likely to have a serious birth defect or developmental disorder. For these and various other reasons, some mothers decide to have an abortion. An abortion is the removal of the embryo/fetus and the **placenta** by a gentle suction device. The device is passed into the uterus through the vagina and cervix. The doctor may inject the cervix with local **anesthesia**, and the woman may have calming medication. After the abortion, there may be some heavier bleeding and cramping for a few days and spotting of blood for several weeks.

When medication is used to end a pregnancy, it is called a **medical abortion.** This option may be used when a woman is less than nine weeks pregnant. A doctor does an examination and blood tests and supervises the medications. One pill ends the pregnancy by blocking **progesterone,** a female hormone that aids pregnancy. Without progesterone, the lining of the uterus breaks down, and the pregnancy cannot continue. A second pill, taken a few days later, will empty the uterus and cause cramping and heavy bleeding. The abortion is complete within four to five hours in more than half of the cases. However, it may take a few days for some women. In about two weeks, the doctor will evaluate the woman's health and check to be sure she is no longer pregnant (Planned Parenthood 2010).

Usually, abortions are performed before 24 weeks of pregnancy. Some states have different rules about the timing of an abortion. Girls under 18 years of age are required to have a parent's permission for abortions in many states. In some cases, a judge may excuse the teen from getting parental consent. A woman's ability to become pregnant in the future is usually not affected by having an abortion.

Some pregnancies end prematurely with the fetus being naturally expelled from the body. This event is called a **spontaneous abortion**, meaning that it happens due to unplanned causes. Some people refer to a **miscarriage** as "losing the baby." This may happen if the fetus is no longer alive, if the mother's body is not able to keep carrying the fetus, or through some accident.

Adoption

Some women decide to go through the pregnancy and release the baby to be adopted after birth. Women may make this choice because they are not prepared to raise a child but have sincere beliefs against abortion. People who want to adopt a baby are evaluated by adoption services or agencies. The agencies can connect people who want to adopt with people who want their baby adopted. The baby's birth parents may take part, to various degrees, in choosing the adoptive parents and being involved in the child's life. Adoption agreements are carefully designed to protect the rights of the child and both sets of parents. Lawyers may be asked to help make sure the adoption takes place legally. Decisions about adoption can involve the biological mother and father and the grandparents. Counselors can assist families with discussing and reaching agreements about these important decisions. Adoption is also discussed in chapter 1, "Environment and Mental Health," in volume 5.

Abandonment

A few people facing pregnancy do not seek support and do not tell others of their condition. These women do not receive proper prenatal care and do not have help facing the challenges of their situation. Sometimes the pregnancy remains a secret, and after delivery occurs the parent or parents do not know what to do. Some may feel unable to care for the baby or may feel that they do not want to keep the baby. In these cases, the baby may be abandoned, or left somewhere by the parent. Babies have died in these instances because they were left in an unsafe place or somewhere they would not receive the proper treatment after birth. In 1998, an estimated 30,800 babies were abandoned in the United States (National Abandoned Infant Assistance Resource Center 2005).

Parents may fear being charged with a crime if they give the baby to the authorities. Safe haven laws have been created to avoid this desperate situation and to save babies' lives. The laws vary from state to state. Babies may be taken to a safe place, such as a hospital emergency room, fire station, or police station. No names will be requested, and the person leaving the infant will not be punished. When the parent leaves the baby, he or she can decide to give up parental rights so that the baby can be adopted by others (Campbell Philipsen 2003).

Family Responses to Pregnancy

A teen's parents, other family members, school personnel, and friends may all have reactions and opinions about a teen pregnancy. The teens' parents may be unhappy about the interruption in the lives they had hoped their children would lead. They may worry about the maturity and ability of their son or daughter to raise a baby. The teens' parents may not have been aware that their child was sexually active. Teens' parents may believe that they will have to take care of the baby; they may or may not be happy with the responsibility. Friends and family may also be surprised to learn of the pregnancy. Some may be excited that a baby will be born; others may realize that a pregnancy can bring difficulty into the teenagers' lives. Pregnant teenagers may be dismissed from some schools or may go to alternative schools during the pregnancy. Dealing with all these different reactions is a large task for expectant teen parents who are also dealing with their own feelings.

Conception and Fetal Development

Pregnancy begins with conception. The female egg is fertilized by the male sperm, and a fertilized egg, or zygote, is formed. The zygote develops and is referred to as an embryo until 8 weeks of development. At this point, the organism is called a fetus until birth. Medical examinations and ultrasounds may be utilized to estimate the age of the fetus. The expected delivery date is often calculated at 40 weeks from the first day of the last menstrual period. Typical gestation from the time of conception is 38 weeks.

Pregnancies are referred to in three time periods, labeled as the first, second, and third **trimesters.** Each trimester lasts approximately three months.

Fetal Development: First Trimester

During the first trimester, the embryo develops from a microscopic group of cells into a fetus and a placenta. The placenta is the organ that develops within the uterus to supply food and oxygen to the fetus through the umbilical cord. By the end of the first trimester, the fetus will have developed a heart and circulatory system; the face, sense organs, and nail beds are also beginning to take shape. The fetus is about two inches long at the end of the first trimester. Toward the end of the first trimester, the baby's heartbeat may be found with a **Doppler**, an ultrasound instrument that amplifies the sound of the heartbeat.

Fetal Development: Second Trimester

In the second trimester, the fetus grows rapidly to eight or nine inches in length and a weight of about two pounds. Muscles and bones are developing, and the lungs are forming. The face is almost fully formed during this trimester, and the eyes are open by the end of the sixth month. The senses of hearing, taste, and vision are functioning.

Fetal Development: Third Trimester

Fetal development comes to completion in the third trimester. The baby can suck her or his thumb, move about, and inhale and exhale **amniotic fluid** to prepare for breathing air after birth. Amniotic fluid is the fluid contained in the amniotic sac surrounding the fetus. This fluid allows the developing fetus to move around, helps its lungs to develop, provides cushioning and protection, and maintains a healthy temperature in the fetal environment. The fetus will now weigh between six and nine pounds, the fingernails are formed, the genitals are developing, the brain and nervous system are fully developed, and organ systems reach full development. For more information and illustrations of stages of pregnancy and fetal development, visit the Women's Health Information website, listed in the resources section at the end of this chapter.

Stages and Symptoms of Pregnancy

The mother may experience different symptoms as the pregnancy progresses through the different trimesters.

Pregnancy: First Trimester

In the first trimester, the mother may have **morning sickness**, a state of nausea or vomiting. It may occur in the morning or at any time during the day. Being pregnant for the first time or having sensitivity to changes in hormone levels and stress may increase the tendency to have nausea. Morning sickness may be relieved by eating early before getting out of bed or having a snack before bed. Eating several light meals throughout the day may help. Saltine crackers or rice cakes are often easy to tolerate. Nausea may be decreased by **sea bands**, elastic wrist bands for seasickness. These bands (available at some dive shops) apply pressure to an acupressure point on the inner wrists. Pregnant women may also experience:

- Fatigue and an increased need for more rest and sleep
- Forgetfulness due to pregnancy hormones, lack of sleep, and having a lot to think about
- Indigestion and **heartburn** (a hot or burning feeling in the upper abdomen near the breastbone)
- Constipation and **flatulence** (excess gas), which may be reduced by eating more fiber, drinking more fluid, and exercising
- Visible veins on the abdomen, breasts, legs
- Thin cloudy vaginal discharge. **Douching** (flushing out the vagina with liquid solutions) is not recommended during pregnancy.

Sexual desire and activity may undergo some changes during pregnancy. Sexual desire may increase or decrease. Many women find that their sexual interest decreases during the physical changes and discomforts of the first trimester. Fears about the baby may affect both parents' attitudes toward sexual activity. Most low-risk pregnancies do not require avoidance of any sexual practices. The health care practitioner will give advice on activities to avoid. Some cramping is normal for pregnant women during or after orgasm.

The pregnant woman's weight and size may not increase much during these first three months because the fetus is very small. Sometimes the pregnancy shape is visible earlier in the pregnancy, especially if the mother has a small build or less abdominal muscle tone. A larger abdomen may also occur with overeating, bloating, or the presence of more than one fetus.

Pregnancy: Second Trimester

In the second trimester, the nausea or vomiting of the first trimester may cease or decline. Breast engorgement may continue, but breast tenderness should decrease. The mother's appetite and energy may increase. Fetal movement should be felt during this part of the pregnancy. Sexual interest may increase in the second trimester because the woman feels better and increased blood flow to the genital area may improve sensation and enjoyment.

Gums may bleed during brushing and be sore due to pregnancy hormones. **Periodontitis** is an infection and inflammation of the bones that support the teeth. This disease is more likely during pregnancy. Periodontitis increases the risk of premature birth (Bobetsis, Barros, and Offenbacher 2006). These serious problems may be avoided with a dental exam and cleaning during pregnancy.

If dental work is needed during pregnancy, it may be best to wait until the second trimester. The safety of local anesthesia during pregnancy has not been proven (American Pregnancy Association 2007a). Using as little local anesthetic (such as novocaine) as possible may be advised. However, enough medication must be used to keep the client comfortable, because stress from pain can also be harmful in pregnancy. If possible, dental procedures requiring more sedation should be delayed until after the baby is born (American Pregnancy Association 2007a).

In the second trimester, other changes may include:

- ***Linea negra***, a dark line running from the navel to the pubic bone.
- Freckles or moles may become darker.
- **Mask of pregnancy** (also known as **chloasma** or **melasma**), a color change across the middle of the face. The "mask" is a patch of darker skin in light-skinned women and a lighter patch in dark-skinned women.
- Leg cramps (may be relieved by rest, stretching the legs, and drinking more fluids).
- Backaches (because of changing body shape and loosening of the pelvic joints in preparation for delivery).
- Sleep problems (because of the pregnancy discomforts).
- Clumsiness (because of swelling, looseness of the joints, and a shift in the body's center of gravity).

- Noticeably larger abdomen. Navel may stick out, and hips may widen.
- Abdominal soreness (from stretching of ligaments supporting the uterus).
- Swelling of legs and enlarged breasts.
- **Hemorrhoids,** swollen veins in the rectal area that may itch, burn, and bleed (may be caused by increased blood flow and pressure from enlarged uterus).

The changes in body image may be difficult to accept, but weight gain is necessary for a healthy pregnancy. However, too much weight gain can increase the risk of diabetes or high blood pressure. Women can work with health care professionals to achieve appropriate weight during pregnancy. Well-fitting maternity clothing and a supportive bra can reduce discomfort.

Pregnancy: Third Trimester

In the third trimester, many of the symptoms already discussed may continue, plus some new symptoms. Fetal movements may become milder than the earlier kicks, as there is less room in the uterus for active movement. The baby may squirm about now and may choose to lie in positions that can cause discomfort to the mother, exerting pressure within her body. The woman may have more frequent urges to urinate with increased pressure from the baby and less space for the bladder inside the abdomen. Urine may leak out under the pressure of heavy coughing or laughing. In the last trimester, the woman may be more uncomfortable and have less energy; interest in sex may decrease.

There may also be shortness of breath late in the pregnancy because of the mother's increased body size and crowding inside the abdomen from the growing baby. This breathlessness may decrease later when the baby drops lower in the pelvis in preparation for delivery. Swelling of the ankles, feet, or hands may be a problem in later pregnancy. Swelling may be reduced by drinking more fluids, moderate exercise, comfortable footwear, and elevating the feet and legs when possible. Take off rings and bracelets before swelling makes removal too difficult.

The mother may feel some brief and scattered **contractions**, called **Braxton Hicks contractions**, in which the uterus hardens for a few minutes and then returns to normal. These are considered normal in pregnancy. Near the end of the pregnancy, vaginal discharge may become heavier and may contain red or pink streaks or more mucus. Breasts may excrete a watery milk-like substance.

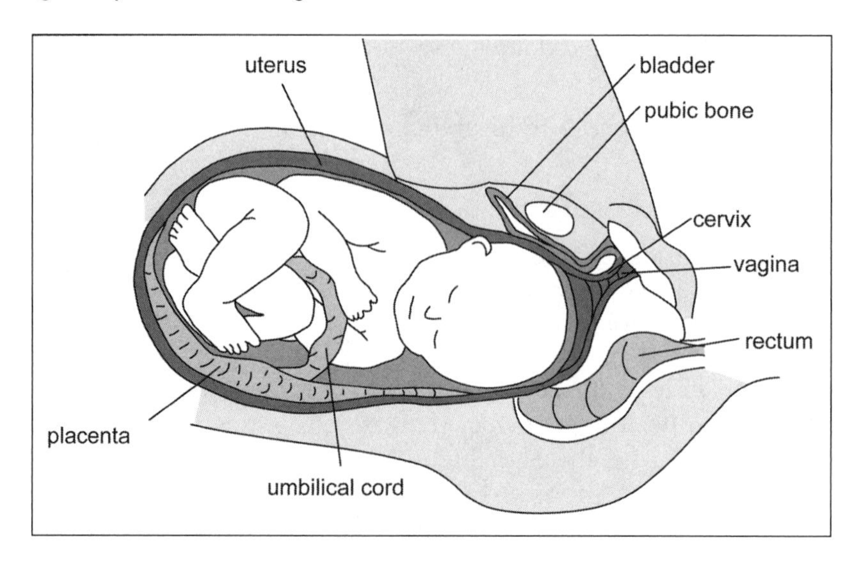

Full-term fetus. *(Sandy Windelspecht)*

By this time, a pregnant woman may be growing very weary of the various discomforts and inconveniences of pregnancy. She may also be very excited that the baby will be arriving soon or more apprehensive at the challenges that the delivery will bring.

Preparing for delivery includes discussing options and preferences with the health care team, readying a place for baby at home, or finishing details for adoption. The mother should pack a bag for the trip to the hospital and get together things the baby will need for the first days of life and the trip home. See the baby equipment section later in this chapter for more information.

Measures for a Healthy Pregnancy

Several measures that pregnant women should follow for a healthy pregnancy include getting more rest and taking time to relax. Be consistent with taking vitamins, keeping doctor visits, eating wisely, and using good hygiene. Exercise with caution but remain physically active. Check with the health care team about any medications, including over-the-counter medications. Many medications are not considered safe during pregnancy.

Reducing Risks in Pregnancy

Some foods to avoid during pregnancy may contain bacteria that can cause severe food poisoning. Other foods to avoid because they may contain bacteria, parasites, or other harmful substances include:

- Raw or rare red meat or poultry
- Raw or uncooked shellfish (oysters, shrimp, mussels, or crab)
- Raw sprouts
- Unpasteurized juices, milk, or cheese
- Raw eggs
- Meat pâtés, deli and processed meats (may contain *listeria* bacteria) (American Pregnancy Association 2010b)

Other foods to avoid may contain harmful substances:

- Swordfish, marlin, and shark (may contain unsafe levels of mercury)
- Liver products (may have unsafe levels of vitamin A)

Several activities must be restricted or avoided in pregnancy. Avoid breathing any toxins, especially paint, solvents, or ammonia. X-rays should be restricted in pregnancy; it is important to inform x-ray technicians of a patient's pregnancy or the possibility of pregnancy. Exposure to extreme heat should be minimized during pregnancy, and physicians may place restrictions on some occupations or activities. Exposure to pesticides should be avoided.

Alcohol must be avoided, as it may lead to a **fetal alcohol spectrum disorder** (FASD). An FASD can cause the baby to have abnormal facial features, low birth weight, intellectual deficits, learning problems, a small head, and problems with the heart, kidneys, or bones (American Pregnancy Association 2010a). According to the Centers for Disease Control and Prevention (2009), there is no safe amount of alcohol and no safe time to drink during pregnancy.

Smoking is also harmful to the baby, and secondhand smoke must also be avoided. Nicotine is shown to cause premature birth and low birth weight (American Pregnancy Association 2008). Many drugs and medications are unsafe in pregnancy, particularly illicit substances. A baby can be born addicted to drugs that the mother uses during pregnancy. Babies who are born addicted may go through dangerous and painful withdrawal symptoms. Use of some substances can also cause the baby to be born early and may result in the baby having a small head, organ difficulties, or brain damage (American Pregnancy Association 2008). For more information on the effects of alcohol, tobacco, and other drugs during pregnancy, see chapters 1, "Types of Substances," and 2, "Substance Use, Abuse, and Chemical Dependency," in volume 4.

Chemicals used in some hair treatments may be harmful to the fetus. Although some health care practitioners say that probably too little is absorbed to cause problems, it may be best to avoid straightening treatments, permanents, and hair colors. The products may not be safe, and hair may not turn out as expected because of pregnancy hormones (American Pregnancy Association 2007b). Skin breakouts may also increase with the hormonal changes of pregnancy. Skin treatments should be approved by the health care team. Accutane and Retin-A are not allowed during pregnancy, and other products may not have been tested for safety.

Tanning beds raise the body temperature and may not be safe during pregnancy. The UV rays can also reduce **folic acid** levels. Folic acid is a vitamin that promotes cell growth in the fetus (American Pregnancy Association 2007c). It is best to avoid belly piercing or any other body piercings during pregnancy. However, if there is already a piercing present, the ring or band may be worn unless the tightness of the expanding pregnant abdomen makes it uncomfortable. Tattoos are to be avoided in pregnancy because of the risk of infection.

Extreme noise should be avoided in pregnancy. Some studies have shown that long-term high levels of noise can increase the risk of hearing loss for the baby. High levels of sound may also lead to early delivery and low birth weight. Research in this area is not yet conclusive; therefore, people should use caution until the effects of noise are better understood. People working in places with high levels of noise may need to work in quieter areas during pregnancy. Excessive noise in everyday life can also be avoided; for example, the radio volume in the car can be reduced, and concert seats should be away from the loudest areas of the auditorium.

It is pointless for a pregnant woman to worry about risks that occurred before she knew she was pregnant. These guidelines are recommended to reduce risks. The baby might not show any ill effects from things the mother did before she knew she was pregnant. Once the woman knows she is pregnant, she may then begin to observe all the safe practices of pregnancy and reduce any further risk to her baby.

Preparing for Birth

Another group of risk factors to consider during pregnancy are those that can lead to **sudden infant death syndrome (SIDS)**. SIDS is the sudden death of an infant under one year of age that cannot be explained by any investigation or autopsy tests. This tragic event is devastating to a family. Most commonly, SIDS is discovered by a parent or caregiver who checks on an infant thought to be sleeping and finds that the baby is dead. The rate of SIDS has fallen remarkably since 1980, secondary to measures taken to reduce risks to infants. Early regular medical care and good nutrition can reduce the risk of premature delivery, which is a major risk factor in SIDS. The use of cocaine, heroin, or cigarettes during pregnancy increases the risk for SIDS. The highest rates of SIDS occur in infants of teen mothers, and this risk increases even more when teens have more than one pregnancy. The rate of SIDS also increases the less time that passes between pregnancies. Therefore, waiting at least one year between pregnancies can lower the risk for SIDS (American SIDS Institute 2010). Further information about infant care measures that can reduce the risk of SIDS can be found in the parenting portion of this chapter.

As pregnancy progresses, many mothers have desires or urges to prepare for the arrival of the baby. They may be involved in preparing their home for the baby: getting supplies and "feathering the nest." Mothers may prepare by learning about caring for the baby and adjusting to changes in the family. Parents and caregivers can take classes in child care, first aid, and childhood emergencies. They can learn cardiopulmonary resuscitation (CPR) for infants and children. Classes in infant feeding, breastfeeding, baby hygiene and diapering, and childhood safety may be available for free at hospitals. Parents feel more prepared by taking classes before the baby's birth. There are also classes for siblings that include older children in the care of the new baby. Information about local CPR and child first aid classes can be found at the American Heart Association and American Red Cross websites, listed in the resources section at the end of this chapter. A video about how to help a choking child can be seen at Learn CPR, listed in the resources section at the end of this chapter.

Classes about childbirth, called Lamaze classes, are very helpful for expectant mothers and fathers. The classes teach methods to stay calm and deal well with labor and train fathers or other coaches to help the mother through the delivery. Breathing exercises and methods to tolerate pain are very helpful to getting through childbirth.

The Pregnancy and Childbirth Health Care Team

Many people work together with pregnant women and their families to support a healthy pregnancy, labor, and delivery. Some of these people include:

- *Obstetrician:* Physician who treats pregnant women and delivers babies
- *Midwife or doula:* Person with training to deliver babies and offer support and advice to pregnant women

- *Anesthesiologist:* Physician who administers and oversees anesthesia
- *Pediatrician:* Physician who assesses and treats babies and children
- *Geneticist:* Specialist in genetic diseases and conditions
- *Nurse practitioner or nurse anesthetist:* Nurses who provide obstetric, pediatric, or anesthesia care
- *Labor and delivery nurses:* Nurses who assess and treat women in childbirth
- *Postpartum nurses:* Nurses who care for mothers and babies after delivery
- *Lactation consultant:* Professionals who teach and support mothers in nursing and feeding concerns
- *Social workers:* Professionals who assist with obtaining resources for mother and baby care and advise in coping and problem solving for the family

Labor and Childbirth

There are several signs that indicate that the baby will soon be born. One early sign may be the passing of the **mucous plug**, a clear jellylike substance that has plugged the cervix during the pregnancy. This plug may be ejected during the beginnings of **dilatation** (opening of the cervix). A pink- or brown-tinged mucous discharge may also be seen in the last days before birth. **Water breaking** refers to the rupture (tearing) of the amniotic sac and the release of amniotic fluid. This may occur without warning and is a sign that labor will probably begin soon. The fluid may come forth in a gush or may leak slowly from the vagina. If the fluid is not clear or if it has a greenish tint, the health care practitioner must be notified right away. This may signal that the baby has experienced distress and had a bowel movement in the uterus. Occasionally labor may begin without the water breaking, and the membranes are sometimes ruptured by health care personnel at the hospital.

Deliveries can go smoothly and both the baby and the mother can be safe even when women do not have assistance from hospital care or health care professionals. In some cultures and in years past, many babies were born with no one to assist the mother. The majority of births occur without complications. In these cases, the baby could have been born at home without difficulties. Most mothers want to be at a hospital or birthing center; they want to be sure that any care that may be needed will be available. When circumstances do not allow for a hospital delivery, things are likely to still go well.

TABLE 3.4.1 **DELIVERING YOUR BABY ALONE**

- Call 9-1-1, unlock your door, and if at all possible find someone to help.
- Try not to push; pant to distract yourself.
- Wash the vaginal area and your hands.
- Lie on a bed or floor (on newspapers or sheets).
- If the baby starts to come out, push each time you feel an urge. This will gradually ease the baby out.
- When it is visible, support the baby's head so that the baby does not suddenly pop out.
- Let the baby come out slowly; don't pull on the head.
- If you see the umbilical cord around the baby's neck, slip it over the baby's head.
- Use both hands to gently hold the head and press it down. Use your abdominal muscles to push out the baby's body. First, one shoulder will come out. Carefully lift the head up and watch for the other shoulder. The rest of the body will follow easily.
- Lift baby to your chest (but do not tug on umbilical cord).
- Wipe baby's nose and mouth.
- If baby isn't breathing or crying, rub baby's back and keep the head lower than the body. If the baby is still not breathing, clear out the mouth with a finger and give two very gentle puffs into mouth.
- Don't pull the placenta out. If it comes out, wrap it up. Hold it above the level of the baby if possible. Do not cut the umbilical cord (wait for help to arrive).
- You and the baby should be seen by health care practitioners (an emergency room or your doctor) right away.

Source: Murkoff and Mazel (2008).

Early Labor

Sometimes women believe that they are in labor but are not. This may be called **false labor.** Braxton Hicks contractions that are a preparation for labor may be mistaken for real labor. Many women have gone to the hospital believing that they are about to deliver the baby, only to learn that it is false labor. Timing contractions to see if they get stronger and closer together is one method to check for true labor. Braxton Hicks contractions often go away if the mother lies down and rests. Real labor pains continue regardless of rest or activity (Women's Health Information 2010).

The doctor or midwife can be called when the mother is having contractions, when the water breaks, or for any symptoms that are of concern. Contractions are a tightening of the muscles in the uterus that act to push the baby out. Contractions are said to feel like menstrual cramps that get stronger over time. During early labor the contractions push the baby against the cervix, and the cervix begins to dilate (the opening expands). The cervix also goes through **effacement** (thins out). Early in labor the mother may have pain in her back as well as cramping and may feel pressure in her abdomen. During this phase the mother should rest and get comfortable. She may want to take a warm shower. Contractions should be timed for how long they last and how much time passes between them. Early labor may last for many hours or for more than a day.

The mother's condition will be assessed when she arrives at the hospital, and a fetal monitor may be applied to the abdomen to check the baby's heartbeat. The vaginal area and the cervix will be examined fairly often by several different members of the health care team to monitor the progress of labor. When labor is progressing very slowly, medicines may be given to cause stronger contractions that will speed up the labor. If the water did not break yet, the health care team may rupture the membranes to release the amniotic fluid.

An exam will be done to check the position of the baby in the uterus. The preferred position for vaginal delivery is with the baby's head down, facing the mother's spine and in the lower part of the pelvis. Sometimes babies are lying sideways (**transverse**) or feet first (**breech**) in the uterus. The health care practitioner may attempt to turn the baby from outside the uterus. If the baby remains in a position that cannot be delivered vaginally, a surgical delivery known as a **C-section** (Cesarean section) may be done.

Several measures may be helpful to ease the discomforts of labor:

- Breathing and relaxation techniques (distract from pains)
- Massage, soothing music
- Applying ice or heat
- Taking a warm bath or shower
- Changing positions
- Taking a brief walk
- Having someone trusted and supportive nearby

Hydrotherapy (therapeutic use of water) is used when a woman goes through labor in a tub of warm water. Hydrotherapy may help women feel physically supported, warm, and relaxed and may make it easier to move and find comfortable positions. However, there are concerns about safety and the risk of complications of delivering a baby in water, also known as **waterbirthing** (Women's Health Information 2010).

Pain relief may be used during childbirth. The health of the baby must also be considered in choosing medications. Table 3.4.2 explains the

TABLE 3.4.2 **TYPES OF PAIN RELIEF FOR CHILDBIRTH**

Benefits	Disadvantages/Side Effects
Opioids (Narcotic Pain Medications)	
• Can make pain bearable; doesn't affect ability to push • Can still get epidural/spinal block after opioids	• Short-acting; doesn't get rid of all the pain • Drowsiness, nausea, vomiting, itchiness • May slow baby's breathing and heart rate if given right before delivery
Epidural and Spinal Block	
• Allows most women to be alert with very little pain during labor and childbirth • Pain relief starts 10–20 minutes after medicine is given • Degree of numbness adjustable throughout labor • With spinal block, pain relief starts right away and lasts 1–2 hours	• Woman can move but might not be able to walk • If blood pressure drops, baby's heartbeat may slow • Backache for a few days after labor • Epidurals can prolong first and second stages of labor. If given late in labor or too much medicine is used, pushing may be difficult. • Increased risk of assisted vaginal delivery
Pudendal Block	
• Only used late in labor, usually right before baby's head emerges • Provides some pain relief while allowing woman to remain alert and able to push	• Baby is not affected; has very few disadvantages

Source: Adapted from Women's Health Information (2010).

different options for pain relief and anesthesia, medications that eliminate sensitivity to pain.

Active Labor

Active labor begins when the cervix is fully dilated and effacement is complete. The cervix usually expands to 10 centimeters (approximately 4 inches). Contractions become much more intense and are about 3–4 minutes apart. This stage of labor may last 30 minutes to 2 hours. The mother will use pelvic muscles to push the baby out during contractions. Breathing techniques may be used to keep the mother calm and to improve her ability to focus on pushing the baby through the birth canal. **Crowning** is when the top of the baby's head is visible. At this point, the mother will be told to push the baby out of the vagina. The doctor may need to make a small cut (**episiotomy**) to enlarge the vaginal opening. This prevents tearing of the tissues in the vaginal area as the baby's head is passed. Many women do not need an episiotomy.

Childbirth

As the baby emerges from the vagina, members of the health care team will ease the baby out of the mother's body. They will assess the baby and ensure that the baby begins to breathe. The placenta will later be expelled from the body in this final stage of labor, and the umbilical cord will be cut. Any episiotomy or vaginal tears will be repaired with stitches. The health care team will continue to monitor the mother for uterine contractions that will shrink the uterus and decrease bleeding from the detachment of the placenta. This process may be aided by massaging the lower abdomen and by breastfeeding.

A C-section is sometimes used to deliver babies. C-sections are done when babies go into distress and must be delivered quickly or when the mother's health will be endangered by a difficult labor. C-sections may be done when there are problems with vaginal delivery or when the mother is having two or more babies. An epidural anesthesia may be used for a C-section so that the surgery is not felt but the mother may remain awake. A **catheter** (tube) will be placed into the bladder to drain urine. The doctor will make an **incision** (cut) through the skin, fat, and muscle of the abdomen. A second incision will then be made to open up the uterus. One doctor will support the baby while another pushes on the abdomen to turn the baby so that the baby can be lifted out of the abdomen. Once the baby is delivered, the umbilical cord is cut and the placenta is removed. The doctor then stitches up the opening in the uterus and closes up the incision in the abdomen. Mothers who have a C-section will be watched for a few hours as they recover from surgery. This procedure is a major surgery, and full recovery will take about six weeks. The mother will need to focus on healing and getting used to her new baby during these weeks.

Postpartum

Postpartum is the period immediately after childbirth. The assessment of the baby and the recovery of the mother are the first issues during the postpartum period. During this time the parents begin to learn about taking care of their baby and begin to get acquainted with their child.

During the postpartum period, sanitary pads will be needed for the bloody discharge that may continue for several weeks. There may be abdominal cramps as the uterus contracts down to its smaller size. Hemorrhoids, constipation, and pain from stitches near the vagina may be a problem. A C-section incision may be tender or painful, making movement difficult. Women who have had a C-section may also notice sharp pains in the shoulder area (related to small amounts of blood that have irritated the diaphragm, sending pain signals to the shoulder area).

Mothers may be very tired after the experience of giving birth. They may also be anxious about the care of their new baby. If the baby is having any difficulties, the new mother can be expected to be preoccupied or worried. Some new mothers may feel down about impending changes or about the end of pregnancy. It is normal to swing between these emotions and elation about their new child. Women can have the **baby blues,** or brief feelings of sadness, fear, or irritability. In some cases, mothers have **postpartum depression.** Postpartum depression can impair the mother's overall functioning and requires prompt treatment.

While still at the hospital, the mother may be taught how to care for the **umbilicus** (belly button) of her baby. Clean water on a cotton ball can be used to clean around the stump of the umbilical cord. This stump will be attached to the baby for about two weeks, at which point it will fall off by itself. This area should be cleaned with each diaper change. The stump needs air, so diapers should be folded down below the navel area.

Some male babies will be circumcised in the first days of life. **Circumcision** is the removal of the **foreskin**—skin around the head of the penis. After circumcision, the penis is kept wrapped in gauze with an ointment to prevent sticking and rubbing against the diaper. The penis is cleaned and the gauze reapplied with each diaper change. This treatment should continue until the area has completely healed. Parents should look into the risks and benefits of circumcision before deciding if their son should

? Did You Know?

Postpartum depression is not the same thing as the baby blues. Women with baby blues may have mood swings, sadness, anxiety, irritability, or trouble sleeping. Symptoms may last a few days to a few weeks. Postpartum depression is more intense and may last up to several months. Symptoms may include problems with appetite, fatigue, insomnia, decreased sexual interest, withdrawal from others, and lack of joy in life. There may be feelings of inadequacy and guilt, thoughts of self-harm, or difficulty bonding with the baby. Symptoms may interfere with the ability to cope with daily pressures and to take care of oneself and the baby.

Postpartum depression may be caused by physical and hormonal changes in the mother's body, emotional changes and challenges, and lifestyle changes. The risk for postpartum depression is higher in mothers with a history of depression, in unstable relationships, during financial difficulties, or when there are other stressors. Treatment may include antidepressant medication, counseling, or hormone therapy.

Postpartum psychosis is a rare condition that may develop within the first weeks after delivery. **Hallucinations**, **delusions**, confusion, and thoughts and attempts to hurt oneself and the baby may be seen. Most mothers are alarmed to see these symptoms and take steps to get treatment and protect themselves and the baby. This condition rarely ends in harm to the baby, but the condition requires immediate medical attention.

Source: Mayo Clinic (2010).

have the procedure. In the Jewish tradition, circumcision is performed in a religious ceremony eight days after birth. The procedure is done by a **mohel** (or **moyle**), a person trained to safely perform this procedure. Circumcision is also discussed in chapter 1 of this volume.

Bonding is the process of forming an emotional attachment with the baby. The bonding process is very important for the baby's development and sense of security and safety. Love and feelings for the baby motivate parents to place the baby's welfare as a priority and to make sacrifices for the baby. It is just as normal for some parents to feel an instant connection with the baby as it is for others to gradually develop this bond. Parents who take longer with this process need not feel guilty or inadequate. For many parents, the ongoing tasks of caring for the baby strengthens the bond. The development of the baby brings more and more reasons to be attracted to loving the baby (Hirsch 2008).

Babies respond to touch, voices, facial expressions, and warmth. Showing affection for the baby comes naturally to some parents. Other parents may not be used to physical affection, or they may fear making mistakes with the baby. Babies respond well to many forms of positive attention. Parents often learn what their baby likes and dislikes. Caregiving tasks offer many chances at interactions. Bathing, feeding, dressing the baby, and preparing for sleep can all be times to bond or show affection to the baby (Hirsch 2008).

Infant Nutrition

Breastfeeding

Research has shown breastfeeding to be the best nutrition available for babies. After delivery, milk ducts in the mother's breasts produce a substance called **colostrum**, a thick yellow- or gold-colored liquid that contains nutrients and fluids for the baby. As the baby continues to nurse, the ducts produce milk. This milk contains all the nutrition the baby needs for the first months of life. The breasts will continue to produce milk in a supply equal to the amount of milk the baby consumes.

The baby and the mother will need time and some trial and error to get used to breastfeeding. Some babies must be stimulated to wake up and nurse. The baby may also have difficulty sucking and may be frustrated at the small amount of liquid that is available at first. The mother may have trouble positioning the baby at the breast and may have problems relaxing into this new experience. She may be anxious about the responsibility of providing nutrition for the baby. The mother may also have problems with nipple soreness, which can be reduced by making sure the baby's mouth covers more than just the tip of the nipple. With patience and some endurance, the baby and mother are usually able to master the tasks of breastfeeding within a few days. Some new mothers consult a **lactation consultant.** These professionals can help teach and support mothers in nursing and feeding concerns. La Leche League, listed in the resources section at the end of this chapter, offers support and information for mothers who want to breastfeed.

Fever and painful lumps or redness in the breast are signs of infection. If this occurs, the woman should seek a doctor's advice. Feeding the baby often to express the milk can help if the breasts become **engorged** (overfull). The discomfort can be treated by applying warm compresses or ice packs. Nipple dryness or cracking may be relieved by rubbing the nipple with breast milk or with a natural moisturizer, such as lanolin. Nursing

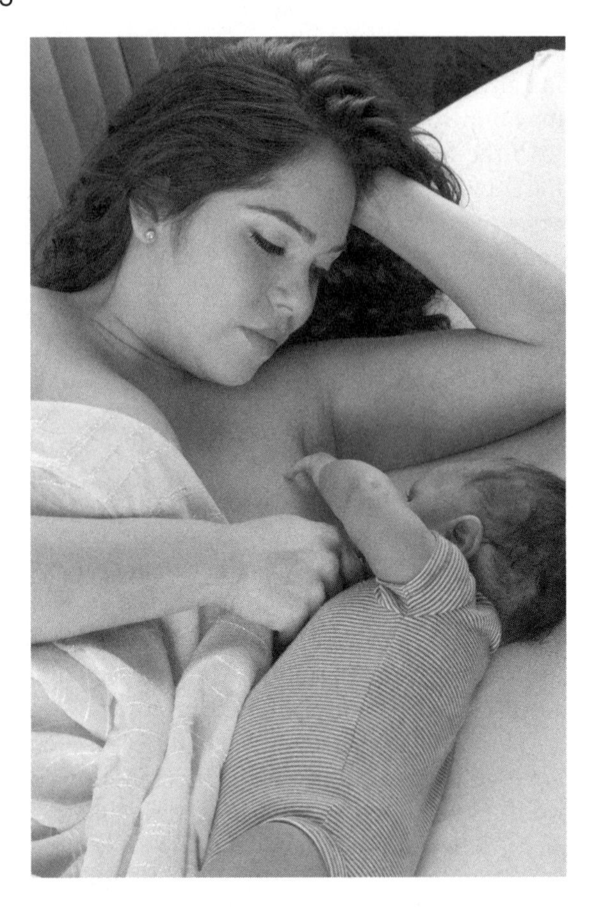

A mother breastfeeding her baby. *(Shutterstock.com)*

mothers need to eat a well-balanced and nutritious diet and stay well hydrated by drinking plenty of fluids.

Some medications must be avoided by nursing mothers, and caffeine and alcohol are usually restricted to small amounts. Many medicines, including over-the-counter (nonprescription) preparations, may pass into the breast milk. A pharmacist can explain which medications may be harmful to the baby. Some foods that the mother eats may produce gastric distress in the baby. Other types of food may be risky because of contaminants, such as fish containing mercury. The health care practitioner or a lactation consultant should be able to give advice about what foods to avoid.

Breastfeeding mothers should ensure that the hospital staff knows not to give the baby any supplemental feedings and to bring the baby for nursing whenever hungry. Babies nurse first from one breast and may need to be patted so they will burp. **Burping** releases any swallowed air and clears more room for food in the stomach. Then the baby is switched to the other breast and is burped again when finished eating. At the beginning of life, babies should be fed 8–12 times a day. This will require the mother to sit with her baby often and is a good opportunity for the mother to get the rest she may need and bond with the baby.

As they grow, babies will take in other foods. They will start with baby cereal and progress on to pureed vegetables, fruits, and meats. The child will move on to more solid foods later. The baby will need less breast milk as this process moves forward, but the milk will continue to be produced to meet the demands of the baby. Many pediatricians recommend that babies continue with some breastfeeding for at least 12 months (Women's Health Information 2011).

There are many advantages of breastfeeding:

- Breast milk is most easily digested (it has no preservatives or additives).
- Breast milk contains antibodies (can protect the baby from infections and allergies).
- Breast milk is free, readily available, and does not require bottles, refrigeration, or heating.
- Breastfed infants are less likely to be victims of SIDS (American SIDS Institute 2010).

When mothers will not be present to breastfeed the baby, milk can be pumped by a hand pump or a gentle electric pump designed for the purpose. This milk can be refrigerated or frozen and later thawed out and given to the baby in a bottle. Even when the milk will not be given to the baby, the mother will want to pump to continue to stimulate the milk supply that her baby will need. Some families decide to give some formula feedings and some breast milk feedings, depending on the needs of the baby and the mother. Breastfeeding also benefits the mother by stimulating the uterus to contract more quickly to prepregnancy size. Some studies have found that maternal weight loss is enhanced by breastfeeding (Women's Health Information 2011). Breastfeeding may reduce a woman's risk of breast cancer and can offset the increased risk of cancer brought on by having a first baby after age 25 (Laino 2007).

Formula Feeding

Some mothers give babies formula feedings. This decision should be carefully weighed while considering the needs of the infant. If the mother will be overwhelmed by the task of nursing, the resultant stress may be a hardship to the mother and the baby. In this case, the decision to use formula may be good for family welfare. Sometimes the mother does not have enough milk for the baby's needs. Some babies do not have a lactating mother available. Whenever formula is used, the health care team will decide what type and amount of formula is best for the child. Cost and convenience of the products can vary. Powder formulas must be mixed with water, and proper storage of formula is important. The WIC program (listed in the resources section at the end of this chapter) is available to help with nutrition and health care for women, infants, and children.

Parenting

Being a parent can be a very difficult and very rewarding task. Children bring many changes in the lifestyle and responsibilities of parents. For teen parents, the presence of the child makes life very different than the life of their peers. Child care requires many sacrifices. It is wonderful to see a child grow and do well; this can be the reward of all the hard work of parenting.

Some new mothers and fathers may not have experience with children. Others may have younger siblings or babysitting experience, leaving them with knowledge about basic child care. In some families and in some cultures, there are different beliefs or attitudes about each parent's role in baby care.

Some girls may grow up dreaming of being a mother. They may play with dolls, imagining how fun it would be to have their own baby. Some girls look forward to lives where they have their own children while also pursuing a career. Other girls may grow up planning a different life, one in which they do not have children and focus only on career, school, or other pursuits. These expectations may be influenced by the way the woman's own family was structured. Many cultures place the mother at the center of responsibility for child care and household tasks. When a woman also has work or school, her time and energy can be overtaxed.

Many men model themselves after their own fathers. This is especially true when the son has admired the father or seen him as a positive influence. However, when fathers have not been present or have been negligent or difficult, the son may use his father as a model of what he does not want to do as a parent. As a result, a new father may emphasize with his child those things he wished for in his own childhood. If a father had few belongings as a child, he may want to give his own child lots of clothes, toys, or other advantages. If the father was teased in boyhood, he may push for toughness in his children to protect them from ridicule. If his parents were excessively strict, a father may risk not being strict enough as a parent himself.

Men who grew up without a father in their life may want to be more available for their own child. However, it may be difficult for them to know how to be present because they grew up without seeing what a good father does. They may vow to be responsible in ways their own fathers were not. Seeking education and advice about how to keep this vow can be helpful. These men can decide to support their children and their children's mothers in ways their own fathers did not. They may do so by providing financial support, helping with household chores, giving emotional support, and being physically present in good times and bad.

A supportive father learns about child care and participates in taking care of his child. Reading about basic child care, practicing with an experienced caregiver, and increasing his confidence can improve the father's skill at taking part in his baby's life. Both parents becoming familiar with safety aspects of the child's care can increase their confidence that they can keep the baby safe. Each parent can improve their relationship with the baby and their sense of competence by spending time alone with the baby. The other parent can then pursue leisure activities. After parents have spent some time on themselves, they may be better able to meet the baby's needs.

Parents may enjoy passing on knowledge or bringing a new experience to their son or daughter. Parents will each have their own strengths and may enjoy applying their skills to enhance their child's life. For example, an athletic mother may be the better parent to practice sports with a child, while a patient father may do best with homework help. Firmer parents may be better at enforcing rules, and insightful parents may be best equipped to understand children's feelings. Listening, flexibility, and the ability to compromise will be helpful when parents disagree about a decision concerning their children.

Discipline

Examples from childhood are hard to resist, because in moments of stress people tend to fall back on familiar responses. For example, parents will remember how they were disciplined as children. Parents who promised themselves never to call a child "stupid" (as their parent called them) may be horrified to find those words slip out when they are faced with a crisis. They may resort to old messages as they frantically search for a way to get through to their child. Avoiding getting into such a desperate state can help parents maintain their resolve against making certain mistakes and allow them to deal more calmly with their children.

Discipline is a way to teach children how to interact with others and with their world. **Punishment**, on the other hand, involves imposing a penalty for a fault or an offense. Decisions about discipline may be based on what a person learned in the past. There are many good approaches to teaching children about right and wrong and about preferred behaviors. Consistency may be the most important aspect of child discipline. This consistency must be seen within each parent and between both parents to have the best results. Taking a stand about consequences for problem behaviors and following through on these decisions can be very effective in disciplining children.

Shaping the behavior of young children involves praising preferred behaviors and avoiding or preventing others, through removing harmful objects and temptations. Many child care experts agree that children of any age should not be hit. Spanking is discouraged by the American Academy of Pediatrics. Spanking can teach children that it is okay to hit others in anger. Spanking can also physically harm the child, gives attention for unwanted behaviors, and make the child afraid of the parent (Pendley 2008). It is very important to never shake a baby, even in play. Shaking can result in bleeding in the brain and death.

Older children should be told what behaviors are wrong and what will happen if the behaviors occur again. Consequences for behaviors should suit the situation whenever possible. The consequence of making a mess can be cleaning it up. The consequences of following through on a household responsibility can be more privileges because the child has proved that he or she can be responsible. Parents can communicate with children about lessons to be learned and may express love and affection as they are imposing the consequences designed to teach the child.

Coparenting and Family Relationships

Coparenting, or shared parenting, involves both parents working together to raise their child, even when the parents are not living together. When the parents do not get along, it can be difficult to communicate about the child. One parent may speak against the other or act in resentful ways about the involvement each parent has. Because the child is a part of both parents, degrading the child's other parent is disrespectful to the child. Focusing negatively on the other parent only makes the coparenting relationship more difficult and less effective.

Parents who are not in a couple relationship will deal with challenges depending on their relationship and the ages and characteristics of their children. When the mother and father can behave as friends, parenting can go well. Infants benefit from time for bonding with each parent.

As toddlers develop separation issues, they may feel more secure with routines involving both parents. Young children may believe that they are the reason for problems in the family. Reassuring contact with both parents can be helpful at this age. Typical child developmental needs should be considered when making coparenting arrangements and custody plans.

When parents work as a team and communicate fully about the children and their activities, the entire family can benefit. Lack of communication between parents can create an opportunity for children to play one parent against the other and create problems. Being able to agree about decisions concerning children is important for coparenting. When both parents accept plans for their child, they can work more smoothly together.

There may be complications for a couple or for coparents if extended families or in-laws do not get along. Parents usually know their children better than anyone else does. Parents also have the most responsibility for raising the children. For these reasons, parents must balance their insight about their families and their respect for extended family members. Teen parents may benefit from advice from more experienced parents. The teen parents may decide not to use this advice, but they can appreciate input. It is important to remain firm on what is best for the children or the family, even when others challenge the decision. Different types of families and parenting arrangements are discussed further in chapter 1, "Environment and Mental Health," in volume 5.

Childhood Health Care

Pediatric (child) health care requires following a schedule of office or clinic visits for well-baby checks to monitor the baby's progress. Additional medical evaluations for illnesses, skin problems, or eating difficulties may occur. Pediatric health practitioners are good sources for answering questions about the child's development, growth, and health status. Children will receive vaccinations on a prescribed schedule (for more information, see chapter 3, "Prevention," in volume 1). The health care practitioner should be promptly contacted if the baby has prolonged diarrhea or vomiting or a fever over 102.2 degrees Fahrenheit. A trip to the emergency room may be advisable in these cases.

Arranging for Health Care for Infants

The choice of a pediatrician for the new baby may be addressed during the pregnancy. Knowing which doctor will be caring for the baby is helpful for planning and advice. Some births with special needs and C-sections require the pediatrician to be present at delivery. The pediatric practitioner usually sees babies one to two weeks after birth to answer questions, check growth rate, and monitor healing of the umbilical cord and circumcision, if applicable.

Childhood Emergencies

In children of any age, difficulty breathing, severe injury, severe pain, serious bleeding, or choking must be evaluated right away. A large cut in the abdomen, chest, or head also requires immediate care. Emergency care is needed for children who lose consciousness (pass out) and for those who have head injuries or seizures. A child with a sudden stiff neck and a fever, rash, and headache may have meningitis and must be seen by a doctor immediately. Emergency evaluations are needed when a child has an electric shock, nearly drowns, is burned, or breathes in smoke. A child who has a bicycle or car accident, a hard fall, or a sports injury should get emergency care, even if the child seems fine after the incident. An ambulance may be needed to get a child to the emergency room. If someone is driving the child to the hospital, it is best to have another person along to tend to the child.

TABLE 3.4.3 **HOW TO HELP A CHILD WHO IS CHOKING**

- Be sure the child cannot speak (a sign that the airway is blocked).
- Stay calm. Have someone call 9-1-1 while you help the child.
- Stand behind the standing child and wrap your arms around the waist.
- Make a fist with your right hand and place the thumb side against the child's abdomen; cover this fist with your left hand.
- Press into the child's abdomen with a quick upward thrust.
- Repeat these thrusts until the object pops out. The child should still be seen by a medical professional.
- If the child passes out, continue efforts to dislodge.
- If pulse or breathing stop, begin CPR.

Source: Yale School of Medicine (2011).

Baby Care

In the first months of life, people must be very careful to wash their hands before contact with the baby. People who are ill should not handle babies. This precaution reduces the risk of spreading cold germs or other infections to babies. Items that may contact the baby's mouth should be washed often. Baby bottles and other feeding supplies require special cleaning processes.

Use hygiene supplies that are designed for infants to care for babies. These products will be free of fragrances and alcohol. Babies' skin is fragile and needs very gentle cleansing. A baby's dry skin also needs protection from harsher products. Because babies' eyes may come into contact with the soap much more often than in adult use, soaps need to be non-stinging or no-tears. Baby clothes and linens should be washed in special detergent to avoid skin irritation.

Bathing

Young babies should be bathed in a small tub or the kitchen sink after the sink is cleaned and all traces of cleanser removed.

- Wash baby with mild baby soap and warm water.
- Use two washcloths, one for the face and another for the body.
- Apply soap to skin, work from the neck down, and save the crotch area for last.
- Rinse soap off.
- Wash hair or the head. Lean head back and pour water over to rinse.
- Support baby's head at all times during the bath to reduce the chance of the head going underwater. Babies can easily breathe water into the lungs or drown in the bath; careful supervision is needed.
- Dry baby thoroughly, diaper, dress, and wrap baby in a blanket.

Baby Clothing

Diapers may be disposable or cloth. The disposable diaper is better at holding fluids away from baby's skin, is less likely to leak, and is more convenient. Cloth diapers do not present the environmental problems of disposable diapers and are less expensive, even with the cost of laundering them. Diaper rashes may occur with both types and may require creams to heal. Diaper barrier ointments may be used to heal or protect the skin. Barrier ointments are more necessary when diarrhea irritates the skin. Talcum powder is usually not recommended for babies, as it may cake up in the genital area. Also, powders can place talc in the air that can be harmful for baby to breathe. Cornstarch (talc-free) powders are available but may also clog in the genital areas (Heller 2010).

While fashionable clothes for baby are often cute and seem irresistible, babies' clothing needs are actually simple. Wardrobes should include t-shirts or one-piece garments, outer knit pants or jeans, socks, nightgowns or footed sleepers, a light jacket or sweater, and knit caps. In colder weather, the baby will need a heavier blanket and a heavier jacket. It is important to choose clothes that are comfortable, safe, appropriate for the weather and climate, and easily cleaned.

Babies do well going without shoes until they begin walking. Socks may be worn for warmth. Shoes must be well fitted and offer proper support for young walkers. Soles should be flexible and soft. The arch of the foot does not form until children are two years old; for this reason, shoes for children under age two should not provide arch support. Shoes should fit well, with about a half inch from the child's toe to the end of the shoe's toe. Open-toed shoes may cause young walkers to trip and are better used when a child is very steady on his or her feet.

By law, nighttime wear must be made of fire-retardant fabrics. When children are unattended in their rooms at night with space heaters or open flames nearby, their clothes are more likely to catch fire. Girls in flowing nightgowns are more at risk. Laws requiring fire-retardant nightwear fabrics and safe household heating have greatly reduced the number of children admitted to hospitals for burns from nightclothes catching fire. The rate of admission is 75 percent less than before these laws were passed in 1972 (Harborview Injury Prevention and Research Center 2010). However, some parents worry that the chemicals used to create fire-resistant sleepwear may be harmful to their children. Nightclothes that do not have the treatment must be sold with the advice to be worn snug, to avoid flowing clothes catching fire. Many children fall asleep in street clothes or use t-shirts for pajamas. Parents must carefully weigh the safety issues of sleepwear.

Child Safety

There are many threats to safety in the child's environment. A list of emergency numbers should be posted in a central place. This list can include how to reach family members, doctors, pharmacies, hospitals, emergency services, and the poison control center. First aid manuals and reminders about how to do child and infant CPR should also be easily accessible. Parents should be trained in how to do rescue breathing and cardiac compressions for CPR and in how to handle a choking emergency.

Household Safety

As babies become more mobile, safety hazards increase. Baby-proofing the living space is an important task. Childproof locks, covers, and other equipment to help make a home safe for children can be purchased in baby stores or discount stores. All toys must be approved for the child's age. Small parts of toys or small household items must be kept out of babies' reach to prevent choking. Parents should also be aware of all the hazards that may harm the children when away from their own home.

Safety with Furniture and Household Items

- Secure heavy furniture and bookshelves to the wall (prevents children pulling over onto themselves).
- Pad sharp edges of tables and furniture (prevents injury if toddler falls against them).
- Remove glass-topped furniture and other breakable items from child areas.
- Secure rugs with nonskid pads.
- Keep recliners in closed position (prevents children from being trapped in workings).
- Store guns outside of the home. If not possible, unload guns and securely lock away, out of children's sight. Store ammunition separately.
- Install smoke detectors and carbon monoxide (CO) detectors with fully charged batteries throughout the home.
- Remove tablecloths (could be pulled down and bring objects down on baby).
- Remove houseplants or flowers that are poisonous. Wild mushrooms, azaleas, daffodils, mistletoe, morning glories, irises, lily of the valley, philodendron, and oleander are poisonous to humans (National Capital Poison Center 2010).
- Do not allow smoking inside a home or car with a child. Smoking is harmful while holding an infant, even outdoors. Research indicates that smoking parents may increase the chances of their children later becoming smokers (Chassin et al. 2008).

Electrical Safety

Electricity can be very dangerous for children. Outlets and appliances are tempting when located at the child's level of vision and within reach. Outlet covers or outlet plate covers can protect the baby from electric shock. Other safety measures include the following:

- Keep irons or other small appliances out of reach of children.
- Tie and secure long electrical cords to walls.
- Ground large appliances, and place televisions, computers, or sound equipment against walls to prevent access to cords.
- Radiators, floor-level heaters, and fireplaces should have childproof screens or covers. Space heaters are dangerous; try to use other types of heaters. If space heaters must be used, place them at least three feet from any items that may pose a fire hazard. (Mondozzi 2009)

Doors and Hazardous Items

- Secure areas that are not safe with childproof doorknob covers.
- Secure exterior or exit doors with a latch out of child's reach.
- Interior locks can become locked, or children can lock themselves in rooms and not be able to open the door. Remove or disable locks, especially in bathrooms.
- Secure windows that are at child level with childproof locks to prevent children from opening windows and falling out.
- Check rails on stairs and balconies for narrow spacing (prevents children's bodies from slipping through). Slats must be close enough to prevent a child getting her or his head stuck between slats. Rails must be stable enough to not give way when leaned or pushed upon.
- Use security gates to block stairs or areas where children may be harmed.
- Keep exercise equipment out of children's reach, especially treadmills or home exercise systems.
- Secure lids on garbage cans.
- Secure doors to outdoor storage (sheds, garages, and barns).
- Lock away and store fuels, paint, and other toxins out of reach.
- Pools in the yard are extremely dangerous. Use locked fencing at least four feet high with a self-closing gate. (Dowshen 2009)

Kitchen Safety

- Use childproof locks on doors of refrigerator, dishwasher, lower cabinets, and drawers.
- Place knives, heavy objects, and hot foods or liquids away from counter edges (prevents them from being pulled down by children).
- Unplug countertop appliances and push to back of counter.
- Remove stove controls (prevents children from turning stove on). Turn cookware handles to back of stove, out of reach.
- Highchairs must include a secure strap; always use the strap.
- Lock up and store out of reach toxins, cleaning products, medications, alcohol, and any harmful substances.
- Keep trash cans locked and out of reach.

Bedroom Safety

- Use infant beds and playpens with slats spaced no more than 2⅜ inches apart (prevents babies from getting their heads trapped between slats).
- Ensure that mattress fits snugly in the crib (prevents trapping baby between crib and mattress). Keep side rails pulled up. Large cutouts in the headboard or footboard and painted baby furniture made before 1974 are not safe, as lead paint was used before that time (Dowshen 2009).
- Keep comforters (sold in crib sets), large stuffed toys, and pillows out of crib (suffocation dangers). Bumper ties should be six inches or less. Remove long ribbons or ties from mobiles or toys. Babies sleep best with small light blankets and fitted sheets.
- Keep wall hangings and window treatments with cords away from the crib, out of baby's reach (prevents children from getting tangled in cords; death can occur from being strangled by the cords).

It is unsafe to place baby carriers on tables or other surfaces where they may fall off if the baby rocks or moves the carrier. At any age, babies must not be left where they can fall. Scooting or rolling over for the first time can happen when a child is left alone for just a moment on the edge of a bed or sofa, resulting in a fall and possible injury. Babies on changing tables need a safety belt and constant hands-on supervision to prevent falls.

 WHAT PEOPLE ARE SAYING **THE BED SHARING CONTROVERSY**

Bed sharing is when infants or young children sleep in the same bed as their parents or caregivers. Cosleeping is when they sleep nearby, in the same room. In many parts of the world, bed sharing is common. Cultures, family beliefs, and social and economic factors influence attitudes about bed sharing, as do opinions about health and safety issues.

Disadvantages of Bed Sharing

Opponents of bed sharing cite concerns about increased risk of SIDS, decreased quality of sleep, increased stress for children and parents, and unhealthy dependence on parents for soothing and to get to sleep. Safety concerns include the chance that a small baby may be smothered by a sleeping adult and concerns that modern bedding is not safe for infants.

Advantages of Bed Sharing

Advocates claim that bed sharing is beneficial, offering protection against SIDS, facilitating breast-feeding, allowing parents to get better sleep, and improving infant bonding with parents.

Is There a Resolution?

The American Academy of Pediatrics (AAP) opposes bed sharing with *very young* babies but encourages cosleeping (Task Force on Sudden Infant Death Syndrome 2005). Some studies found that the risk of SIDS among bed-sharing infants to be higher, but only with mothers who smoked. Other studies found an increased risk of SIDS with bed sharing among infants with nonsmoking mothers, but only when infants were younger than 11 weeks of age, mothers had consumed alcohol or were overtired, or when there were more people in the bed with the infant. Many studies have found a reduced risk of SIDS with cosleeping.

The AAP concludes that there is no single risk factor for SIDS and makes several recommendations for safe infant sleeping:

- Infants should sleep on their backs (supine position) rather than on their stomachs (prone) or sides.
- Don't smoke during pregnancy.
- Use a firm sleeping surface; never have an infant sleep on a couch, water bed, or soft surface.
- Keep soft objects and loose bedding out of the crib and away from the sleeping infant.

- A separate bed in the same room is recommended.
- An infant should not be in bed with a parent or caregiver who is overtired or has used substances that could impair alertness.
- Consider using a pacifier at nap time or bedtime.
- Avoid overheating the infant.

Source: Task Force on Sudden Infant Death Syndrome (2005).

Bathroom Safety

Bathrooms contain many potential hazards for young children:

- Never leave babies or young children unattended in bathtub. Children can drown in only a few inches of water; therefore, buckets, puddles, and fountains can all be dangerous if babies fall into them head-first.
- Keep toilet lids down and latched with a childproof lock (prevents drowning in the toilet bowl and injuries by a dropped seat or lid).
- Use bathtubs with nonskid surfaces or adhesives on tub bottom.
- Use bathtub faucet covers (prevents injury from child's head hitting faucet).
- Secure bathroom drawers and cabinets with childproof latches.
- Turn down water heaters to below 120 degrees Fahrenheit (Mondozzi 2009).
- Bathroom outlets need ground fault circuit interrupters (prevents electrocution from wet appliances).
- Unplug hair dryers and other grooming appliances and store them out of reach.
- Store out of reach and lock up razors and sharp objects, toxic cleaning products, grooming substances, medications, and any harmful substances.

Other Child Safety Issues

Pets in the home can pose a danger to a baby and must be supervised. Even the gentlest pet can sit on, lick, or otherwise interact unsafely with a child. A baby should not be left unobserved when with other young children. Children may not feed or lift the baby safely, and they may drop the baby. Adults who will watch the baby need to be carefully informed about the baby's level of mobility, ability to eat and drink, and any relevant individual traits.

Babysitters need a level of maturity to make sound decisions in an emergency. Additionally, knowledge of first aid, relief of choking, and infant CPR are desirable in caregivers. The constant mindfulness of all people in the home is important to ensuring the safety of children.

Baby Equipment

Babies must travel in a car seat whenever in any vehicle. Infant car seats must be securely belted into the seat in the back seat facing backwards until the baby has reached at least 1 year of age. Strap in the baby and the car seat exactly as stated in instructions from the car seat manual. Older children will need booster seats from age 4 until age 10 or 12, depending on local or state laws (SafetyBeltSafe U.S.A. 2007). Regulations for infant and child car seats vary by state. Guidelines for your state can be found at the Governors Highway Safety Association (GHSA) website, listed in the resources section at the end of this chapter.

Babies can add a lot of luggage to an overnight trip unless there is a room set up for them where they are going. A safe place to sleep, such as a portable crib, is important. The baby will also need a safe area for feeding and bathing, safe toys, proper clothing for the climate, and measures to stay safe in another's home.

Strollers or baby carriers may be useful when going out with the baby. Babies must be securely fastened and should never be left alone in a stroller. Highchairs in restaurants must have a secure strap to hold the baby. Some highchairs accommodate infant carriers, but caution should be used to ensure stability in a busy place where chairs can be bumped by others.

Grocery store carts may pose safety problems. Infants may remain in infant car seats or carriers if they are designed to attach securely to the grocery cart. Older babies and toddlers may sit in the small basket seat with a lap belt securely fastened, but adults should never step away from the cart. Padded grocery covers are available for comfort and hygiene, but the cart safety strap must still be used. Children should never stand up in the bottom or top part of the cart, as this unstable weight can cause the cart to tip over and cause serious injury.

All products that are used for babies must be kept in good working order. At times, child equipment is recalled for safety issues. Government or product websites or the U.S. Consumer Product Safety Commission website (listed in the resources section at the end of this chapter) should be regularly checked for any recalls of child equipment.

The Diaper Bag

For day trips outside the home, a diaper bag can be prepared with:

- Foods and fluids for baby, along with bottles, cups, spoons
- Extra diapers, baby wipes, diaper disposal bags
- Extra clothes, extra baby hat
- Plastic bags for soiled clothing or diapers
- Blanket/changing cloth, hand sanitizer
- Extra pacifiers, burping cloths, bibs
- A few toys, baby pain relief, diaper ointments

Toys

Buying toys for a baby can be a fun activity. However, a baby's need for toys is often not as great as families may think:

- Toys that give practice with motor skills are recommended.
- Soft or huggable toys may provide comfort.
- Toys with sounds, lights, textures, or colors help babies develop and use their senses.
- Very young babies prefer high-contrast stimuli, such as black and white toys (Hamer 1990).

Babies often play with a number of objects, some of which may not be safe:

- Small toys or items that may go in baby's mouth can cause choking.
- Some toys may contain lead, other metals, or chemicals. These may harm the baby if chewed on.
- Objects with sharp edges may cut a baby.
- Long cords from toys may strangle a baby.
- Very large or heavy objects may pose a smothering threat.
- Babies should only play with toys or objects that are labeled as safe for their age.

Rolling **baby walkers** (also known as wheelie walkers) have a sling for the baby to sit in so that the baby's feet touch the floor. The babies may roll the walkers around the room, allowing them to be more mobile. Since brakes became required to prevent injury from the walkers rolling down stairs, walkers have become safer (Consumer Reports 2006).

Some parents choose to avoid walkers because their safety is somewhat controversial.

As they grow older, children can play with toys that allow them to imitate roles or occupations that they see in adults. Cooking with toy pots, working with toy tools, or caring for baby dolls can spark children's imagination and teach useful skills. Books are great sources for enjoyment and lifelong learning. Older children progress in learning to interact and play with others. Parents and caregivers can model showing respect for others. Praising children for using language to express their feelings and wants reinforces these habits.

Developmental Milestones

As they grow, children begin to use new skills, such as taking a first step, smiling, rolling over, or crawling for the first time. These skills are called **developmental milestones**. Children develop at different rates, and the age at which a child may exhibit a certain skill will vary. Parents who are concerned about a child not reaching a milestone should consult with their health practitioner. Practitioners will monitor milestones at health care assessments during the child's early life. Developmental milestones for different ages are described at the Centers for Disease Control and Prevention website, listed in the resources section at the end of this chapter.

Around one year of age, children may begin taking steps. Each time they succeed in their efforts, parents can show their pleasure and excitement. When the child falls, parents should not make a fuss. By minimizing the fall and moving past it, parents are attending only to the preferred behavior, that of success toward walking. This method of rewarding preferred behavior and ignoring undesired behaviors is used over and over in parenting. For example, parents may respond with excitement or praise when a child says an actual word but pay no attention to nonsense syllables. Because of the rewards attached, the child begins to use the word that was praised. In toilet training, a child's efforts to use the toilet are causes for much excitement and complimenting. Toileting accidents are treated as unimportant. A child is more likely to continue a behavior when praise and positive attention are received. Negative attention or punishments are less likely to promote a desired behavior.

Child Care

Some mothers or fathers stay home throughout the day to care for the child; others may work outside the home. When both parents work outside the home, other family members may be available to provide child care at the child's home or the family member's home. A schedule can sometimes be worked out for several family members, indicating when they are available to take care of the baby.

Some families hire in-home help with the baby: a sitter or a nanny. These workers usually come in to the home during the workday. In some cases, the caregiver is given housing within the family's home. Babies and older toddlers may also be cared for at day care centers or nurseries. Day care centers may serve only a few children or may hold classes for several levels of preschool children. People using day care services must decide how often the baby will attend and what hours the baby will be present. Some state regulations limit the number of hours on a given day that a baby may be left in day care. Parents must consider day care location and what they can afford. They may seek assistance with costs. Much thought can go into selecting which day care option is best for the family's needs.

Some families are concerned about the safety of leaving a child in the care of others. Most day care sites are open to people dropping in to check on the care of their children at any time. Others allow parents to view the children and their care using video cameras within the center. Word of mouth and a good reputation may indicate that quality care is given. State agencies inspect and certify child care centers; parents may ask about the center's official licensing. Asking for references may give insight into how other parents rate the center.

Choosing a day care facility often involves a number of questions about how the place functions and what it has to offer. Parents should be permitted to visit unannounced anytime the center is open. Does the center have written policies and scheduled activities, and are these followed by the staff? Is there enough staff, and are they trained well? It is important to be comfortable talking with staff about the child and about the center's function (American Academy of Pediatrics 2010). More information about choosing a child care center can be found at the American Academy of Pediatrics website, listed in the resources section at the end of this chapter.

Stranger Safety

Babies are not likely to meet strangers without a loved one near. Still, it is important for adults to be aware of possible problems that can arise. Do not allow a stranger to hold the baby unless you are sure you can stay close and control the encounter. Do not announce your plans to people around you, and be aware of people who approach you. Criminals may try to take advantage of a person distracted by children. Be aware and avoid dangerous areas. Never leave a baby unattended in a car, even to walk from the car to pay at a gas station window. **Carjacking**—stealing a car from the driver—can occur with the baby still inside the vehicle. If someone asks for your keys, take the baby out of the car as you give the person the keys.

As children get older, they must learn not to talk to or take anything from strangers. They must be taught not to get into anyone's car or go off with anyone they do not know for any reason. A family password can be used if another adult is sent to pick them up. Children may wear a parent's phone number on their clothes in crowds and should be taught to seek out a police officer anytime they become lost.

Other Responsibilities for Parents

Parents are expected to provide for their children financially. It can be very challenging for teens to balance school, work, and all the expenses of caring for themselves and a child. Many teens are able to rely on their own parents or others for help with housing, expenses, transportation, and insurance. However, family members may no longer be willing or able to cover these expenses for teens who have become parents. In these cases, the teens will need to plan a budget and secure their own sources for income, insurance, and providing for other needs.

Teen parents will need to consider child care options and costs as well as work schedules that can maximize their time to care for the baby. Employment that offers benefits such as paid sick days, savings plans, and health insurance for the employee and family are preferable to jobs with no benefits. Typically, part-time employment has no or limited benefits.

Health insurance can be obtained individually and is important for healthy people as well as those with chronic illnesses. A healthy person may have an accident or illness that amounts to very costly medical bills. With health insurance, the individual pays only a portion of the medical expenses. More information about the types, costs, and benefits of health insurance can be found at the TeensHealth website, listed in the resources section at the end of this chapter.

Health insurance is also available from government sources for people of very limited income or those with serious disabling conditions. There are also government programs to provide food and medication to children. The Children's Health Insurance Program (CHIP) provides coverage for millions of uninsured children in the United States (Centers for Medicare and Medicaid Services 2011). Contact local Medicaid and Medicare offices for information about low-cost health insurance for children and adults.

Dealing with the many costs of supporting oneself and a child requires careful planning. A place to live, utility bills, food costs, taxes, telephone

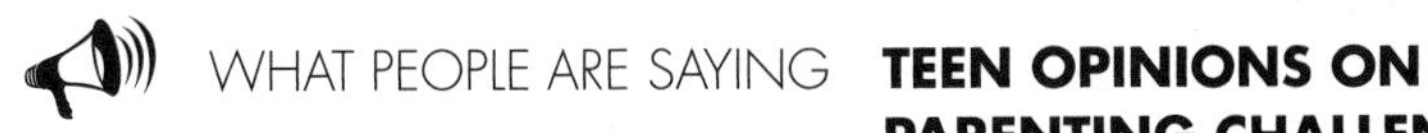

TEEN OPINIONS ON PARENTING CHALLENGES

What are some of the challenges of being a teen parent and trying to finish high school?

- "Being a parent is a more than full-time job, and unless the grandparents are willing to care for the child while the parents finish their education, then I don't know how they could possibly balance school and a small child." ES, age 20, California
- "Being a teen parent most obviously takes away time that one could be studying or participating in extracurriculars, but it also puts financial pressure on a parent that could lead them to drop out of school in order to pursue a job." KK, age 19, Kentucky
- "You are no longer in charge of your own schedule, and many of your other friends can no longer relate and sympathize with you." KK, age 18, Louisiana
- "Money would be a big challenge of being a parent while going to school. It would be hard to balance school, taking care of a child, and a job." KG, age 19, Texas

fees, clothing, household supplies, home or vehicle repairs, and emergency savings are just some of the items that need to be covered by one's income. This list does not include any entertainment or less essential expenses such as music, electronics, dining out, and gifts for oneself or others. It is also important to plan for the future when considering a budget, including funds for one's own or children's college expenses and funds for one's retirement years—however far away retirement may seem. An example of a single parent's budget can be found at the Single Parent Alliance and Resource Center, listed in the resources section at the end of this chapter.

Resources

Websites, Help Lines, and Hotlines

American Academy of Pediatrics
Choosing a child care center: http://www.healthychildren.org/english/family-life/work-play/Pages/Choosing-a-Childcare-Center.aspx

American Heart Association
Find a local CPR or first aid class: http://www.heart.org/HEARTORG/classConnector.jsp?pid=ahaweb.classconnector.home#

American Red Cross
Find local infant and child CPR classes: http://www.redcross.org/portal/site/en/menuitem.d229a5f06620c6052b1ecfbf43181aa0/?vgnextoid=648946a80f2bb110VgnVCM10000089f0870aRCRD&vgnextchannel=aea70c45f663b110VgnVCM10000089f0870aRCRD

Centers for Disease Control and Prevention (CDC)
Developmental milestones: http://www.cdc.gov/ncbddd/actearly/milestones/index.html

Centers for Medicare and Medicaid Services
The Children's Health Insurance Program: http://www.cms.gov/LowCostHealthInsFamChild/

Governors Highway Safety Association (GHSA)
Child passenger safety laws (by state): http://www.ghsa.org/html/stateinfo/laws/childsafety_laws.html

La Leche League
Breastfeeding information, support, and resources: http://www.llli.org/resources.html

Learn CPR, University of Washington School of Medicine
CPR information, video demonstrations, and choking information for infants, children, and adults: http://depts.washington.edu/learncpr/index.html

National Abandoned Infant Assistance Resource Center
Resources related to children who are abandoned, or at risk of abandonment, and their families: http://aia.berkeley.edu/information_resources/abandoned_infants.php

National Highway Traffic Safety Administration (NHTSA)
Child Safety: Which Car Seat Is Right for Your Child?
http://www.nhtsa.gov/Safety/CPS

Single Parent Alliance and Resource Center
Sample Single Parent Budget Worksheet: http://www.singleparent411.org/documents/sparc_budget.pdf

TeensHealth from Nemours

Finding Low-Cost Medical Care: http://kidshealth.org/teen/infections/stds/lcost_medcare.html

Health Insurance Basics: http://kidshealth.org/teen/your_body/medical_care/insurance.html

Navigating the Health Care System: http://kidshealth.org/parent/_cancer_center/treatment/healthcare.html#a_Navigating_the_Health_Care_System

U.S. Consumer Product Safety Commission

Infant/Child Product Recalls (not including toys): http://www.cpsc.gov/cpscpub/prerel/category/child.html

Women, Infants, and Children (WIC)

A government nutrition program for women, infants, and children: http://www.nutrition.gov/nal_display/index.php?info_center=11&tax_level=2&tax_subject=394&topic_id=1767&placement_default=0

Women's Health Information

Stages of Pregnancy: http://womenshealth.gov/pregnancy/you-are-pregnant/stages-of-pregnancy.cfm

Videos

Learn CPR. 2011. *First Aid for a Choking Child.* University of Washington School of Medicine. http://depts.washington.edu/learncpr/videodemo/choking-child-video.html.

Further Reading

California Highway Patrol. 2009. "4 Steps for Kids." In *California Vehicle Restraint Laws: Infants and Small Children.* April. California Office of Traffic Safety. http://www.chp.ca.gov/community/pdf/ca_vr_laws.pdf.

Murkoff, Heidi, and Sharon Mazel. 2008. *What to Expect When You're Expecting.* 4th ed. New York: Workman.

Nourie, Cory E. 2009. "Health Insurance Basics." TeensHealth from Nemours. March. http://kidshealth.org/teen/your_body/medical_care/insurance.html.

References

American Academy of Pediatrics. 2010. "Choosing a Child Care Center." June 11. http://www.healthychildren.org/english/family-life/work-play/Pages/Choosing-a-Childcare-Center.aspx.

American Pregnancy Association. 2007a. "Dental Work during Pregnancy." February. http://www.americanpregnancy.org/pregnancy health/dentalwork.html.

American Pregnancy Association. 2007b. "Hair Treatment during Pregnancy." April. http://www.americanpregnancy.org/isitsafe/hairtreatments.html.

American Pregnancy Association. 2007c. "What's a Sun Goddess to Do during Pregnancy: Pregnancy and Tanning." February. http://www.americanpregnancy.org/pregnancyhealth/tanning methods.html.

American Pregnancy Association. 2008. "Using Illegal Drugs during Pregnancy." October. http://www.americanpregnancy.org/pregnancyhealth/illegaldrugs.html.

American Pregnancy Association. 2010a. "Alcohol Use in Pregnancy." http://www.americanpregnancy.org/pregnancyhealth/alcohol.html.

American Pregnancy Association. 2010b. "Is It Safe while Pregnant?" http://www.americanpregnancy.org/isitsafe/.

American SIDS Institute. 2010. "Reducing the Rate of SIDS." http://sids.org/nprevent.htm.

Bobetsis, Yiorgos A., Silvana P. Barros, and Steven Offenbacher. 2006. "Explaining the Relationship between Periodontal Disease and Pregnancy Complications." *Journal of the American Dental Association* 137 (Suppl. 2): 7S–13S. http://jada.ada.org/cgi/content/full/137/suppl_2/7S.

Campbell Philipsen, Nayna. 2003. "Abandoned-Baby Laws." *Journal of Perinatal Education* 12(2): 41–43. doi:10.1624/105812403X106829. http://www.ncbi.nlm.nih.gov/pmc/articles/PMC1595144/.

Centers for Disease Control and Prevention. 2009. "Alcohol Use in Pregnancy." August 24. http://www.cdc.gov/ncbddd/fasd/alcohol-use.html.

Centers for Medicare and Medicaid Services. 2011. "The Children's Health Insurance Program." U.S. Department of Health and Human Services. May 24. http://www.cms.gov/LowCostHealth InsFamChild/.

Chassin, Laurie, Clark Presson, Dong-Chul Seo, Steven J. Sherman, Jon Macy, R. J. Wirth, and Patrick Curran. 2008. "Multiple Trajectories of Cigarette Smoking and the Intergenerational Transmission of Smoking: A Multigenerational, Longitudinal Study of a Midwestern Community Sample." *Health Psychology* 27(6): 819–828. doi:10.1037/0278-6133.27.6.819.

Consumer Reports. 2006. "A Baby Walker That's Not Acceptable." December 8. http://news.consumerreports.org/home/2006/12/a-baby-walker-t.html.

Dowshen, Steven. 2009. "Taking Care of Your Grandchildren." KidsHealth from Nemours. May. http://kidshealth.org/parent/positive/family/grandkids.html#.

Hamer, Russell D. 1990. "What Can My Baby See?" *Parents' Press* 11(2) (November). http://www.ski.org/Vision/babyvision.html.

Harborview Injury Prevention and Research Center. 2010. "Fire and Burn Injury Interventions: Flammable Fabrics Act." University of Washington. http://depts.washington.edu/hiprc/practices/topic/fireburns/fabricslaw.html.

Heller, Jacob L. 2010. "Talcum Powder Poisoning." National Library of Medicine. January 27. http://www.nlm.nih.gov/medlineplus/ency/article/002719.htm.

Hirsch, Larissa. 2008. "Bonding with Your Baby." KidsHealth from Nemours. February. http://kidshealth.org/parent/pregnancy_newborn/communicating/bonding.html.

Laino, Charlene. 2007. "Breastfeeding Cuts Breast Cancer Risk." WebMD. Breast Cancer Health Center. http://www.webmd.com/breast-cancer/news/20070417/breastfeeding-cuts-breast-cancer-risk.

Lucille Packard Foundation for Children's Health. 2011. "Common Tests during Pregnancy." http://www.lpch.org/DiseaseHealthInfo/HealthLibrary/pregnant/tests.html.

Mayo Clinic. 2010. "Postpartum Depression." June 3. http://www.mayoclinic.com/health/postpartum-depression/DS00546.

Mondozzi, Mary. 2009. "Household Safety: Preventing Burns, Shocks and Fires." KidsHealth from Nemours. May. http://kidshealth.org/parent/firstaid_safe/home/safety_burns.html#.

Murkoff, Heidi, and Sharon Mazel. 2008. *What to Expect When You're Expecting*. 4th ed. New York: Workman.

National Abandoned Infant Assistance Resource Center. 2005. "Boarder Babies, Abandoned Infants, and Discarded Infants." Fact Sheet.

December. http://aia.berkeley.edu/media/pdf/abandoned_infant_fact_sheet_2005.pdf.

National Capital Poison Center. 2010. "Even Plants Can Be Poisonous." http://www.poison.org/prevent/plants.asp.

Pendley, Jennifer S. 2008. "Disciplining Your Child." KidsHealth from Nemours. October. http://kidshealth.org/parent/positive/talk/discipline.html.

Planned Parenthood. 2010. "Abortion." http://www.plannedparenthood.org/health-topics/abortion-4260.asp.

SafetyBeltSafe U.S.A. 2007. "FAQ: Frequently Asked Questions." July 24. http://www.carseat.org/Resources/FAQs.htm.

Storck, Susan. 2010. "Gestational Diabetes." National Center for Biotechnology Information, U.S. National Library of Medicine. September 11. http://www.ncbi.nlm.nih.gov/pubmedhealth/PMH0001898/.

Task Force on Sudden Infant Death Syndrome. 2005. "The Changing Concept of Sudden Infant Death Syndrome: Diagnostic Coding Shifts, Controversies Regarding the Sleeping Environment, and New Variables to Consider in Reducing Risk." *Pediatrics* 116(5): 1245–1255. doi:10.1542/peds.2005-1499. http://aappolicy.aappublications.org/cgi/reprint/pediatrics;116/5/1245.pdf.

Wiener, Laura. 2007. "Thirteen Signs You May Be Pregnant." Parents.com. http://www.parents.com/pregnancy/signs/symptoms/signs-you-may-be-pregnant.

Wind, Rebecca. 2010. "Following Decade-Long Decline, U.S. Teen Pregnancy Rate Increases as Both Births and Abortions Rise." Guttmacher Institute. News Release. January 26. http://www.guttmacher.org/media/nr/2010/01/26/index.html.

Women's Health Information. 2006. "Pregnancy Tests Fact Sheet." April 1. http://www.womenshealth.gov/publications/our-publications/fact-sheet/pregnancy-tests.cfm#c.

Women's Health Information. 2010. "Healthy Pregnancy: Labor and Birth." September 27. http://womenshealth.gov/pregnancy/childbirth-beyond/labor-birth.cfm#b.

Women's Health Information. 2011. "Why Breastfeeding Is Important." August 4. http://www.womenshealth.gov/breastfeeding/why-breastfeeding-is-important/#top.

Yale School of Medicine. 2011. "How to Help a Choking Child." http://www.yalemedicalgroup.org/stw/Page.asp?PageID=STW000550.

Glossary

abortion: The removal of the embryo/fetus and the placenta by a gentle suction device.

amniocentesis: A procedure in which a needle is placed into the pregnant uterus and fluid is drawn for testing.

amniotic fluid: The fluid contained in the amniotic sac surrounding the fetus; allows the developing fetus to move around, helps its lungs to develop, provides cushioning and protection, and maintains a healthy temperature in the fetal environment.

anesthesia: Medications that eliminate sensitivity to pain.

artificial insemination: The process of using a small tube to insert sperm into the uterus through the cervix to fertilize an egg.

baby blues: Brief feelings of sadness, fear, or irritability after the birth of a baby.

baby walker: A rolling device with a sling for the baby to sit in so that the baby's feet touch the floor, allowing the baby to roll the walker around the room; also known as wheelie walker.

bonding: The process of forming an emotional attachment.

Braxton Hicks contractions: Brief and scattered hardening of the uterus for a few minutes before returning to normal; considered normal in pregnancy, these often precede actual labor.

breech: A baby lying with the feet lowest in the uterus; born feet first.

burping: The baby's release of any swallowed air, which clears room for food in the stomach.

carjacking: Stealing a car from the driver, usually by threatening harm with a weapon.

catheter: A tube placed into the bladder to drain urine.

chloasma: *See* **mask of pregnancy**.

circumcision: The removal of the foreskin.

colostrum: Thick yellow- or gold-colored liquid that contains nutrients and fluids and is present before breast milk.

conception: When the pregnancy begins; when sperm from the male fertilizes or joins with the egg of the female.

contraction: A tightening of the muscles in the uterus; acts to push the baby out during childbirth.

coparenting: Shared parenting; both parents working together to raise their children, including when parents do not live together.

crowning: When the top of the baby's head is visible through the vagina during delivery.

C-section: Surgical delivery of a baby; Cesarean section.

delusions: False beliefs.

developmental milestones: New skills, such as taking a first step, smiling, rolling over, or crawling for the first time.

dilatation: Gradual opening or expanding of the cervix.

discipline: A way to teach children how to interact with others and with their world.

Doppler: An ultrasound instrument used to hear a baby's heartbeat.

douching: Flushing out the vagina with liquid solutions.

effacement: Thinning out of the cervix.

embryo: The fertilized egg or zygote up to eight weeks of development.

engorged: Overfull.

episiotomy: A small cut to enlarge the vaginal opening during childbirth.

false labor: Symptoms that lead women to believe they are in labor when they are not.

fetal alcohol spectrum disorder (FASD): Problems in the baby resulting from exposure to alcohol during pregnancy; may lead to abnormal facial features, low birth weight, intellectual deficits or learning problems, a small head, and problems with the heart, kidneys, or bones.

fetus: An unborn or developing baby; from eight weeks of development until birth; compare with embryo.

flatulence: Excess gas in the digestive tract.

folic acid: A vitamin that promotes cell growth in the fetus.

foreskin: The skin around the head of the penis.

gestational diabetes: A condition in pregnant women who develop elevated blood sugar.

hallucination: A false visual, auditory, smell, taste, or tactile perception.

HcG: Human chorionic gonadotropin.

heartburn: A feeling of burning in the upper abdomen, near the breastbone; indigestion.

hemorrhoids: Swollen veins in the rectal area that may itch, burn, or bleed.

human chorionic gonadotropin (HcG): A hormone that is produced when the fertilized egg implants in the uterus and is present in a pregnant woman's blood and urine.

hydrotherapy: Therapeutic use of water, including going through labor in a tub of warm water.

incision: A cut or opening made with a scalpel or surgical knife.

in vitro fertilization: A procedure in which eggs are taken from a woman and sperm are taken from a man and then combined in a laboratory dish to achieve fertilization, after which the embryos are implanted in the uterus.

lactation consultant: A person who teaches and supports mothers in nursing and breastfeeding concerns.

linea negra: A dark line that runs from the navel to the pubic bone of a pregnant woman.

mask of pregnancy: Color change across the middle of the face during pregnancy, a darker patch of skin in light-skinned women and a lighter patch in dark-skinned women; also known as chloasma or melasma.

medical abortion: When medication is used to terminate a pregnancy.

melasma: *See* **mask of pregnancy**.

miscarriage: The end of pregnancy when the fetus dies from unplanned causes; also known as spontaneous abortion.

mohel: A person trained to safely perform a circumcision in a religious ceremony; moyle.

morning sickness: A state of nausea or vomiting during pregnancy.

moyle: *See* **mohel**.

mucous plug: A clear jellylike substance that plugs the cervix during pregnancy.

ovulation: Release of an egg from the ovary.

ovum (pl., ova): Female egg.

periodontitis: Infection and inflammation of the bones that support the teeth.

placenta: The organ that develops within the uterus to supply food and oxygen to the fetus through the umbilical cord.

postpartum: The period immediately after childbirth.

postpartum depression: A mental health disorder occurring shortly after delivery with sad or irritated mood, decreased functioning, and difficulty coping with life pressures.

postpartum psychosis: A rare and serious condition that impairs the new mother's perception of reality and may bring thoughts of harming herself or the baby.

pregnancy: The condition in which there is an offspring developing in the mother.

progesterone: A female hormone that aids pregnancy.

punishment: A penalty for a fault or an offense.

sea bands: Elastic wrist bands that, with a small button, apply pressure to an acupressure point on the inner wrists and decrease sensations of nausea.

sexual intercourse: When the penis is placed in the vagina.

SIDS: Sudden infant death syndrome.

spontaneous abortion: The loss of a fetus due to unplanned causes; also known as a miscarriage.

sudden infant death syndrome (SIDS): The sudden death of an infant under one year of age, unexplained by any investigation or autopsy tests.

transverse: A fetus lying sideways in the uterus; may cause problems with delivery, necessitating a C-section.

trimester: A three-month period; pregnancy is divided into three trimesters.

ultrasound: A test that uses high-frequency sound waves to produce pictures of the inside of the body.

umbilicus: The navel or belly button.

water breaking: The rupture or tearing of the amniotic sac and the release of the amniotic fluid.

waterbirthing: Delivering a baby in water.

zygote: A fertilized egg.

About the Authors

Georganna Leavesley, PhD, is a registered nurse and a licensed clinical psychologist. Dr. Leavesley has a bachelor of science degree in nursing from Texas Christian University in Fort Worth, Texas, and a master of science degree in nursing from the University of Texas at Austin. She has a master of arts degree and a doctoral degree in clinical psychology from the University of Houston, University Park. Dr. Leavesley evaluates and treats clients as a full-time private practitioner of clinical psychology and is also an instructor of mental health nursing at Our Lady of Holy Cross College in New Orleans. She has more than 30 years of clinical experience and has lectured and written on a wide variety of topics. Her areas of expertise and interest include depression, coping with medical illness, chronic pain, symptom management, geropsychology, and dementia.

Yvette Malamud Ozer is a clinical psychology PhD student at the California School of Professional Psychology/Alliant University in San Francisco. Her research and practice interests include neuropsychology, culturally appropriate assessment, neurodevelopmental disabilities, psychopharmacology, and resilience. She has a master's degree in clinical child/school psychology from California State University, East Bay, and a certificate in substance abuse counseling from the University of California Berkeley Extension. She is coauthor of the *Encyclopedia of Emotion* (Greenwood/ABC-CLIO, 2010).

Contributors

Rebecca Malamud Ozer is interested in social justice issues, including women's rights and LGBT issues.

Harley Hosford is an undergraduate studying at Berkeley City College until transferring to a four-year university, where he will be studying biomechanical engineering.

Index

Boldface page numbers refer to volume numbers. A key appears on all verso pages. An italicized *t* following a page number indicates a table. An italicized *f* following a page number indicates a figure.

12-step groups, **3**:36, **4**:81, 106

Abandonment
  divorce and feelings of, **5**:11
  response to pregnancy, **3**:185
  safe haven laws, **3**:185
Abortion, **3**:183–184
  laws regarding minor consent, **3**:151
  medical, **3**:194
  PID and, **3**:161
  spontaneous (miscarriage), **1**:18, **2**:21, **3**:161, 184, **4**:57, 60
    medications and risk of, **4**:57
Abrasion, **1**:141, 156, 160
Absolute physical activity intensity, **2**:149–150
Abstinence,
  food abstinence, **2**:115
    See also Anorexia mirabilis
  from substances, **4**:106–107
  sexual abstinence, **3**:129–132
    effectiveness as birth control method, **3**:145
    Teen Opinions on, **3**:130
    versus asexuality, **3**:52, 95
    virginity and, **3**:78–81
    See also Sexual abstinence
Acculturation, **5**:44–46
Acid rain, **1**:14
Acne, **1**:91–92
  and body dysmorphic disorder, **2**:124
  and consumerism, **5**:55
  steroids and, **4**:29, 51–52
Acquaintance or date rape, **3**:110–111
  date rape drugs, **3**:112, **4**:8, 10, 23
Acute disease, **1**:35
Acute injury, **1**:156, **2**:162
Adaptive behavior, **5**:143–144, 158
  and coping, **5**:82
  intellectual disability and, **5**:143–144
  versus maladaptive behavior, **5**:158
Adderall, **4**:20–21
ADHD medications (stimulant), **4**:20–21
Adjustment
  adolescence and, **3**:34
  difficulties, **1**:63, 68
  disorders, **5**:104
  stresses associated with, **5**:11, 13–15
Adoption, **1**:3, **3**:184, **5**:16–17
  birth family, **5**:16
  closed adoption, **5**:16–17
  open adoption, **5**:17
  resources, **5**:219
Adrenaline (epinephrine)
  for anaphylaxis, **1**:55, 182
  as neurotransmitter, **4**:45
  fight-or-flight response and, **5**:78
  stimulants and, **4**:47–48
  stress and, **5**:78–79
Adulterant, **4**:26, 56–57
Adulterated product, **2**:20

1: Health Basics
2: Nutrition and Physical Fitness
3: Sexual Health and Development
4: Alcohol, Tobacco, and Other Drugs
5: Mental and Emotional Health

Aerobic
  capacity, **2:**150
  energy system, **2:**170
  exercise, **2:**148, 150, 152–155, 160, 161, 162, 170, 180
Aftershock, **1:**168
Age of consent
  for abortion, **3:**151, 184
  for birth control or sterilization, **3:**145, 149–152
  for health care, **3:**149–152
  for sex, **3:**82–84, 109, 149–150
    age-gap provisions, **3:**82
    by U.S. state, **3:**83*t*
Agonist-antagonist drug treatment, **4:**84
AIDS. *See* HIV/AIDS
Air pollution, **1:**13–17
  asthma and, **1:**56, **2:**31
  emphysema and, **1:**57
  fossil fuels and, **1:**22
  mining and, **1:**24
  protection from, **1:**15–16
Air quality, **1:**15, 17, 22, 56, 166
  air quality index (AQI), **1:**15
Airborne
  allergen, **1:**55–56
Al-Anon, **4:**110
Alateen, **4:**110
Alcohol, **4:**3–8
  calories in, **2:**2, 42
  ethanol, **4:**3
  poisoning, **4:**6, 114
Alcohol use
  abuse and, **3:**103, 107
  Alcoholics Anonymous (AA), **4:**81, 106
  Al-Anon, **4:**110
  Alateen, **4:**110
  Antabuse (disulfrum), **4:**83–84
  binge drinking, **2:**24, **4:**6–8, 108, 114
  breastfeeding and, **3:**202, **4:**10–11, 61, 62
  cancer and, **1:**68, **4:**97
  central nervous system (CNS) and, **4:**4
  consumption, **4:**4
  contraindications, **4:**6
  as coping strategy, **5:**86, 155
  and dehydration, **2:**170
  detoxification (detox) from, **4:**80–81
  driving, and, **1:**127–128, 130, 136, 137
    impaired driving, **4:**7–8
  effects of, **4:**4–6
    effects on body, **4:**50–51, 97
    effects on brain, **4:**47, 49, 97
    masking effects, **4:**74
  family and, **4:**64–65
  fetal alcohol spectrum disorders (FASD), **3:**191, **4:**61, **5:**143, 146–147
  gastritis and, **1:**45
  hallucinations, **4:**5
  heart disease and, **1:**52–54, 97
  hard liquor, **4:**4
  the liver and, **1:**47, **4:**50, 97
  minimum drinking age, **4:**68–70
    Teen Opinions on, **4:**68
  pedestrians, and, **1;**139
  personal relationships and, **3:**76, **4:**66
  problems associated with, **4:**6
  proof, **4:**3–4
  rape and, **3:**112
  Rethinking Drinking (NIAAA), **4:**104
  sexual behavior and, **3:**95–96, 149
  size of standard drink, **4:**4, **4:**5*t*
    U.S. standard drink equivalents, **4:**5*t*
  sleep and, **1:**7
  social implications of alcohol abuse, **4:**66–67
  social norms and, **5:**44
  stroke and, **1:**64
  vehicle use and, **1:**139, 153–154
    impaired driving, **4:**7–8
  and weight concerns, **2:**24
  and wellness, **1:**1, 5
  withdrawal from, **4:**5, 9, 80
  See also Driving under the influence (DUI), Driving while intoxicated (DWI)
Alcoholics Anonymous (AA), **4:**81, 106
All-cause mortality rates, **2:**147

Allergies, **1**:14, 54–56
  allergen, **1**:22, 26, 55–56
  allergy shot, **1**:55
  anaphylaxis, **1**:54–55,182, 184, **2**:30, 42
    EpiPen, **1**:55, 182
  biological pollutants and, **1**:24
  drug allergies, **1**:55
  food allergies, **1**:55, **2**:30–32, 35
    peanut allergy, **2**:30
  latex allergy, **3**:141, 142
  pests and, **1**:26, 94
  pets and, **1**:25
  hives, **1**:55
  smoking and, **4**:13
  to tattoos or piercings, **1**:97–98, **3**:27, 29
  to vaccinations, **1**:106
Alzheimer's disease, **1**:62–64, **5**:106
  health care options for the elderly, **1**:63–64
American Personal Responsibility in Food Consumption Act (2005), **2**:62
American Psychologist, **5**:57
Amnesia, **5**:106
  Rohypnol and, **4**:10, 23
  sleep-related eating disorder (SRED) and, **2**:120–130
Amniocentesis, **3**:181–182
Amniotic fluid, **3**:186, 194, 196
Amphetamines, **4**:19–20, 24, 46–47, 50, 53, 59
  breastfeeding and, **4**:62–63
  cardiovascular system and, **4**;50, 53
  nervous system and, **4**:51, 53
  oral health and, **4**:52
  pregnancy, use during, **4**:59
  stroke and, **1**:54
  variants of, **4**:17
  for weight loss, **3**:25
Amps (amperes), **1**:178–179
Anaerobic energy system, **2**:170
Analgesics, **3**:12, 16, 17, 161, 197–198, 217, **4**:2, 40, 50, 58*t*, 66, **5**:166
  See also Opioids
Anaphylaxis, **1**:54–55,182, 184, **2**:30, 42
Androgyny, **3**:38–39, 52, 85
Anemia, **1**:68–69
  anorexia, and, **2**:119
  breastfeeding infants, and, **4**:62
  chromium picolinate and, **2**:180
  eating disorders and, **2**:119, 129
  iron, **2**:27
  sickle cell, **1**:3, 69
  steroid use, and, **4**:27–28
Anesthesia, **2**:94, 95, **3**:16, 17, 29, 184, 188, 194, 198
Anger, **5**:77, 86–93
  abuse and, **3**:102–103, 109
  causes of anger, **5**:86–87
  health problems related to anger, **5**:87
  management, **5**:77, 80, 86–93
  road rage, **1**:131
  steroid rage, **4**:31
  temper and mood, **5**:87
  violence, **5**:87
  when to get help with your anger, **5**:90*t*
Anger management, **5**:77, 80, 86–87
  strategies, **5**:87–89
  benefits of managing anger, **5**:87
  compromise, **5**:89
  dealing with someone else's anger, **5**:91–93
  vulnerability, **5**:89
  walking away, **5**:87–88
Angina, **1**:51
Anorexia
  athletica, **2**:123–124
  mirabilis, **2**:115
Anorexia nervosa, **2**:108, 110, 113–115, 116–119, **5**:103
  cognitive behavioral therapy (CBT), **2**:118
  death and, **2**:117
  Karen Carpenter and, **2**:117, 118*f*
  Pro-anorexia (pro-an) websites, Teen Opinions on, **2**:119
  risk factors, **2**:26, 112
  signs and symptoms of, **2**:119
  treatment of, **2**:117–118
Antibodies, **1**:54, 106, **3**:203
Antidepressants, **2**:118, 121, 122, **3**:200, **5**:116, 166
  interactions with other medications/ substances, **4**:21
  pregnancy, use during, **4**:58*t*
Antigens, **1**:106
Antioxidants, **2**:8–9, 36
Antipsychotics, **2**:118, **5**:116, 166
  use during pregnancy, **4**:58t

1: Health Basics
2: Nutrition and Physical Fitness
3: Sexual Health and Development
4: Alcohol, Tobacco, and Other Drugs
5: Mental and Emotional Health

Antisocial behavior, **5**:35
Anxiety, **5**:101, 105
- anticipatory anxiety, **5**:125
- anxiety disorders, **5**:105, 123–129
- avoidance, **2**:126, **3**:76, **5**:105, 123, 124, 125, 127, 128, 133
- bullying and, **5**:28
- compulsions, **2**:113, 121–125, 127–129, **5**:126–127
- dental anxiety, **1**:105
- drug/alcohol use and, **4**:6, 15, 19, 20, 21, 24, 48
- drug/alcohol withdrawal and, **4**:5, 9, 13, 22, 23, 44
- eating disorders, and, **2**:111, 113, 121, 124, 129–130
- generalized anxiety disorder (GAD), **5**:127
- medications and, **4**:8, 40
- performance anxiety, **5**:125
- postpartum depression and, **3**:199–200
- response prevention, **5**:126
- self-esteem and, **5**:3
- separation anxiety, **5**:101
- social phobia, **5**:125
- stress and, **5**:79
- symptoms of anxiety, **5**:124
- test anxiety, **5**:124–125
- *See also* Obsessive-compulsive disorder (OCD), Posttraumatic stress disorder (PTSD)

Anxiolytics, **4**:40, 58, **5**:166
- use during pregnancy, **4**:58

Appendix/Appendicitis, **1**:59
Apple shape, **2**:69
Arrhythmia, **1**:51–52, **2**:97, 129
Art therapist, **1**:36
Arthritis, **1**:67, **2**:45, 65, **4**:27
- osteoarthritis, **1**:67
- rheumatoid arthritis (RA), **1**:67

Asbestos, **1**:13, 17, 88
Asexuality, **3**:34, 35, 51, 52, 95
Asperger's syndrome, **5**:100, 144–145
Aspiration, **1**:42, **2**:129
Assertive communication, **5**:31, 90, 91, 158
Assistive technology, **1**:38, **5**:141
Association of Professional Piercers (APP), **3**:29
Asthma, **1**:14, 22, 25, 26, 27, 56
- food allergies and, **2**:30
- glucosamine and, **2**:181
- obesity and, **2**:66
- smoking and, **4**:13, 49, 55

Athletic supporter, **1**:155, 159
Atkins
- diet, **2**:88–91
- Robert, **2**:89*f*

Attention deficit hyperactivity disorder (ADHD), **5**:101, 135–137
- associated problems, **5**:136
- criteria/symptoms, **5**:136
- facts/myths, **5**:135, 137
- FASD and, **5**:147
- hyperactivity, **4**:20, **5**:101, 136–137, 147
- impulsivity, **4**:49, 60, **5**:35, 87, 101, 136
- in adults, **5**:136
- inattention, **4**:4, **5**:101, 136
- learning disabilities and, **5**:137
- medications for, **4**:19, 20–21, 52, 58
- prevalence, **5**:135

Autism spectrum disorders (ASD), **5**:144–145
- Asperger's syndrome, **5**:100, 144–145
- autism, **5**:100, 144–145
- pervasive developmental disorders (PDDs), **5**:100–101, 144
- vaccines and, **1**:107

Autoimmune, **4**:27

Baby care, **3**:209–218
- baby clothing, **3**:209–210, 216
  - nightclothes, **3**:210
- baby equipment, **3**:216–218
  - baby walkers, **3**:217–218
  - diaper bag, **3**:217
- baby powder, **1**:88, **3**:210
- bathing, **3**:201, 209, 215
- bed sharing controversy, **3**:214–215

diapers, **3**:199, 209–210, 217
feeding
breastfeeding, **3**:201–203
formula feeding, **3**:203–204
infant nutrition, **3**:201–203
Prader-Willi syndrome, **2**:128
healthcare, finding, **3**:207–208
hygiene, **3**:193, 209
safety, **3**:210–216
babysitters, **3**:215–216, 218–219
bathroom, **3**:212, 215
bedroom, **1**:145, **3**:213–215
doors, **3**:212–213
electrical, **1**:146–147, **3**:212
emergency numbers list, **3**:210
exercise equipment, **3**:212
furniture and household items, **1**:19, 164, **3**:211–215
guns, **3**:211
hazardous items, **1**:20, **3**:212
household, **3**:211–216
houseplants/flowers, **3**:211
older children, **3**:193, 215–216
pets, **3**:215
pools, **3**:212
windows, **3**:212, 213
shoes, **3**:210
skin care, **1**:93, **3**:199, 209–210
sudden infant death syndrome (SIDS), **1**:107, **3**:192–193, 214–215, **4**:55, 58
toys, **1**:19, **3**:211, 213, 217, 218
See also Child health care
Bacteria, **1**:17, 26, 38, 39, 40, 42–45, 48–49, 88, 89, 90, 92, 98, **2**:21, 22, 23, **3**:24, 29, 190, **4**:52, 55
cellulitis, **4**:52
Chlamydia trachomatis, **3**:156–157
dental health, and, **1**:101, 103, 104
E. coli, **1**:44
Gonorrhea (*Neisseria gonorrhoeae)*, **3**:158–159
Listeria moncytogenes, **2**:22, **3**:191
Pelvic Inflammatory Disease (PID), **3**:161
pneumonia (*Mycoplasma pneumonia)*, **1**:43
pneumococcal disease, **1**:49
salmonella, **2**:22
staphylococcus, **1**:49, **3**:24
streptococcus, **1**:39, **3**:24, 182
Syphilis (*Treponema pallidum)*, **3**:161–162
tetanus (*clostridium tetani)*, **1**:108–109
tuberculosis (Mycobacterium tuberculosis), **1**:43, **2**:21
typhoid, **1**:17
viruses and, **1**:26
yeast and, **1**:39
Barbecue, fire hazards, **1**:148
Basal metabolic rate (BMR), **2**:71
Behavioral teratogenicity, **4**:57
Bicycle
accident, **3**:208
environment and, **1**:16, 22
exercise, as, **2**:155
helmets, **1**:140–141
levels of prevention, illustration, **1**:85
safety, **1**:140–141
Bile, **1**:59
Biliopancreatic diversion, **2**:93–95
Binge drinking, **2**:24, **4**:6–8, 100, 108, 114
Binge eating (compulsive eating), **2**:115, 121–124, **5**:103
age of onset, **2**:121
health risks, **2**:121
signs and symptoms, **2**:122*t*
statistics, **2**:121
treatments, **2**:122
Biological
child, **1**:3
family, **5**:16
parent, **1**:3, **3**:184
Biological hazard, **1**:24
Biological pollution, **1**:24–27
dust mites, **1**:26–27
pests, **1**:19–20, 26, 94, 101
pets and, **1**:25
viruses and bacteria, **1**:26
volatile organic compound (VOC), **1**:27
See also Mold and mildew
Biological sex, **3**:38, 40, 48, 51, 85
Biopsy, **1**:47, 68, **3**:161
Bipolar disorder, **2**:126, **5**:109, 112–114
medications during pregnancy, **4**:58
Birth control. *See* Contraception (birth control)
Bisexuality, **3**:34–35, 49, 51, 85
eating disorders, and, **2**:113

1: Health Basics
2: Nutrition and Physical Fitness
3: Sexual Health and Development
4: Alcohol, Tobacco, and Other Drugs
5: Mental and Emotional Health

Blind study, **5**:60
Blindness, **1**:23, 48, 60, 176, **3**:156, 162
night blindness, **2**:16
Bloating, **2**:92, 120, 124, 129, **3**:21, 179, 188, **4**:50
Blood, **1**:67
red blood cells, **1**:67–71, **2**:9, 11, 27, **4**:27
T cells, **3**:152
in urine, **1**:44, **3**:180
white blood cells, **3**:152
Blood diseases, **1**:67–71
anemia, **1**:68,69, **2**:27, 119
leukemia, **1**:68,
sickle cell disease, **1**:3, 69–71,70*f*, **3**:182
Blood pressure, **1**:3, 19, 52–54, 60, 61, 109–112, 177, 181, **2**:12, 24, 65, 69, 75, 92, 93, 119, 146, 157, 160, 175, **3**:24, 182, 189, 197, **4**:9, 10, 12, 20, 21, 23, 24, 28, 29, 48, 50, 53, 57, **5**:78, 79, 87
sleep and, **1**:6, 7
See also Hypertension
Blood sugar, **1**:60, 65, 109, 111, **2**:4, 8, 12, 94, 95, 133, 160, 170–173, 181, 182, **4**:28, 53, 57
diabetes and, **1**:3, 59–60, 65, 109, 111
Blood transfusions, **1**:68, 70–71, **2**:23, **3**:152
Blood-borne diseases, **1**:98, **4**:26, 30
See also Hepatitis, HIV/AIDS
Body image, **2**:108–112, 134–135, **3**:25, **5**:40
body dysmorphic disorder (BDD), **2**:124–125, **4**:30
body modifications, **3**:26–30
body size expectations (unrealistic), **2**:112*t*, **5**:50
Botox injections, **3**:26, **5**:56
breast augmentation surgery, **3**:9, **5**:56
cosmetic surgery, **2**:111, **3**:8, 9, 17, 26, 48, **5**:56
eating disorders and, **2**:115, 119
Hornby, Lesley (Twiggy), **2**:108, 109*f*
the media and, **2**:110,111, **3**:25, 97, **5**:1, 5, 47–49
muscle dysphoria, **2**:125–126
negative body image dangers, **2**:111
college students with negative body image, **2**:110
peer pressure, **2**:108
plastic surgery and, **2**:111
preadolescents and, **2**:109–110
pregnancy and, **3**:189
self-esteem and, **2**:109,110
social environment and, **5**:47–49
subjectivity and, **2**:108
teens and, **2**:29, 65, 109–110, **3**:97
Teen Opinions on media and body image, **2**:111
unrealistic societal ideals of, **2**:108–109, 112
Body lice, **1**:94
Body mass index (BMI), **1**:11, 110, **2**:63,67–69, 75, 93–96, 108, 112, 134
BMI calculator, **2**:70
formula, **2**:67
Body mechanics, **1**:162
Body piercings, **1**:97–99, **3**:26, 28, 29–30, 85, **5**:2
Association of Professional Piercers (APP), **3**:29
female circumcision (FGM) and, **3**:16
hepatitis and, **1**:46
HIV and, **3**:152, 155
keloids, **1**:98, **3**:29
pregnancy and, **3**:192
Teen Opinions on, **3**:27
Body size expectations (unrealistic), **2**:112*t*, **5**:50
Body washing, **1**:86–88, 100, 176
Boils (furuncles), **1**:49, 50
Bone marrow, **1**:67, 71, **4**:56
transplants, **1**:69, 71
Botox injections, **3**:26, **5**:56
Bovine spongiform encephalopathy (BSE), **2**:22–23
Bowel

disease, **1**:58
movements, **1**:10, 58, 114, **2**:92, 170, **3**:159, 194
obstruction, **1**:57–58
See also inflammatory bowel disease (IBD)
Brain and nervous system diseases, **1**:15, 19, 47–49, 62–66, 68, 90, **2**:21
AIDS dementia, **3**:154, **5**:109
Alzheimer's disease, **1**:62–64, **5**:106
bovine spongiform encephalopathy (BSE), **2**:22–23
Creutzfeldt-Jakob (mad cow) disease, **2**:22–23
dementia, **1**;54, 62, 63, 66, **3**:154, 162, **5**:106, 152
toxoplasma gondii, **2**:22–23, **3**:154
See also Encephalitis, Meningitis, Multiple sclerosis (MS), Parkinson's disease, Prions, Seizure disorder (epilepsy), Stroke (cerebrovascular accident), Syphilis
Breach, **1**:169
Breasts, **3**:5–9, 20, 21, 22, 44, 49
augmentation surgery, **3**:8, 9, 26, **5**:2, 56
cancer, **1**:68, 69, 110, 111, **2**:65, **3**:7, 9, 203
engorgement, **3**:188, 201
gynecomastia, **3**:6, **4**:29, 31
mammograms, **3**:7
self-examination , **1**:111, **3**:7
Breastfeeding, **3**:201–203
advantages of, **3**:203
as birth control method, **3**:133, 135
coffee drinking, **4**:62
colostrum, **3**:201
contraception and, **3**:135, 138, 141–143
frequency of, **3**:203
medications and, **3**:202, **4**:57–58
nutrition and, **2**:27, 71
substance use and, **4**:61–63
alcohol, **4**:10–11, 61–62
barbiturates, **4**:10, 62
heroin, **4**:62
marijuana, **4**:11, 62
methamphetamine, **4**:62, 63
PCP, **4**:62
See also La Leche League, Lactation consultant, Smoking
Breast milk
disease transmission through, **3**:152
Brockovich, Erin
case study, **1**:21
photograph, **1**:20
Bronchi, **1**:40, 54
Bronchitis, **1**:39, 40, 57, **4**:12, 13, 49, 55
Brownell, Kelly, **2**:126
Bruxism, **4**:52
Bulimia nervosa, **2**:110, 113, 114–115, 120–121, 127, 133, 134, **5**:103
death from, **2**:121
signs and symptoms of, **2**:120
treatment for, **2**:121
Bullying, **3**:69, 85, 101, 114, **5**:2, 26–30, 45, 89–90,
causes, **5**:29–30
coping with, **5**:31–32
cyberbullying, **5**:2, 27–29
Teen Opinions on, **5**:29
hate incidents and, **3**:53, 101 **5**:30
LGBTQI and, **3**:42, 51, 53, 85, **5**:27
Phoebe Prince case, **5**:31
suicide and, **3**:51, **5**:28–29
Buprenorphine, **4**:84
Burns, **1**:97, 177–178, **3**:208, 210, **4**:52, 60
chemical, **1**:88, 181
ear candles and, **1**:90
fireworks and, **1**:149
first-degree, **1**:97
major, **1**:178
minor, **1**:177
poisoning and, **1**:181
second-degree, **1**:97
sunburn, **1**:22, 95, 97
third-degree, **1**:178

Caffeine, **4**:19, 21, 47
breastfeeding and, **3**:202, **4**:21, 62
breast soreness and, **3**:6
dehydration and, **2**:29, 170
dietary supplements and, **2**:42
in energy drinks, **2**:44
ephedra, use with, **2**:97, 98, 184, **4**:21
PMS and, **3**;23
sleep, and, **1**:7, **4**:21, **5**:102
in sports supplements, **2**:178, 180*t*

1: Health Basics
2: Nutrition and Physical Fitness
3: Sexual Health and Development
4: Alcohol, Tobacco, and Other Drugs
5: Mental and Emotional Health

Calcium
absorption of, **2**:9, 21, 26, 28
bone health and, **1**:109, **2**:14, 26, 175, **4**:28
deficiencies, **2**:18, 75, 176
dietary sources of, **2**:11, 77*t*
dietary supplements, **2**:45*t*, 179
functions of, **2**:11, 26–27
lead absorption and, **1**:19recommended dietary intake, **2**:27*t*
Calories
comparisons, **2**:85*t*, 87
empty, **2**:3
expended (burned), **2**:150, 153
food energy, **2**:2
estimating daily needs, **2**:25–26, 70–73, 72*t*, 80–81, 86
See also Kilocalorie
Cancer, **1**:4, 13, 14, 17–19, 21, 61, 67–69, 88, 110–112, **2**:65, 69, 75, 153, 176, 182, 183, **3**:15, 46, 146, 154,160, **4**:6, 14, 27, 31, 52, 55, 67, 97, **5**:79
antioxidants and, **2**:9
biopsy, **1**:47, 68, **3**:161
breast, **1**:68, 69, 110, 111, **2**:65, **3**:7, 9, 203
bone marrow transplants, **1**:69, 71
cervical, **1**:108, 110, 115, **3**:159–160
chemotherapy, **1**:68
deaths, **1**:67–68, 69, 95, **4**:13, 27
exercise and, **1**:11, **2**:161
children and, **1**:68
Kaposi's sarcoma, **3**:154
liver cancer, **1**:46, 68, **2**:65, **4**:29
lymphoma, **3**:154
malignant tumors, **1**:68
marijuana and, **4**:15, 55
ovarian, **1**:68, 88, **3**:46
radiotherapy, **1**:68–69, 95
skin cancers, **1**:23, 69, 95–97, 111, **2**:28
smoking and, **1**:4, 68, **2**:179, 182, **4**:12, 13, 15, 44, 49, 55
stomach, **1**:45, **4**:14, 55
testicular, **1**:69, 111–112, **3**:14, 46, **4**:53
Carcinogens, **1**:13, 17–19, 27, 68, 88, **4**:12, 14
Cardiopulmonary resuscitation (CPR), **1**:51, 178, 179, 180, 182, **3**:193, 208, 211
Cardiovascular
disease, **1**:51–54, **2**:64, 65*t*, **4**:12, 24, 50, 53, 55, 67, **5**:106
health, **2**:147, 148, 153, 161
risk, **2**:90, **4**:12, 50, 53
system, **1**:51, **2**:153, **4**:24, 50
Carotenodermia, **2**:14
Carpenter, Karen, **2**:117, 118*f*
Carrier (of disease or genetic trait), **1**:69–70, **3**:84
Case studies
Amber (transgender discrimination and sources of support), **3**:43
Brockovich, Erin, **1**:20*f*, 21
bullying (Phoebe Prince), **5**:31
conflict of interest (Jesse Gelsinger), **5**:58
Hurricane Katrina, **1**:171, 172*f*
infant killed by methamphetamine in breast milk, **4**:63
Gelsinger, Jesse, conflict of interest, **5**:58
methamphetamine and breastfeeding, **4**:63
overhydration and teens, **2**:168
Prince, Phoebe (bullying), **5**:31
sexting in Washington state, **5**:53–54
Cataracts, **1**:23, **4**:28
Cellulite, **2**:97
Cellulitis, **4**:52
Centers for Disease Control and Prevention (CDC), **1**:106, 107, 108, 145, **2**:22, 24, 30, 62, 64, 67, 70, 145, 148, 164, **3**:191, 218, **4**:113, **5**:10, 59, 82, 119–120,122
Central nervous system (CNS), **4**:4, 8, 10, 14, 19–25, 45, 47, 61, **5**:164, 166
Cerebellum, **4**:47

Cerebral cortex, **4**:47
Cerebrovascular accident (CVA), **1**:22, 52–54, 64–65, 70, 104, 109, **2**:24, 64, 65*t*, 69, 75, 97, 160, **4**:12, 19, 50, 51, 53, 67, **5**:109, 117
Cerumen, **1**:90
Chancre, **3**:162
Chaplain/pastoral counselor, **1**:37
Cheeseburger Bill (American Personal Responsibility in Food Consumption, 2005), **2**:62
Chemical accident, **1**:165, 176–177
Chemical emergency. *See* Chemical accident
Chemotherapy, **1**:68
Child health care, **3**:193, **5**:15
  arranging for infants, **3**:207–208
  developmental milestones, **3**:218
  emergencies, **3**:45, 193, 207, 208, 210–211, 216
    how to help a child who is choking, **3**:208*t*
  vaccinations, **1**:46, 108, 116, **3**:207
  See also Baby care
Children's Health Insurance Program (CHIP), **3**:220
Chiropractor, **1**:36
Chlamydia, **1**:110, **3**:146, 156, 163
Choking, **1**:42, 178, 182, **3**:211, 216, 217
  choking child, helping, **3**:193, 208, 211
  choking game, **5**:117–118
  inhalants and, **4**:32
Cholesterol, **1**:51, 52, **4**:26
  in foods, **2**:33, 88
  high cholesterol, **1**:52–54, 60, 64, **2**:75
  levels, **2**:90, 175, **4**:29, 43
  screening, **1**:109, 110
Chronic diseases and disorders, **1**:12, 35, 50–71
  chronic infections, **1**:46
    upper respiratory infections, **1**:38, 39–44, 48
    urinary tract infections, **1**:44–45, 64, **2**:129, **3**:141, 153, **5**;152
  chronic insomnia, **1**:8, **2**:129
  chronic pain, **1**:3, 67, **5**:109
  digestive, endocrine, and urinary system diseases, **1**:58–62
  liver disease, **1**;46–47, **3**:153, **4**:6, 50–51, 56
  respiratory system diseases, **1**:54–58
  See also Bronchitis, Chronic obstructive pulmonary disease, Crohn's disease, Cystic fibrosis, Dementia, Diabetes, Emphysema, Heart disease, Hepatitis, Hypertension, Kidney disease, Multiple sclerosis (MS), Musculoskeletal system diseases, Parkinson's disease, Seizure disorder, Sickle cell disease
Chronic obstructive pulmonary disease (COPD), **1**:56–57, **2**:146
Chronic substance use, **4**:48–49, 51, 52
  alcohol, **4**:50, 97
  coffee, **4**:62
  See also MDMA (Ecstasy)
Circadian rhythm, **1**:8
Circumcision, **3**:11, 14–17
  female genital mutilation (FGM), **3**:15–17
  male circumcision, **3**:11, 14–15, 199–200, 208
    as human rights issue, **3**:17–18
Cirrhosis, **1**:46, **2**:65, **4**:6, 51
Cliques, **3**:32, 43, 68, 69, **5**:44
Club drugs, **4**:10, 22–25
  breastfeeding and, **4**:60
  See also GHB (Xyrem), Ketamine, LSD, MDMA (Ecstasy), Methamphetamine, Rohypnol (roofies)
CNS depressants, **4**:8–10
  abuse potential and tolerance, **4**:10
  barbiturates, **4**:8
  benzodiazepines, **4**:8–9, 10
  depressant club drugs, **4**:10
  effects of, **4**:8
  GHB (Xyrem), **3**:112, **4**:10
  Nembutal, **4**:8
  pregnancy and nursing, use during, **4**:10–11
  psychosis and, **4**:9
  Rohypnol, **3**:112, **4**:10
Coca-Cola, **4**:22
Cocaine, **4**:19, 20, 22, 46, 50, 59
Coca leaves, **4**:19, 40
CocoaVia health snacks, **2**:36

1: Health Basics
2: Nutrition and Physical Fitness
3: Sexual Health and Development
4: Alcohol, Tobacco, and Other Drugs
5: Mental and Emotional Health

Cognitive
  abilities, **1**:62
  changes, **1**:66, **3**:1, 18, 24–25, 31*t*, **5**:17
  deficits, **2**:129, 164, **5**:146
  development, **2**:128, **5**:23
  distractions, **1**:136
  function, **1**:54, 62, **4**:48, 78, **5**:106, 139, 143, 164
Cognitive-behavioral therapy (CBT), **2**:118, 121, 122, 125, 131–134, **4**:82, 83, **5**:84, 85–86, 111–112, 116, 156–159
Coitus interruptus, **3**:133
Colostrum, **3**:201
Combustible, **1**:147–148
Communication skills, **3**:109, **5**:18–19, 22, 41
Compensatory
  Behaviors, **5**:103
  learning strategies, **5**:139
Complex carbohydrates, **2**:3–4, 18, 170, 175
Conceptual skills, **5**:143
Concerta (methylphenidate), **4**:20–21
Concussion, **1**:157–158, **2**:164–166, **5**:117
  dangers of, **1**:158, **2**:164
  frequency, **2**:164–165
  high-risk groups, **2**:164*t*
  leading causes, **2**:164*t*
  recovery from, **2**:165
  warning signs and symptoms, **2**:166*t*
Condoms, **1**:46, **3**:14, 90, 91–94, 132–134, 139–141, 145–147, 149, 152, 155–156, 159–162
  dealing with objections to, **3**:91*t*
  female condom, **3**:139, 142, 145
  talking about, **3**:91–94
Conduct disorder (CD), **5**:101
Confidentiality, **1**:113, **5**:157
  adoption and, **5**:16–17
  and mental health treatment, **5**:157
  minors and health care, **1**:113, **3**:150–152, **5**:157
  and sources of support: **5**:119, 157
Conflict of interest, **5**:58, 59
Consciousness, loss of, **1**:42, 47, 54, 65, 152, 157, 158, 168, 178, 179, 180, 181, 182, **2**:166, **3**:208, **4**:4, 6, **5**:117, 148
Consent
  for abortions, **3**:151, 184
  for health care, **3**:149–152
  inability to give, **1**:182, **3**:17, 111
  informed, **5**:58
  sexual, **3**:77–78, 89–90, 111–112, 150
    legal age, **3**:82, 83*t*
    sex without consent, **3**:109
  for sterilization, **3**:145
  See also Age of consent, Rape/sexual assault
Constipation, **1**:10, 57, 66, 68, 114, **2**:45, 89, 91, 92, 119, 120, 124, 129, **3**:179, 187, 199, **4**:22, 25, 50, **5**:167
Consumer Reports, **2**:43, 179
Consumerism, **5**:55–56
Contraception (birth control), **3**:132–146, **5**:49
  abstinence as, **3**:129–130, 145
  artificial methods, **3**:136–146
    barrier birth control, **3**:24, 132, 139–144, 141–143*t*
      cervical cap, **3**:140, 143
      condoms, **3**:91*t*, 132, 133, 139, 140, 141, 145, 149
      diaphragm, **3**:24, 139, 140, 141, 145
      female condom, **3**:139, 142, 145
      spermicide, **3**:139, 140, 143, 144
      sponge, **3**:24, 140, 142, 144
    intrauterine device (IUD), **3**:139, 145, 161
    medications, **3**:133, 136, 137–138*t*, 139, 150
      birth control pills, **3**:132, 133, 136, 137, 145
      implant, **3**:136, 138
      morning-after pill (emergency contraception), **3**:136, 138, 145

patch, **3**:136, 145
ring, **3**:136, 145
birth control shot, **3**:137, 145
choosing, **3**:132–133
effectiveness of methods, **3**:145*t*
methods of, **3**:132*f*
natural methods, **3**:133–136
breastfeeding as, **3**:135
calendar method, **3**:135, 145
coitus interruptus, **3**:133, 145
fertility awareness-based, **3**:133–135, 145
outercourse, **3**:133, 134
rhythm method, **3**:133
sex during menstrual period, **3**:135–136
withdrawal, **3**:133, 145
sterilization, **3**:144–145
Control group, **5**:60
Controlled studies, **5**:60
Coparenting and family relationships, **3**:206–207
Coping, **5**:82–83
with abuse, **5**:31–32
with body changes, **2**:123
with bullying, **5**:31–32
with changes of adolescence, **3**:24
with chronic pain, **1**:67
with depression, **5**:120
with divorce, **5**:10, 13–14
emotion-focused coping, **5**:83
family and, **5**:9
with hate crimes, **5**:31–32
with illness, **1**;57, 62
support for families/caregivers **1**;57, 62
with learning disabilities, **5**:139–142
with loss, **5**:129, 132, 134, 155
mechanisms, **3**:102, 200
problem solving, **5**:83
problem-focused coping, **5**:83–84
skills, **5**:84, 116, 118
strategies, **5**:86, 116, 118
with stress, **5**:9, 10, 77, 82–86, 155
with substance use, **4**:102–106, 111
types of coping behavior, **5**:83
Coronary artery disease (CAD), **1**:51–52
Corticosteroids, **4**:2, 27
side effects, **4**:28–29
Cosmetic surgery, **2**:111, **3**:8, 9, 17, 26, 48, **5**:56
Labiaplasty, **3**:17
Teen Opinions on, **3**:8
See also Circumcision, Plastic surgery
Counselors, **1**:37, **2**:131, **3**:69, 76, 100, 108–110, 184, **4**:82, 106, **5**:15, 103, 161, 163
family, **5**:11
financial, **5**:82
grief, **5**:134
nutritional, **2**:121, 131, 133
pastoral, **1**:37
peer, **5**:84, 85
school, **1**:12, 163, **3**:51, 86, 109, 114, 117, **4**:79, 100, 103, 104, 115, **5**:15, 33, 38, 125, 157, 163, 164
Cow's milk, **2**:21, 27, 30, 78, 183, **3**:5
Creutzfeldt-Jakob disease, **2**:22–23
Crohn's disease, **1**:58, **2**:95
Cross-dressing, **3**:40–41
Cryotherapy, **3**:161
Culture
acculturation, **5**:44–46
expectations about appearance, **2**:63, 125, 134
bathing habits and, **1**:86
circumcision and, **3**:14, 16
cultural influences, **5**:44–46
dating and marriage and, **3**:70, 73, 74, **5**:18, 43, 46
eating disorders and, **2**:107, 134
emotion, experience and expression of, **5**:113, 131
family and, **1**:3, **5**:9, 18
gender roles and, **3**:39–40, 107, 204
homophobia and, **3**:35, 86
identity and, **3**:31–33
individuality and, **3**:30–32, **5**:46
influences on wellness, **1**:2–3
parenting and, **3**:204
personal space, **5**:44
rites of passage and, **3**:19
sex and, **3**:77, 79, 81
subcultures, **1**:2
substance use and, **4**:11, 14, 16–17, 40, 70–73, 76, 108, **5**:18
suicide and, **5**:120, 122
taboos, **3**:84, 87, 88

1: Health Basics
2: Nutrition and Physical Fitness
3: Sexual Health and Development
4: Alcohol, Tobacco, and Other Drugs
5: Mental and Emotional Health

Cuticle, **1**:86
Cyclothymia, **5**:113
Cystic fibrosis, **1**:57, **3**:182
Cystitis, **1**:44–45

Dairy products, **2**:3, 39
allergies, **1**:55
calcium and, **2**:27
Crohn's disease and, **1**:58
the food pyramid, and, **2**:18
lacto-ovo vegetarians, **2**:176
micronutrients in, **2**:9–11*t*
and tuberculosis (TB), **2**:21
unpasteurized, and HIV, **3**:154
Deaths
from accidents, **1**:127
motor vehicle, **1**:127, 135, 175, 179, **4**:7
alcohol-related, **4**:6, 7, 66, 97
All-cause mortality rates, **2**:147
Alzheimer's disease, complications, **1**:64
from animal bites, **1**:184
cancer, **1**:67–69, 95, **4**:13
dehydration and, **2**:14
from dietary/sports supplements, **2**:42, 97, 98, 180, 184
diets and fasting, related to, **2**:89, 115
disasters, natural, **1**;171, 174
eating disorders, **2**:108, 114, 117, 121, 122, 124, 133
electrocution, **1**:147, 179
encephalitis, **1**:47
energy-drink related, **2**:44
fires, **1**:145
fireworks, **1**:149
from foodborne illness, **2**:22
head injury (TBI) and, **1**:158, **2**:164, 165, **3**:206, **5**:147–148
heat-related, **1**:22, 168, **4**:24
heart disease and, **1**:51
homicide, **1**:179, **4**:31, 64
hypoglycemia and, **1**:60
infectious disease-related, **1**:70, 105, **3**:146, 155, 159, 162
influenza, **1**:40
melanoma, **1**:69, 95
meningitis, **1**:48
poisoning, **1**:164
renal (kidney) failure, **1**:60–62
self-injury/risk-taking behaviors, **5**:115, 117–118
sickle cell disease, **1**:70
skin cancer, **1**:95
substance use related, **1**:139, 164, **4**:6, 10, 19, 23, 24, 25, 32, 40, 52, 63, 64, 66, 67, 97, **5**:168
sudden infant death syndrome (SIDS), **1**:107, **3**:192–193, 214–215, **4**:55, 58
suicide, **4**:31, 64, **5**;31, 119–123
tuberculosis (TB), **1**:43
violence, **4**:31, **5**:38
water-related, **1**:151, 152
workplace, **1**:179
Defensiveness, **3**:93, **4**:115, **5**:86, 88, 92, 93, 159
Defibrillation, **1**:51–52
Dehydration, **1**:61, 88, **2**:7, 8, 14, 29, 88, 89, 94, 95, 120, 129, 133, 147, 167, 169–171, 175, 181–182*t*, **4**:53
Delirium, **4**:10, 23, **5**:106, 152
Delusions, **2**:125, **3**:200, **4**:30, 32, **5**:149–153
Delusional disorder, **5**:152–153
Dementia, **1**:54, 62, 63, 66, **3**:154, 162, **5**:106, 152
Dental care
costs, **1**:37, 38, 105
emergency, **1**:185
HIV and, **3**:152, 155
pregnancy and, **3**:188
team, **1**:37
Dental health, **1**:101–105
bad breath (halitosis), **1**:103–104, **4**:52
bleaches, **1**:102–103
braces, **1**:37, 104–105, 155
brushing, **1**:101–105, **2**:71, **3**:188
cavities, **1**:18, 38, 101–102, 105

dental anxiety, **1**:105
dental caries, **1**:101
erosion, **2**:46, 129, **4**:52
FASD and, **5**:147
flossing, **1**:102, 103
fluoride and, **1**:18, 101, 102
gingivitis, **1**:104
hygiene, **1**:37, 101–104, **4**:52
injury, **1**:185, **2**:127
orthodontic appliances (braces), **1**:104–105, 155
periodontitis, **1**:37, 104, **3**:188
plaque, **1**:103–104
retainer, **1**:105
screenings, **1**:110
sensitivity, **1**:102, 103, **2**:120
tartar, **1**:104
tooth decay, **1**:18, 101–102, 105, **2**:120, **4**:52
stages of, **1**:102*f*
dental treatments (special), **1**:104
Depression, **2**:146, **5**:108–112
abuse and, **3**:106, 107
ADHD and, **5**:136, 137
bullying, **5**:28
causes of, **5**:109–110
clinical depression, **5**:108
coping and, **5**:82, 120
eating/weight and, **1**:11, **2**:65, 81, 111
eating disorders and, **2**:111, 113, 120, 121, 122, 124, 125, 126, 130
encephalitis and, **1**:47
hormones and, **3**:24
LGBT and, **3**:37, 42, 51
loss and, **5**:133, 135
major depressive disorder (MDD), **2**:125, 126, **5**:108,
medications and, **3**:137, **4**:2, 8–9, 20, 22, 58, **5**:166
multiple sclerosis (MS) and, **1**:66
negative thinking and rumination, **5**:110–112
Parkinson's disease and, **1**:66
pellagra and, **2**:16
postpartum, **3**:199–200, **5**:152
premenstrual (PMS), **3**:22
risk of, **5**:110
self-esteem and, **5**:3, 5
sexual harassment and, **3**:116
sleep and, **1**:7
stress and, **5**:79, 87
substance use and, **4**:4, 6, 8–10, 13, 19, 20, 21, 22, 24, 30, 44, 48, 109
types of, **5**:108–109, 112–114
violence and, **5**:33
Dermatologist, **1**:92, 99
Development
child to adult transition, **3**:18–19
individual differences, **3**:18
rites of passage, **3**:19
stages of adolescence, **3**:18
menstruation (the period), **3**:3, 20–24
when to seek medical advice about, **3**:22*t*
See also Menarche, Menopause
puberty, **3**:19–20
in females, **2**:25, 29, 109–110, **3**:2, 5–6, 20, 77, 84, **5**:6
hormones, **1**:99, **3**:6, 20, 24, 84, 129, **5**:109
in intersex individuals, **3**:43–50
in males, **2**:25, **3**:6, 20, 77, 84, **4**:27
physical changes and, **1**:88, 99, **2**:25, 109, **3**:19–20, **5**:6
transgender individuals and, **3**:40
self-image and self-esteem, **3**:25–26, **5**:6
body modifications, **1**:97–99, **3**:26–30, **5**:2, 114
piercings, **1**:46, 98–99, **3**:16, 26, 28–30, 85, 152, 155, 192, **5**:2, 114
tattoos, **1**:97–99, **3**:26–30, 152, 155, **5**:2, 114
Teen Opinions on, **3**:27
eating disorders, **3**:25
self-consciousness, **2**:117, 126, **3**:26, **5**:24, 44, 56
social, emotional, and cognitive changes, **3**:24–34
culture and family, **2**:125, 134, **3**:30–32, **5**:9, 18, 45–46
dating, **3**:34, 70–72, 73, 78, 81, 84, 86, 95–96, 112–113, **4**:7, **5**:22, 45–46, 48
emotional and cognitive changes, **3**:24–25
the five I's of adolescent development, **3**:30, 31*t*

1: Health Basics
2: Nutrition and Physical Fitness
3: Sexual Health and Development
4: Alcohol, Tobacco, and Other Drugs
5: Mental and Emotional Health

Development (*continued*)
friendships, **1**:2, **2**:161, **3**:32–34, 68–69, 74, 84, **5**:4, 21–25, 52
changes in, **3**:34
growing within the context of, **5**:22
identity and, **2**:135, **3**:25, 26, 30–33, 50, 52, 70, 75, 84, 85, 87, 88, 100. **5**:5, 8, 9, 16, 17, 19, 22, 25, 34, 55, 130
peer orientation, **3**:32
privacy and, **1**:113, **3**:33, 34, 89, 151
sexual identity, **3**:33, 75, 84, 85, 87
social and emotional changes, **3**:30–34
roles within family, **3**:33–34
See also Gender identity; Intersex; LGBTQI, Sexual orientation, Transgender
Developmental disabilities, **5**:107, 142–149
See also Autism spectrum disorders (ASD), Intellectual disabilities/ mental retardation, Pervasive developmental disorders (PDDs)
Developmental milestones, **3**:218
DHA (dihydroxyeacetone), **1**:97
Diabetes, **1**:3, 59–60, 54, 109, 111, **2**:160, **4**:53
blood sugar, **1**:3, 59–60, 65, 109, 111
comorbidity/risk, **1**:61, 64, 104, **2**:24, 64, 68, 69, 75,121, 176, **3**:157, 189, **5**:109
complications, **1**:59–60, 93, 103
costs (estimated), **2**:146*t*
diagnosis/screening, **1**:109, 110, 111, **2**:24
exercise and physical activity, **1**:11, **2**:160
genetics and, **1**:3, 60
gestational, **1**:59, **3**:182
heart disease and, **1**:52, 60
hypoglycemia, **1**:60
insulin, **1**:59–60, 111, **2**:4, 10, 12, 128, **3**:182, **4**:53
ketoacidosis, **1**:60
obesity and, **1**:11, 109, **2**:64, 65*t*, 93, 96
prediabetes, **1**:59
sleep and, **1**:7
stress and, **5**:79
substance use and, **4**:6, 21,53
treatment for, **1**:60
types of, **1**:59
vision and, **1**:60
Diagnostic and Statistical Manual of Mental Disorders (DSM), **2**:116, **3**:37, **5**:100
Diagnostic criteria, **2**:122, 123, 126, 127, **4**:42–44, 78, **5**:100, 102, 108, 136, 139, 140, 143, 145, 149, 152
Diagnostic labels, **2**:116, 130, **3**:37, **5**:135–136, 140, 141, 148
stigma associated with, **2**:63, 116, **3**:49, **4**:109, **5**:110, 140, 141, 142
Teen Opinions on, **5**:142
Dialectical behavior therapy (DBT), **5**:116
Dialysis, **1**:61–62, 61*f*
Diarrhea, **1**:39, 40, 58, 68, 100, 114, **2**:16, 22, 91, 95, 120, 124, 170–171, 181, **3**:24, 153, 154, 161, 179, 180, 207, 210, **4**:20, 25, 60, 62, 84, **5**:167
See also Runner's diarrhea
Diet pills (stimulant), **2**:84, 117, **3**:25, **4**:19, 20, 50, 52, 58*t*, **5**:56
Dietary Guidelines for Americans, **2**:16–19, 74–76
Dietary supplements, **1**:23, **2**:18, 28, 32, 42–46, 63–64, 97–99, 125, 128, **4**:30, 31, 61, **5**:116, 141, 167, 168
Consumer Reports (2010) on, **2**:179
contamination, **2**:43, 179
criticism of, **2**:177
Dietary Supplement and Nonprescription Drug Consumer Protection Act (2006), **2**:42–43, 177
Dietary Supplement Health and Education Act (DSHEA, 1994), **2**:21–22, 42, 177

energy drinks, **1**:7, **2**:41, 44, 177, **4**:21, **5**:167
ephedra, **2**:97, 98, 184, **4**:21
evaluating, **2**:183*t*
need for, **2**:43–44, 128
popular supplements
pros and cons of, **2**:45–46
used by athletes, **2**:177–178
regulation of, **2**:20–22, 42–43, 177
safety of, **2**:42, 98*t*, 99, 177, 180–182*t*
summary of claims, evidence, and safety, **2**:180–182*t*
weight-loss supplements, **2**:64, 84, 97–99, 177, **4**:21
See also Selenium toxicity, Sports supplements
Dietitian/nutritionist, **1**:36, **2**:25, 70, 71, 82, 89*f*, 131, 175, 176
Diets
Atkins, **2**:88–91
detox diet, **2**:91
dieting, **2**:14, 26, 70, 75, 83, 108, 110, 112, 116, 117, 122, **5**:48, 56
fad diets and weight-loss aids, **2**:4, 63, 84, 87–91, 108, 113
high-fiber low-calorie diets, **1**:58, 109, **2**:88–89
high-protein diets, **2**:88, 90, 91, 173–175, 178, 181
ketogenic, **1**:65
low-calorie, low-fat diet, **2**:45, 86, 88, 90, 91, 93, 99
low-carbohydrate higher-fat diets, **1**:52, 65, **2**:4, 90–91
special diet for learning disabilities, **5**:141
vegetarian, **2**:17, 26, 44, 46, 119, 175–177
very low-calorie liquid diets and fasting (VLCLD), **2**:88–91, 122
wonder diets, **2**:88
Digestive, endocrine, and urinary system diseases, **1**:58–62
appendicitis, **1**:59
diabetes, **1**:59–60
renal (kidney) failure, **1**:60–62
See also Crohn's disease, Diabetes, Food intolerance, Gallstones, Kidney disease
Digestive system, **1**:17, 40, 45, 55, 58–59
Digestive system infections
giardia, **1**:17
hepatitis, **1**:17, 45–47, **4**:26, 56, 60
See also Gastritis, Hepatitis, Gastroenteritis
Disasters, **1**:165–176
chemical accidents or attacks, **1**:165, 176–177
earthquakes, **1**:142, 165, 166–168, 174, **5**:80, 127
emergency supplies, **1**:165–166, 171, 175
extreme heat, **1**:22, 142, 165, 168–169, **2**:168, **3**:191
family emergency planning, **1**:166–167
fires, **1**:14, 22, 148, 165, 166, 173–175
floods, **1**:22, 24, 25, 134, 142, 144, 165, 169, 171, 173
hurricane, **1**:22, 134, 165, 166, 169–172, 173, **5**:127
landslide, **1**:165, 169, 172–173
nuclear, **1**:20, 165, 174, 176
terrorist attacks, **1**:165, 175, 176, **5**:127
thunderstorms and lightning, **1**:152, 169, 173–174
tornadoes, **1**:165, 166, 169, 173
tsunami, **1**:165, 166, 174
winter storms, **1**:175
Discipline (professional specialty), **1**:35
Discipline
parenting and, **3**:102, 106, 205–206, **5**:12, 30
self-discipline, **2**:24, 126
Diseases and treatment
acute disease, **1**:35
blood and systemic diseases, **1**:67–71
brain and nervous system diseases, **1**:62–66
cardiovascular system diseases, **1**:51–54
heart disease, **1**:51–54
infectious disease, **1**:38–39
inheritable disease, **1**:35
See also Allergies, Alzheimer's disease, Appendix/appendicitis, Arrhythmia, Asthma, Blood and systemic diseases, Brain and nervous system diseases, Cancer, Cerebrovascular accident (CVA), Heart disease, Infectious disease, Kidney disease, Pandemic

1: Health Basics
2: Nutrition and Physical Fitness
3: Sexual Health and Development
4: Alcohol, Tobacco, and Other Drugs
5: Mental and Emotional Health

Dissociative disorders, **5:**107, 149
Disulfrum (Antabuse), **4:**83–84
Divorce/separation, **5:**10–12
coping with, **5:**10, 13–14
feelings of abandonment, **5:**11
DNA (deoxyribonucleic acid), **1:**68, **2:**12, **3:**13
Domestic violence, **3:**37, 68, 101, **4:**65, **5:**11, 32, 37, 110, 127
See also Abusive relationships
Double-blind study, **5:**60
Douching, **3:**156, 187
Doula, **1:**2, **3:**193
Down syndrome, **5:**145–146
See also Developmental disabilities, Intellectual disabilities/mental retardation
Dreams, **1:**8–9
Drinking water, **1:**17–18
Driving under the influence (DUI), **1:**130, 135, 139, **4:**7–8, 66, 69, 75, 98, 110, 114
Driving while intoxicated (DWI), **1:**130, 135, 136, **4:**7–8, 49, 61, 64, 77, 110
Dronabinol, **4:**14
See also Marijuana
Drugs, types of
alcohol, **4:**3–8
club drugs, **4:**10, 22–25
CNS depressants, **4:**8–10
hallucinogens, **4:**16–19
inhalants, **4:**31–32
ketamine, **4:**10, 17, 23, 50, 60
marijuana, **4:**14–16
opioids, **4:**25–26
prescription medications, **4:**2–3
steroids, **4:**26–31
stimulants, **4:**19–22
tobacco, **4:**11–14
See also Alcohol, Alcohol use, Club drugs, CNS depressants, Hallucinogens, Inhalants, Marijuana, Opioids, Prescription medications, Steroids, Stimulants, Tobacco
DSHEA law, **2:**42
Duodenum, **2:**93–94, 96
Dust mites, **1:**26–27
Dysfunctional
behaviors/interactions, **5:**116
thinking, **5:**116
Dyslipidemia, **4:**53
See also Cholesterol

Ear infection, **1:**39, 90–91
Earthquakes, **1:**167–168
Eating disorders, **5:**103
anorexia mirabilis, **2:**115
anorexia nervosa, **2:**108, 116–119
binge eating (compulsive eating), **2:**121–122
body image, **2:**108–112
bulimia nervosa, **2:**120–121
cognitive behavioral therapy (CBT), **2:**118, 133
Diagnostic and Statistical Manual of Mental Disorders (DSM-IV-TR) on, **2:**116
eating disorders not otherwise specified (EDNOS), **2:**122–130
anorexia athletica, **2:**123–124
body dysmorphic disorder (BDD), **2:**124–125
common types of, **2:**123
examples of, **2:**122–123
muscle dysmorphia, **2:**125–126
night eating syndrome (NES), **2:**129–130
orthorexia nervosa, **2:**126–127
pica, **2:**127–128
Prader-Willi syndrome, **2:**123, 128–129
sleep-related eating disorder (SRED), **2:**122, 129–130
medical issues associated with, **2:**129*t*
overview of, **2:**112–115
classifications of eating disorders, **2:**113

deaths from, **2**:114
history of, **2**:115–116
risk factors, **2**:112–113
prevention of, **2**:134–135
sexual orientation and, **2**:113
statistics on, **2**:113–115
treatment, **2**:130–133
cognitive behavioral therapy (CBT), **2**:131–132
family therapy, **2**:132
health care team, **2**:130–131
interventions, **2**:131
treatment goals, **2**:132–134
See also Anorexia nervosa, Binge eating (compulsive eating), Body image, Bulimia nervosa, Refeeding syndrome
Eating habits, **1**:10–11
Eating, healthy
coupon and recipe websites, **2**:35*t*
Dietary Guidelines for Americans, **2**:16–19, 74–76
Dietary Reference Intakes (DRIs), **2**:15
for adolescents and young adults, **2**:27*t*
eating out tips, **2**:40–42
farmers' markets, **2**:37
Food Guide Pyramid, history of, **2**:16–19
food labels, **2**:35–36
generally recognized as safe (GRAS) ingredients, **2**:20
grocery shopping
by the aisle, **2**:34*t*
on a budget, tips for, **2**:33*t*
marketing methods and, **2**:32–34
MyPyramid/MyPlate, **2**:16–18, 17*f*, 73, 74
nutrition in America, **2**:23–25
packaging and, **2**:34
Poison Squad, **2**:20
Recommended Dietary Allowances (RDA), **2**:14–16
Recommended Nutrient Intake (RNI), **2**:14
shelf life, **2**:20
supermarket savvy, **2**:32–40
See also Antioxidants; Cow's milk; Dairy products; Dietary supplements; Eggs; Food allergies; Food safety; Foodborne illness; Meats, poultry, fish, and deli; Nutrition and adolescent needs; Nutrition basics, Organic and natural foods, Produce
Ecosystems, **1**:12
Ecstasy (X, MDMA), **4**:17, 19, 20, 50, 51
Ectomorph, **2**:69
Ectopic pregnancy, **3**:161
Eggs (chicken)
allergies, **1**:106, **2**:30, 31
food safety, and, **1**:165, **2**:39, **3**:154, 191
nutrients/nutritional value, **2**:5*f*, 9–13*t*
vegetarian diet and, **2**:176
Ejaculation, **3**:11–13, 45, 89, 133, 139, 140, 141, 144, 177
nocturnal emission, **3**:12
See also Preejaculate, Premature ejaculation
Electrical shock, **1**:178–179
Electrocautery, **3**:161
Electrocution, **1**:147
Electrolysis, **1**:88
Electronic waste (e-waste), **1**:18
Elimination disorders, **5**:101
Embryo, **3**:3, 4, 9, 21, 177, 183, 186
Emotional
management skills, **3**:31, **5**:22, 116
regulation, **3**:24, 25
Emphysema, **1**:14, 57–58, **4**:12, 44, 49, 55
Encephalitis, **1**:22, 47, 65
Endocrine system, **1**:58, **4**:53
Endomorph, **2**:69
Endorphins, **5**:88, 115
Energy drinks, **2**:44
Environment
steps to protect, **1**:16–17
wellness and, **1**:3–4
Environmental fitness, **1**:12–27
biological pollution, **1**:24–27
Brockovich, Erin, **1**:20*f*, 21
electronic waste (e-waste), **1**:18
environmental protection, **1**:16–17
oil spills, **1**:21
pesticides, **1**:12, 15, 16, 17, 19–20, 26, 27
pollution, **1**:12–15

1: Health Basics
2: Nutrition and Physical Fitness
3: Sexual Health and Development
4: Alcohol, Tobacco, and Other Drugs
5: Mental and Emotional Health

Environmental fitness (*continued*)
sunlight and ultraviolet rays, effects of, **1**:22–23
See also Air pollution, Asbestos, Biological pollution, Fuel emissions, Lead, Noise pollution, Particle pollution, Radioactive pollution, Radon, Smog, Soil pollution, Thermal pollution, Uranium, Water pollution, Work or study environment pollution
Ephedra (ephedrine) use, **2**:97, 98, 184, **4**:21
Epidemic, **1**:39
Epididymitis, **3**:156
Epilepsy. *See* Seizure disorder
Epiphyses, **2**:162
Episiotomy, **3**:198
Eugenics, **3**:145
Euphemism, **5**:45
Exercise, **1**:11–12
Exercise and physical activity
ABCs of exercise, **2**:148–154
barriers to exercise and safety issues, **2**:157–161
benefits of exercise, **2**:145, 147
bones and, **2**:149
Compendium of Physical Activities, **2**:153
components, **2**:149
duration, **2**:149
endurance exercises, **2**:148
frequency of, **2**:149
Haskell, Bill, on, **2**:153
heart disease and, **2**:152
individualized exercise plan, **2**:150
injuries related to sports, **2**:162–166
injury related to exercise, **2**:147–148
Institute of Medicine of the National Academies (IOM) on, **2**:152
intensity level, **2**:149, 151
jogging, **2**:150
maximal heart rate method, **2**:150, 151*t*
metabolic equivalent (MET), **2**:153–154
moderate exercise, **2**:74, 146–148, 150, 152, 154, 155*t*, 157, 160–161
overload principle, **2**:151–152
percentage of people exercising, **2**:145–146, 148
Physical Activity Guidelines for Americans, **2**:154
relative physical activity intensity, **2**:150
resistance exercises, **2**:148–149, 153, 155
secondary lifestyle, cost of, **2**:146–148
signs and symptoms of intolerance to, **2**:156*t*
sore muscles, **2**:157
special exercise considerations for
individuals with cancer, **2**:161
individuals with diabetes or heart disease, **2**:160
individuals with disabilities, **2**:160
pregnant women, **2**:161
specificity principle, **2**:153
sports nutrition, **2**:167–176
target heart rate, **2**:150
types of exercise, **2**:148
vigorous exercise, **2**:155
weight-bearing exercise, **2**:148–149, 153
See also Absolute physical activity intensity, Aerobic, Dietary supplements, Injury related to exercise, Muscle building, Sports injuries, Sports nutrition, Sports supplements
Explicit, **5**:43, 160
sexually explicit, **3**:96, **5**:27, 49–52
See also Autism spectrum disorders (ASD), Social norms
Extreme heat, **1**:168–169
Eyes
Akanthemoeba keratitis (AK), **1**:100
anaphylaxis and, **1**:182
cataracts, **1**:23
color and hepatitis, **1**:46
diabetes and, **1**:60

exams, **1**:110
health, **1**:89–90
hygiene, **1**:89–90
irritation, from
chemical accident, **1**:176–177
mold, **1**:25
pollution, **1**:14, 24
volatile organic compounds (VOC), **1**:27
lice and, **1**:93–94
macular degeneration, **1**:23
movements in sleep, **1**:6, 8
protection
during natural disasters, **1**:166
in sports, **1**:155
from sun, **1**:23
retinopathy, **1**:97
sickle cell disease and damage, **1**:70
stye, **1**:49
UV rays, damage from, **1**:23

Fainting, **1**:179–180
Falls, **1**:180
precautions, **1**:160–161
Family therapists, **5**:162
Feces, **2**:23, **3**:154
Federal Food, Drug, and Cosmetic Act (FD&C Act), **2**:21
Feeding and eating disorders, **5**:101
Fetal alcohol spectrum disorders (FASD), **3**:191, **4**:61, **5**:143, 146–147
Fiber, dietary sources of, **2**:79*t*
Field, Allison E., **2**:75
Fingernails, **1**:86
Fire safety, **1**:144–145
barbecues, **1**:148
electrical hazards, **1**:146–147
fireworks safety, **1**:149–150
heating hazards, **1**:147
high-rise buildings and, **1**:146
household fire safety, **1**:145–146
kitchen fire hazards, **1**:147–148
outdoor residential fire hazards, **1**:148
personal fire safety, **1**:148
school and workplace fire safety, **1**:150–151
smoking safety, **1**:150
First aid, **1**:177–185
home first aid kits, **1**:177
lacerations (cuts), **1**:180–181
poisoning, **1**:181–182
snake, animal, and insect bites, **1**:182–185, 183*f*
tooth injury or loss (accidental), **1**:185
See also Anaphylaxis, Burns, Choking, Electrical shock, Fainting, Falls, Fractures (broken bones), Nosebleeds
Fistula, **1**:58
Flammable, **1**:144, 148, 149
Floods, **1**:22, 24, 25, 134, 142, 144, 165, 169, 171, 173
levees and, **1**:169
Flora, **3**:157
Flu. *See* Influenza
Fluoride, **1**:18, 101, 102
Folic acid, **1**:109, **2**:10*t*, 45*t*, **3**:192
Folliculitis, **1**:49
Food
availability/access to, **1**:4, **2**:24, 25, 32, 6
contamination, **1**:15, 19, 20, 21, 24, 26, 46, 85, 164–165, **2**:20–23, 35, 38–39, 43, **3**:154, 190–191, 202
ethnic food, **1**:2
fast food / junk food, **1**:1, **2**:6, 24, 25, 40, 41,42, 61, 62, 74, 85*t*, **5**:61
labels, **2**:14, 33, 35–36, 40, 74, 87
nonperishable, **1**:166, **2**:20
organic and natural, **1**:19, **2**:40
perishable, **2**:20
See also Food allergies, Food intolerance, Food safety, Foodborne illness
Food allergies, **1**:55, **2**:30–32
Food Guide Pyramid, history of, **2**:16–19
Food intolerance, **1**:55
Food safety, **1**:164–165
Laws, history of, **2**:19–23
Foodborne illness, **2**:22–23, 39
Organisms causing, **2**:22, 50
Formication, **4**:52
Fossil fuels, **1**:22
Foster care, **5**:14–16
Fractures (broken bones), **1**:180
Frozen pizza comparison, **2**:87

1: Health Basics
2: Nutrition and Physical Fitness
3: Sexual Health and Development
4: Alcohol, Tobacco, and Other Drugs
5: Mental and Emotional Health

Fuel emissions, **1**:14
Fungal infections, **1**:92–95
  athlete's foot, **1**:92
  jock itch (tinea cruris), **1**:92–93
  ringworm, **1**:93
Fungi, **1**:38

Gall bladder, **1**:59
Gallstones, **1**:59
Gambling and gaming (pathological), **5**:153–155
Gangs, **5**:33–37
  antisocial behavior and, **5**:35
  central elements,**5**:34
  community and school factors, **5**:36–37
  dealing with, **5**:36–37
  demographics, **5**:34–35
  drug trafficking, **5**:34
  effects on community, **5**:34
  gang names, **5**:34
  girls and, **5**:36
  members, personal characteristics of, **5**:35–36
  organized crime and, **5**:34
  prevalence, **5**:37
  quitting gangs, **5**:36
  turf, **5**:34
  violent crimes and, **5**:33, 34
  why people join gangs, **5**:36, 37
  youth gangs, **5**:34
  See also Juvenile delinquency
Gastric bypass procedures, **2**:93–96
  EndoBarrier Gastrointestinal Liner, **2**:96
  lap-band adjustable gastric banding (LAGB), **2**:93, 94–95
  Roux-en-Y bypass (RNY), **2**:94*f*, **2**:95
  sleeve gastrectomy, **2**:95
  types, **2**:93
  vertical banded gastroplasty, **2**:95
Gastritis, **1**:45
Gastroenteritis (stomach flu), **1**:40
Gay. *See* LGBTQI, Sexual orientation
Gay-straight alliance (GSA), **3**:42, 51–52
Gender
  gender roles and socialization, **3**:39–40
  gender identity, **3**:38–42
  masculinity-femininity spectrum, **3**:38–39
  transgender, **3**:40–42
    challenges and support, **3**:42, 43
    dressing/cross-dressing, **3**:40–41
    female-to-male (FTM), **3**:40
    Hester, Rita and, **3**:42
    male-to-female (MTF), **3**:40
    sexual orientation and, **3**:40
  transvestite, **3**:40
  See also Intersex
Genderqueer, **3**:52
  See also Gender, LGBTQI, Sexual orientation
Generalized anxiety disorder (GAD), **5**:127
Genetics, **1**:3
  diabetes and, **1**:3, 60
  learning disabilities and, **5**:139
Genital candidiasis, **3**:156–157
Genital herpes, **3**:146, 157–158
Genital warts, **3**:160–161
Germs, types of, **1**:38
Gestational diabetes, **1**:59, **3**:182
GHB (Xyrem), **4**:10, 22–23, 50, 51
Global warming, **1**:21–22
Gonorrhea, **3**:146, 158–159
Gonzalez, Tony, **2**:176
Granuloma, **4**:56
Greenhouse effect, **1**:21–22
  Greenhouse gases, **1**:21
Grief, **5**:131–135
  bereavement, **5**:131
  dealing with, **5**:134–135
  emotions and, **5**:132–133
  the grieving process, **5**:132
  myth concerning, **5**:133
  personal growth and, **5**:132
  physical symptoms of, **5**:133
  positive emotions from, **5**:132
  warning signs of, **5**:135*t*
  See also Loss

Group B streptococcus (GBS), **3**:182
Guillain-Barré Syndrome (GBS), **1**:107
Gynecomastia, **3**:6, **4**:29, 31

H1N1 virus, **1**:41
Haffner, Debra, **3**:30
Hair, **1**:99–101
  dandruff, **1**:99
  follicles, **1**:49
  head lice, **1**:93, 99–101
Hallucinations, **3**:200
Hallucinogens, **4**:16–19
  amphetamine variants, **4**:17
  dangers of, **4**:18, 19
  disassociation, **4**:17
  DMT, **4**:17
  DOM, **4**:17
  effects of, **4**:17–18
  examples, **4**:16
  flashbacks, **4**:18
  ketamine (Special K), **4**:10, 17, 23, 50, 60
  medical use, **4**:18–19
  mescal cactus, **4**:17
  peyote, **4**:17
  phencyclidine (PCP, angel dust), **4**:17
  poisonous, **4**:19
  religious use, **4**:16, 17
  synesthesia, **4**:17
  trips, **4**:17–18
  See also Club drugs, MDMA (Ecstasy), LSD, STP
Hand washing, **1**:39, 50, 85–86, 86*f*, 89, 93, **3**:209, **5**:126
  fingernails, **1**:86
Haskell, Bill, **2**:153
Hate crimes and hate incidents, **3**:101
  bullying and, **5**:30
  hate incident, **5**:27, 30
Health, definition, **2**:2
Health care teams, **1**:35–37
  for childbirth, **3**:193–194
  dental, **1**:37
  for eating disorders, **2**:130–131
Health insurance, **1**:4, 37–38, **3**:220
  children's, **3**:220
Health quizzes, **5**:61
Health screenings and medical visits, **1**:109–116
  gynecological examinations, **1**:114–115
  health care examinations, **1**:112
  health care practitioner, talking with, **1**:113
  health screens, **1**:109–112
    screening recommendations, **1**:110*t*
  laboratory tests and diagnostic procedures, **1**:113–114
  medical visits, **1**:112–116
  pap smears, **1**:110, 115, **3**:159
  personal health care record, **1**:116
  self-examinations for health screening, **1**:111
    breast self-exam, **1**:111, **3**:7
    skin self-exam, **1**:111
    testicular self-exam, **1**:111–112, **3**:14
  symptoms not to be ignored, **1**:114
  See also Medical care, paying for
Hearing
  deafness, **1**:145
  hard of hearing, **1**:145
  loss, **1**:23, 39, 48, 90, 109, **3**:192, **5**:146, 147
Heart, diagrams of, **1**:53*f*
Heart disease, **1**:7, 11, 14, 15, 21, 40, 51–54, 60, 61, 62, 64, 104, 109, **2**:5, 6, 9, 24, 45, 64, 68, 69, 75, 81, 90, 121, 145, 146, 152,160, 176, 180, 182, **4**:21, 50, 55, 67, **5**:79, 80, 87
  congenital, **1**:52–53
  coronary artery disease (CAD), **1**:51–52
  electrocardiogram (EKG), **1**:52
  exercise and, **2**:152,160
  family behaviors and, **1**:52
  heart attack (myocardial infarction; coronary), **1**:51
  heart failure, **1**:52
  heart transplant, **1**:52
  prevention, **1**:52
Heartburn, **2**:124, **3**:187
Heat stroke, **1**:168, **2**:169, 184, **4**:53
Heimlich maneuver, **1**:178
Hemorrhage, **1**:184, **2**:46, **3**:17, **5**:117
Hepatitis, **1**:17, 45–46, **3**:146, **4**:56
  hepatitis A, **1**:46
  hepatitis B, **1**:46
  hepatitis C, **1**:47, **4**:56
Hernia, **3**:12
Heroin, **4**:46, 50, 51, 59–60, 62

1: Health Basics
2: Nutrition and Physical Fitness
3: Sexual Health and Development
4: Alcohol, Tobacco, and Other Drugs
5: Mental and Emotional Health

Herpes simplex, **3**:157
Herpes zoster, **3**:157
Hester, Rita, **3**:42
Heterosexism, **3**:35–36, 50
Hippocampus, **4**:47
HIV/AIDS
  anal sex and, **3**:152
  dementia and, **3**:154
  diagnosis of, **3**:153
  diseases associated with, **3**:153–154
  early symptoms of HIV, **3**:153
  emotional toll of, **3**:154–155
  health measures for, **3**:154
  HIV transmission, **3**:152
  Kaposi's sarcoma and, **3**:154
  men who have sex with men, **3**:155
  medications, **3**:153, **3**:154
  pets and, **3**:154
  prevention of, **3**:155
  progression from HIV to AIDS, **3**:155
  safe sex, **3**:146, 148
  salmonella and, **3**:154
  steroid use, **4**:30
  substance use, and, **4**:54, 55–56
  T cell destruction, **3**:152, 155
  testing for, **3**:164
  toxoplasmosis and, **2**:22–23, **3**:154
  unprotected sex and, **3**:152
Hives (urticaria), **1**:55
Homophobia, **3**:35, 86
  internalized homophobia, **3**:37
Homosexuality, **3**:37–38, 85
  See also Sexual orientation, LGBTQI
Hormones, **1**:58, **2**:26, 27, **3**:22
  adrenaline (epinephrine), **1**:55, 182, **4**:45, 47, **5**:78, 79
  androgens, **3**:3, 4*t*, 10, 13*t*, 44, 46, 47, **4**:27
  depression and, **3**:24, **5**:79, 109, 113, 152
  estrogen, **3**:3, 4*t*, 20, 21, 136, **4**:53
  follicle-stimulating hormone (FSH), **3**:20
  gonadotropin-releasing hormone (GnRH), **3**:20
  human chorionic gonadotropin (HcG), **3**:180
  insulin, **1**:59–60, 111, **2**:4, 10, 12, 128, **3**:182, **4**:53
  intersex conditions and, **3**:44–49
  leptin, **2**:113
  luteinizing hormone (LH), **3**:20
  melatonin, **1**:8, **4**:45
  oxytocin, **5**:79
  progesterone, **3**:3, 4*t*, 136, 184
  puberty and, **1**:99, **3**:6, 20, 24, 84, 129, **5**:109
  replacement therapy, **3**:40, 46, 200, **4**:27
  sex drive and, **3**:95, 129, **4**:51
  sex hormones, **2**:128, **3**:4*t*, 13*t*,
  substance use and, **4**:53
  testosterone, **3**:10, 13*t*, 20, **4**:53
  transgender and, **3**:40, 41, 48, 51
  thyroid, **2**:13, 117, **3**:21, **5**:106
  weight and, **1**:11
Hornby, Lesley (Twiggy), **2**:108, 109*f*
Hospice, **5**:134
Human chorionic gonadotropin (HcG), **3**:180
Human papillomavirus (HPV), **1**:49, 108, **3**:146, 159–161, 163
Human reproductive system, **3**:1–17
  female reproductive system, **3**:2–9, 2*f*
    anatomy, **3**:4–5
    androgens, **3**:3
    cervix, **1**:115, **3**:3, 4, 11, 20, 44, 139–140, 143–144, 156, 158, 160, 163, 177, 183, 194, 196, 198
    cilia, **3**:4
    clitoris, **3**:2–3, 5, 15–16, 45, 46, 48
    endometrium, **3**:3, 4
    estrogen, **3**:3, 4*t*, 20, 21, 136, **4**:53
    fallopian tubes, **3**:3, 4, 11, 144, 161
    fimbria, **3**:4
    glans, **3**:5
    hymen, **3**:3, 5, 78–79
    labia, **3**:2–3, 5, 15, 17, 45
    menstrual cycle, **3**:4
    mons pubis, **3**:2, 3

ova (egg), **3**:1, 3, 4, 9–11, 20–21, 130, 136, 139–140, 144, 177–180, 185
ovaries, **1**:88, **3**:3, 4, 20, 21, 46, 144, 180
pelvis, **3**:2, 3, 161, 189, 196
urethra, **1**:44–45, 87, **3**:3, 5, 158, 163
vagina, **1**:39, 87, 88, 112, 114–115, **3**:2–5, 11, 20, 21, 23, 24, 44, 46, 133, 134, 136, 139–142, 146, 159, 160, 161
vulva, **3**:2, 5, 133, 134, 140, 152, 159, 160
See also Menstruation (the period)
genitals, **1**:155, **3**:1, 12, 29, 30, 41, 42, 44–49, 52, 87, 115, 130, 134, 146, 157, 186
male reproductive system, **3**:9–17, 10*f*
anatomy, **3**:13*t*
cilia, **3**:13
epididymides, **3**:9–11, 13*t*, 14, 156, 159
erection, **3**:11–12, 140, 142
flaccid penis, **3**:12
foreskin, **1**:87, **3**:11, 13, 14, 15, 140, 199
glans, **1**:87, **3**:11, 13, 14, 15
inguinal hernia, **3**:12
pelvis, **3**:156
penis length, **3**:12
prostate, **1**:68, 69, **2**:65, 182, 183, **3**:9, 11, 13, 156, **4**:29
scrotum, **1**:93, 112, **3**:9, 10, 12, 13*t*, 14, 45, 156
semen, **1**:46, **3**:3, 11, 13*t*, 89, 134, 139, 140, 144, 152
seminal vesicles, **3**:9, 11, 13*t*
sperm, **3**:1, 4, 9–11, 13, 20, 21, 45, 130, 133–135, 139, 140, 144, 177–179, 185, **4**:27, 29
testicles, **1**:111–112, **2**:128, **3**:9–14, 156, 159, **4**:29, 53
self-exam, **1**:111, **3**:14
torsion (rupture), **3**:12
urethra, **1**:44, **3**:9, 11, 13, 45, 158, 163
vas deferens, **3**: 9–11, 13*t*
See also Breasts, Circumcision, Gynecomastia
Humidifier, **1**:27, 40
Hurricane, **1**:22, 134, 165, 166, 169–172, 173, **5**:127
categories of, **1**:170
hurricane warning, **1**:172
hurricane watch, **1**:172
Katrina, **1**:171
meteorologists and, **1**:169
Saffir-Simpson Hurricane Wind Scale, **1**:170*t*
See also Levees
Hydration, **1**:89, 103, **2**:167–170
See also Dehydration, Sports nutrition
Hydrocele, **1**:112
Hygiene
body washing, **1**:86–88, 100, 176
dental, **1**:101–103
depilation, **1**:87–88
ears, **1**:90
eyes, **1**:89–90
face, **1**:88–89
fingernails, **1**:86
hand washing, **1**:39, 50, 85–86, 86*f*, 89, 93, **3**:209, **5**:126
illnesses caused by poor hygiene, **1**:100*t*
shaving, **1**:87–88
skin, **1**:88
Hymen, **3**:3, 5, 78–79
Hyperinsulinemia, **4**:53
Hyperkalemia, **2**:128
See also Potassium
Hypertension, **1**:52, 53–54, 62, 64, 109, 111, **2**:24, 44, 64, 92, 97, **4**:53, 58
Hypoglycemia, **1**:60, **2**:160
Hypokalemia, **2**:128
See also Potassium
Hypomania, **5**:113
Hypothalamic-pituitary-gonadal axis, **4**:29
Hypothermia, **1**:152, 175, 178
Hysterectomy, **3**:144

Idiom, **5**:45, 144
See also Autism spectrum disorders (ASD), Culture,
Ileum, **2**:93, 94
Illicit drug, **3**:191, **4**:31, 41, 61, 64, 65, 66, 108, 109
See also Substance use, abuse, and dependence
Illnesses caused by poor hygiene, **1**:100*t*

1: Health Basics
2: Nutrition and Physical Fitness
3: Sexual Health and Development
4: Alcohol, Tobacco, and Other Drugs
5: Mental and Emotional Health

Immune deficiency, **1**:15, 106, **3**:134, 152, **4**:26
See also HIV/AIDS
Immunity, **1**:3, 55, 106–108, **2**:4, 8, 27, 32, **3**:159, 162
Immunization (vaccinations), **1**:105–109
allergies and, **1**:106
antibodies, **1**:106
antigens, **1**:106
fear of, **1**:106–107
meningococcal, **1**:108
repeating, **1**:107
schedule for children and teens, **1**:108*f*
side effects, **1**:106
tetanus, **1**:108–109
travel and, **1**:108
Impetigo, **1**:49
Implicit, **5**:43
See also Social norms
Import and Drugs Act (1848), **2**:20
Impulse control, **4**:47, **5**:87, 116, 118
Impulse control disorders, **5**:104–105
Impulse purchases, **2**:33, 34, 35
Incest, **3**:84, 102, 110
Infection
body piercing and, **1**:98–99
ear infections, **1**:90–91
tattoos and, **1**:97–98, **3**:26–29
Infectious disease, **1**:38–39
H1N1 virus, **1**:41
infecting organisms, **1**:38
preventable through vaccination, **1**:49*t*
stomach flu, **1**:40–42
substance abuse and, **4**:54, 56
See also Bronchitis, Encephalitis, Gastritis, Hepatitis, Influenza, Meningitis, Methicillin-Resistant Staphylococcus aureus (MRSA), Pneumonia, Staph infections, Tuberculosis (TB), Upper respiratory infection (URI), Urinary tract infections (UTI), Walking pneumonia
Infertility, **1**:21, **2**:64, **3**:44, 46, 49, 146, 148, 156, 159, 161, **4**:53
See also In Pregnancy
Inflammatory bowel disease (IBD), **1**:58
Influenza (flu), **1**:38, **1**:40–42
Inhalants, **4**:31–32, 50, 51
effects of, **4**:32
huffing, **4**:32
nitrates, **4**:32
nitrous oxide (N_2O), **4**:32, 55
pregnancy and, **4**:32
toxicity, **4**:31
types, **4**:31–32
Inheritable disease, **1**:35
Injury related to exercise, **2**:147–148
injury prevention strategies for sports, **2**:158–159*t*
in team sports, **2**:161–162
tips for reducing chance of injury, **2**:157–158
Insomnia, **1**:8, **2**:129
Insulin, **1**:59–60, 111, **2**:4, 10, 12, 128, **3**:182, **4**:53
Intellectual disabilities/mental retardation, **5**:100, 143–144
Rosa's Law, **5**:148–149
terminology, **5**:148
See also Adaptive behavior, Developmental disabilities
Intelligence, **5**:100, 139, 143
Intersex, **3**:42–50
causes of, **3**:44
definition, **3**:42
frequency of intersex conditions, **3**:47*t*
versus gender identity or sexual orientation, **3**:48
"hermaphrodite," use of term, **3**:49
puberty and, **3**:43–50
treatment of intersex conditions, **3**:47–48
types of intersex conditions, **3**:44–46
5-alpha-reductase (5ARD) deficiency, **3**:44
androgen insensitivity syndrome (AIS), **3**:44
aphallia, **3**:45
clitoromegaly, **3**:45

congenital adrenal hyperplasia (CAH), **3**:45
hypospadias, **3**:45
Klinefelter syndrome, **3**:45
MRKH (Mayer Rokitansky Kuster Hauser syndrome), **3**:46
micropenis, **3**:45
ovotestes, **3**:46
partial androgen insensitivity (PAIS), **3**:46
Swyer syndrome, **3**:46
Turner syndrome, **3**:46
virilization, **3**:44, **3**:47
See also Hormones, Karyotype
Intertrigo, **1**:93
I-statements, **4**:112

Jaundice, **1**:46, **4**:58*t*
See also Hepatitis
Joint dislocation, **1**:156, **2**:162
Jordan, Michael, **2**:67
Journal of the American Medical Association (JAMA), **5**:57
The Jungle (Sinclair), **2**:20
Jutel, Annemarie, **2**:75
Juvenile delinquency, **5**:34–36

Karyotype, **3**:44–46
Ketamine (special K), **4**:10, 17, 23, 50, 60
Ketoacidosis., **1**:60
Ketogenic diet, **1**:65
Ketones, **1**:65, **2**:88, 91
Ketosis, **2**:88
Khat, **4**:21–22
Kidney
disease, **1**:52, 54, 60–62, 69, 103, **2**:45–46, 120, 175, **3**:153, **4**:6, 29, 51, 53, **5**:168
transplant, **1**:62
renal (kidney) failure, **1**:52, 60–62, **2**:44, **4**:51
Kinsey Heterosexual-Homosexual Rating Scale, **3**:34, 35*t*
Korsakoff's syndrome, **4**:6

La Leche League, **3**:201
Lacerations (cuts), **1**:180–181
Lactation consultant, **3**:194, 201, 202
Lacto-ovo vegetarians, **2**:176
Landslides, **1**:165, 169, 172–173
Lap-band adjustable gastric banding (LAGB), **2**:93, 94–95
Lead, **1**:13, 15, 19, **2**:43, 127, 179, **3**:213, 217
Learning
problems, **1**:19, 48, **3**:107, 191, **4**:10, 20, 23, 24, 32, 45, 47, 48, 49, 51, 53, 57, 59, 61
sleep and, **1**:7
style, **3**:33
Learning disabilities, **4**:61, **5**:137–142
ADHD and, **5**:137
causes, **5**:139–140
compensatory learning strategies, **5**:139
coping with, **5**:139–142
diagnosis of, **5**:139
environmental toxins and, **1**:19, **5**:139
genetics and, **5**:139
nonverbal learning disabilities, **5**:138
nutrition and, **5**:139, 141
verbal learning disabilities, **5**:137–138
Leaves
cannabis sativa, **4**:9, 15
coca, **4**:19, 40
hallucinogenic, **4**:17
khat, **4**:21–22
tobacco, **4**:13
Lesbian. *See* LGBTQI
Lesion, **1**:91, 92, 95, 111, **3**:154, 162, **4**:51
Lethargy, **1**:47, **2**:119, **5**:148
Levees, **1**:169, 171
LGBTQI (lesbian, gay, bisexual, transgender, queer or questioning, intersex)
A: asexual or ally, **3**:52–53
ally, **3**:41, 43, 52–53
asexual, **3**:34–35, 41, 52–53, 95
coming out, **3**:41, 50–51, 86
I: intersex, **3**:**3**:42–50, 52
in the closet, **3**:50
LGB: sexual orientations, **3**:51
outing someone, **3**:41
Q: questioning or queer, **3**:52
queer, **3**:50, 52, 85
questioning, **3**:50, 52, 86
T: gender identity, **3**:51–52
Safe Space stickers, **3**:51
Trevor Project, **3**:51
See also Sexual orientation, Gender identity, Intersex, Transgender

1: Health Basics
2: Nutrition and Physical Fitness
3: Sexual Health and Development
4: Alcohol, Tobacco, and Other Drugs
5: Mental and Emotional Health

Libido, **3**:52, 95
Librium, **4**:8
Lice, **1**:93–94, 99–101
body lice, **1**:94
head lice, **1**:93, 99–101
pubic lice (crabs), **1**:93–94
Limbic system, **4**:45–46
nucleus accumbens, **4**:45
reward system, **4**:45–48, **5**:24
ventral tegmental area (VTA), **4**:45–46
Loss (grief and), **3**:75. **5**:14, 99, 103, 107, 108, 109, 120, 127–135, 155
ambiguous loss, **5**:130
anticipatory loss, **5**:130
disillusionment, **5**:130
suicide and, **5**:119, 131
survivor guilt, **5**:131
See also Grief
Lozenge, **1**:40
LSD (lysergic acid diethylamide), **4**:17, 22, 24–25, 48–50, 52, 53, 60, **5**:151
See also Club drugs, Hallucinogens
Lumbar puncture (spinal tap), **1**:47

Macular degeneration, **1**:23, **2**:182
Major depressive disorder (MDD), **2**:125, 126, **5**:108, 110
See also Depression, Mood disorders
Maladaptive behavior, **4**:82, **5**:158
Malignant tumors (cancerous growths), **1**:68
Mammograms, **1**:111, **3**:7
Manic episode (mania), **5**:109, 112–114, 152
Marijuana, **4**:9, 14, 50, 51, 59, 62
cancer and, **4**:15
combined with other drugs, **4**:16
common names for, **4**:15
dronabinol (Marinol, Norvir, Cesamet), **4**:14
as food, **4**:14
hashish (hash), **4**:15
long-term problems of, **4**:15
medical marijuana, **4**:9*f*, 14
psychoactive effects/properties of, **4**:14, 15
secondhand smoke and, **4**:16
THC (delta-9-tetrahydrocannabinol), **4**:9, 14, 47
Masturbation, **3**:87–89, 96, 134, **5**:50
benefits of, **3**:87–88
facts or myths about, **3**:88
frequency, **3**:89
taboos, **3**:87
Maximal oxygen uptake (VO_{2max}), **2**:150
MDMA (Ecstasy), **4**:17, 19–20, 22–24, 48–54, 59
Meats, poultry, fish, and deli, **2**:38–39
the Media, **5**:46–50
body image and, **2**:107–109, 110, 111, 134, **3**:25–26, **5**:40, 47–49
consumerism, and, **5**:55–56
critical thinking and, **5**:1, 57–61
relationships and, **5**:46–49
obesity/weight, and, **2**:61–62, 134
self-image and self-esteem, **3**:25–26, **5**:4–5, 40
sexual behavior and, **5**:46
sexual orientation and, **3**:35, 85–86
sexualized media, **3**:97–98, **5**:49–50
social norms and, **5**:40, 46
substance use and, **4**:69, 70–71, 76, 79
and wellness, **1**:4–6
See also Pornography
Medical care, paying for, **1**:37–38, 116
Melanoma, **1**:69, 95
Memory
impairment, **4**:6, 8, 10, 23, 24, 30, 48, 49, 51
loss, **1**:64, 66, 157, **5**:106, 118, 152
problems, **1**:8, 19, 47, 48, 54, 64, 68, **2**:166, **3**:154, **4**:32, 44, 45, 47, 65, **5**:106, 168
See also Amnesia
Menarche, **2**:109–110, **3**:19, 20–21
Meninges, **1**:48
Meningitis, **1**:48–49, **1**:48*f*, 107–108, **3**:208
Menopause, **3**:21

Menstruation (the period), **3**:3, 20–24
amenorrhea, **2**:119, 124, 129
birth control and, **3**:133–136, 143
intersex conditions and, **3**:44, 49
irregular, **2**:120, 129, **3**:21, 161
length of, **3**:21
menstrual cramps, **3**:21–22, 88, 137
ovulation, **3**:21, 133, 134–136, 139, 180, 181*f*
premenstrual syndrome (PMS), **3**:22–23, **5**:140
sanitary products, **3**:23–24
moon cup, **3**:23
pad (sanitary napkin), **3**:23
panty liner, **3**:23
tampons, **3**:23–24
steroids and, **4**:28
toxic shock syndrome (TSS), **3**:24
when to seek medical advice about, **3**:22*t*
Mental health disorders
adjustment disorders, **5**:104
delirium, dementia, amnesia, and other cognitive disorders, **5**:106
dissociative disorders, **5**:107
eating disorders, **2**:29, 63, 65, 81, 107–143, **3**:25, 37, **4**:30, **5**:49, 100, 101, 103, 109, 115
general medical condition, due to a, **5**:106
mood disorders, **2**:126, 129, **5**:105, 109, 112–114, 152, 158, 165
See also Bipolar disorder, Cyclothymia, Depression, Hypomania, Major depressive disorder (MDD)
other conditions that may be a focus of clinical attention, **5**:103–104
personality disorders, **5**:104, 115, 121
sexual and gender identity disorders, **5**:103
sleep disorders, **1**:7, **2**:122, 129–130, **4**:8, 10, 20, 22, **5**:102
See also Insomnia
somatoform and factitious disorders, **2**:125, **5**:107
See also Eating disorders/Body dysmorphic disorder (BDD)
substance-related disorders, **1**:104, 113, **2**:93, 113, 121, 125, **3**:25, 37, **4**:39–94, **5**:49, 87, 106, 109, 115, 121, 123, 124, 151, 165, 168
child and adolescent mental health disorders, **5**:100–102
Rett's syndrome, **5**:100, 144
conduct disorder (CD), **5**:101
elimination disorders, **5**:101
feeding and eating disorders, **5**:101
oppositional defiant disorder (ODD), **5**:101
separation anxiety, **3**:207, **5**:101
stereotypic movement disorder, **5**:101
tic disorders, **5**:101, 126
delusional disorder, **5**:152–153
diagnosis of mental health disorders, **1**:62, **2**:122, 125, 126, 127, **4**:42–44, 78, **5**:61, 100–107, 108, 109, 124, 126, 136, 139, 140, 145, 149, 152, 161
See also Attention deficit hyperactivity disorder (ADHD), Autism spectrum disorders, Depression, Developmental disabilities, Diagnostic criteria, Diagnostic labels, *Diagnostic and Statistical Manual of Mental Disorders* (DSM), Down syndrome, Fetal alcohol spectrum disorders (FASD), Gambling and gaming (pathological), Grief, Impulse control disorders, Intellectual disabilities/mental retardation, Learning disabilities, Loss, Pervasive developmental disorders (PDDs), Schizophrenia, Suicide
Mental health disorders, treatment for, **5**:156–161
behavior therapy, **2**:128, **4**:82, **5**:145, 147, 156–158
cognitive-behavioral therapy (CBT), **2**:118, 121, 122, 131–132, **4**:82, **5**:84, 85–86, 111, 112, 116, 156, 158–159
confidentiality and, **5**:157
dialectical behavior therapy (DBT), **5**:116

1: Health Basics
2: Nutrition and Physical Fitness
3: Sexual Health and Development
4: Alcohol, Tobacco, and Other Drugs
5: Mental and Emotional Health

Mental health disorders, treatment for (*continued*)
family therapy, **2**:118, 131, 132, 133, **5**:15, 156
group therapy, **2**:118, 121, 133, **5**:156, 164
individual therapy, **2**:118, 121, 131, 133, **5**:156, 157, 164
medications for mental health, **5**:164–168
addiction and, **5**:166–167
common classes, **5**:166
neurotransmitters and, **5**:165–166
pharmacotherapy, **2**:131, **5**:164
polypharmacy, **5**:168
psychotropic medications, **4**:2, **5**:164–166
risk factors, **5**:168
safety, **5**:167–168
for self-injurious behavior, **5**:116
side effects, **5**:167
See also Analgesics, Antidepressants, Antipsychotics, Anxiolytics, CNS depressants, Sedative-hypnotics, Stimulants, Tranquilizers
mental health practitioners
counselors, **1**:37, **2**:131, **3**:69, 76, 100, 108–110, 184, **4**:82, 106, **5**:15, 103, 161, 163
family therapists, **4**:80, **5**:161–162
nurses, **1**:35–36, 112, **2**:131, **3**:109, 194, **4**:80, 104, 118, **5**:33, 161–163
other mental health professionals, **5**:163
psychiatrists, **1**:36, **2**:130, **4**:80, **5**:100, 122, 136, 161, 162
psychologists, **1**:36, **2**:131, **4**:1, 80, 82, 104, **5**:33, 83, 100, 136, 139, 151, 153, 161–162
school-based mental health professionals, **1**:12, 37, 163, **3**:51, 86, 109, 114, 117, **4**:79, 100, 103, 104, 115, **5**:15, 33, 38, 125, 157, 163–164
school psychologists, **3**:51, 109, 114, **4**:115, **5**:15, 139, 163–164
social workers, **1**:36, **2**:131, **3**:194, **4**:80, 104, **5**:15, 161–163
See also Counselors
motivational interviewing, **4**:82–83
other factors in therapy, **5**:160–161
psychodynamic therapy, **5**:116, 156, 159
self-harming behaviors, treatments for, **5**:115–116
self-help methods and peer support, **1**:57, 62, **3**:42, 53, 155, **4**:80, 81, 110, 115, **5**:13, 15, 17, 134, 155, 159–160
supportive therapies, **5**:156–157
talk therapy: *See* Psychotherapy
Teen Opinions on supporting friends or family with mental health issues, **5**:160
treatment plan, **5**:157
types of therapy, **5**:156–157, 161–164
Mesomorph, **2**:69
Metabolic equivalent (MET), **2**:153–154
Metabolic
abnormalities, **2**:133, **3**:45
balance, **2**:129, 133
illnesses associated with obesity, **2**:65*t*
rates, **2**:86, 152, 153, 156
system, **4**:53
See also Aerobic energy system
Metabolic syndrome, **4**:53
Metabolize, **1**:47, **2**:6, 10*t*, 133, 171, 172, **4**:50, 74
Methamphetamine, **4**:19–20, 20, 24, 53, 62
meth mouth, **4**:52
Methicillin-Resistant Staphylococcus aureus (MRSA), **1**:49–50
Methylene chloride, **1**:27
Methylphenidate (Concerta, Ritalin), **4**:20, 21
“Metrosexual,” **3**:38
Microcephaly, **5**:146
See also Fetal alcohol spectrum disorders (FASD)

Midwife, **3**:193, 196
Mild traumatic brain injuries (MTBI). *See* Concussion
Ministroke. *See* Transient ischemic attack (TIA)
Minors, **1**:113, **3**:17, 26, 82, 96, 102, 150–152, **4**:68, 69, 76
See also Abortion; Age of consent; Confidentiality; Consent; Sexual activity, legal issues pertaining to
Miscarriage (spontaneous abortion), **1**:18, **2**:21, **3**:161, 184, **4**:57, 60
Medications and risk of, **4**:57
Mohel (or moyle), **3**:200
See also Circumcision
Mold and mildew, **1**:13, 19, 24–25, 56
Monogamy, **3**:72–73, 90, 145
Mood, **5**:87
mood swings, **2**:120, **3**:24, 121, 179, 200, **4**:8, 28, 30, 48, 77, **5**:86, 109, 115, 123, 140
Mood disorders, **2**:126, 129, **5**:105, 109, 112–114, 152, 158, 165
Morphologic teratogenicity, **4**:57
Motivation
depression and, **5**:108
exercise and, **1**:12
grief and, **5**:135
marijuana use and, **4**:49
and social norms, **1**:2
stress and, **5**:78
Motivational interviewing, **4**:82–83
Motor vehicle safety, **1**:127–128
ATV safety, **1**:139
cell phone usage while driving, **1**:135–136
courtesy, **1**:131–132
distractions, **1**:135
cognitive, **1**:136
manual, **1**:137
visual, **1**:137
driving
defensive, **1**:130–131
designated driver, **1**:137–138
precautions, **1**:129–130
safe driving tips, **1**:130
education and licensure, **1**:128–129
how to handle
brakes, failure of, **1**:143
car fire, **1**:133–134
foggy or extra-sunny conditions driving, **1**:144
gas pedal malfunction, **1**:143
rainy-day driving, **1**:143–144
snow, sleet, and ice driving, **1**:142
tire blowout, **1**:143
vehicle submersion (underwater), **1**:134
motorcycle/moped safety, **1**:139
passenger safety, **1**:137–138
passengers and, **1**:136
speed, **1**:132
vehicle maintenance, **1**:132–133
See also Water safety
Multiple sclerosis (MS), **1**:66, **4**:27, **5**:109
Muscle building, **2**:178
See also Exercise and physical activity
Muscle dysmorphia, **2**:125–126
Musculoskeletal system diseases, **1**:67, **2**:65*t*, **4**:51
Music therapist, **1**:36
Myelin, **1**:66, **4**:51
See also Multiple sclerosis (MS)
MyPyramid/MyPlate, **2**:16–18, 17*f*, 73, 74
Myths/facts about
abusive relationships, **3**:107
ADHD, **5**:135, 137
grief, **5**:133
masturbation, **3**:88
rape myth, **5**:50
substance use, **4**:73–74, 114
suicide, **5**:122
teen sexual intercourse, **3**:131
violence, **5**:32
vitamin D, **2**:28

Narcotics, **3**:197, **4**:25, 50
Narcotics Anonymous (NA), **4**:81, 106
Narcolepsy, **4**:10, 20, 22
Nar-Anon, **4**:110
National Center for Victims of Crime (NCVC) website, **5**:33
National Health and Nutrition Examination Survey (NHANES), **2**:64, 75
National Institutes of Health (NIH), **2**:15, 76, 179, **5**:59

1: Health Basics
2: Nutrition and Physical Fitness
3: Sexual Health and Development
4: Alcohol, Tobacco, and Other Drugs
5: Mental and Emotional Health

National Institute on Alcohol Abuse and Alcoholism (NIAAA), **4**:66, 77, 79
National Institute on Drug Abuse (NIDA), **4**:73, 77, 97, 104
Negative attribution, **5**:111
Negative thinking and rumination, **5**:110–112, 123
Neglect, **2**:132, **3**:102, **5**:14, 86, 115, 127
Nembutal, **4**:8
Nervous system, **1**:62, **4**:4, 45, 51, **5**:164
  activation, **1**:23
  function, **1**:17
  infectious diseases of, **1**:47–49
    encephalitis, **1**:47
    meningitis, **1**:48–49, 48*f*
  damage, **1**:14, 19, 27
  diseases of, **1**:62–66, 108–109
  See also Alzheimer's disease, Stroke (cerebrovascular accident), Seizure disorder (epilepsy), Multiple sclerosis (MS), Parkinson's disease
Neuron, **4**:45–48, **5**:18
  receptor, **4**:25, 45–48
  peripheral nervous system, and, **4**:45
  reuptake, **4**:45
  synapse, **4**:45–48
  transporter, **4**:45, 47–48
Neurotransmitter, **4**:45–48, 53, **5**:88, 110, 165–166
  adenosine, **4**:45, 47
  amino acids, **2**:4, 6*t*, 10, 11, 177–178, 180, **4**:45
    aspartate, **4**:45
    GABA (gamma-aminobutyric acid), **4**:45, 47
    glutamate, **4**:45, 48
    glycine, **2**:6, **4**:45
  histamine, **1**:54, **4**:45
  monoamines, **4**:45
    acetylcholine, **4**:45
    adrenaline (epinephrine), **1**:55, 182, **4**:45, 47, **5**:78, 79
    dopamine, **4**:45–48, **5**:151
    melatonin, **1**:8, **4**:45
    norepinephrine, **4**:45, 47–48
    serotonin (5-HT), **2**:10, 113, **4**:45, 47–48
  peptides, **4**:45
  endorphins, **5**:88, 115
Newsweek, **5**:57
Nicotine, **4**:12–13, 22, 50, 51, 83
  gum, **4**:12
  dependence, **4**:12
  replacement therapy for teens, **4**:83
  See also Smoking, Tobacco
Night eating syndrome (NES), **2**:129–130
Nits, **1**:94, 100–101
Noise
  and boater's fatigue **1**:154
  extreme noise, **3**:192
  pollution, **1**:12, 23–24
Nontraditional families, **5**:9, 10, 21
Nonverbal
  behavior, and culture, **5**:44
  communication, **5**:115, 138, 144
  learning disabilities, **5**:138
  social cues, **3**:24–25, **5**:144
Nosebleeds, **1**:54, 181, **4**:28
Nuclear
  blast, **1**:176
  disasters, **1**:20, 165, 174, 176
Nurse practitioner, **1**:36
Nurses, **5**:162–163
Nutrients, **1**:10
  See also Recommended Nutrient Intake (RNI), Nutrition basics, Weight management
Nutrition, preventing disease through, **1**:109
Nutrition and adolescent needs, **2**:25–30
  anemia, **2**:27
  calcium, **2**:26–27, 28
  caloric requirements, **2**:25–26
  dietary reference intakes for adolescents and young adults, **2**:27*t*
  fluid consumption, **2**:27–28
  growth, **2**:26
  growth patterns, **2**:29

iron, **2**:27, 28
protein, **2**:26
puberty, **2**:25, 29
Spotlight on What Teens Eat, What They Need, **2**:29, 49
vitamin D myth, **2**:28
See also Anemia, Nutrition basics
Nutrition basics
amino acids, **2**:4, 6*t*, 10, 11, 177–178, 180
essential, **2**:4, 6*t*
nonessential, **2**:4, 6*t*, 10
carbohydrates, **2**:170–173
complex, **2**:3–4, 18, 170, 175
dietary carbohydrates, **2**:3
simple, **2**:3, 170
dietary protein, **2**:5*f*, 26
diet-induced thermogenesis (DIT), **2**:6
essential nutrients, **2**:3
essential trace minerals, **2**:8
fats, **2**:4–6, 7t, 173
bad, **2**:5
dietary, **2**:4, 7*t*
good, **2**:6
monounsaturated, **2**:5
saturated, **2**:5
trans, **2**:5
fatty acids, **2**:4
essential fatty acids (EFAs), **2**:4
polyunsaturated, **2**:5
generally recognized as safe (GRAS) ingredients, **2**:20
hydrogenation, **2**:5
kilocalorie (kcal), **2**:2
macronutrients, **2**:2, 3
energy provided by, **2**:2*t*
micronutrients, **2**:7
functions, **2**:9–13*t*
minerals, **2**:3
oxygen bomb calorimeter, **2**:2
vitamins, **2**:7–8
fat-soluble, **2**:8
water soluble, **2**:8
vitamins and minerals, **2**:175
deficiency, **2**:15, 16
water, **2**:6–7
See also Antioxidants, Calcium, Eating healthy, Fad diets and weight-loss aids
Nutrition in America, **2**:23–25
Nutritional comparison of fast foods, **2**:85*t*

Obesity, **1**:7, 11, 52, **2**:61–66, 65–66*t*, 74
asthma and, **2**:66
diabetes and, **1**:11, 109, **2**:64, 65*t*, 93, 96
diseases associated with, **2**:65–66*t*
National Health and Nutrition Examination Survey (NHANES), **2**:64
Saguy, Abigail C., on, **2**:62–63
Sassi, Cecchi, and Devaux on, **2**:63
See also Diets, Overweight, Weight management
Obsessive-compulsive disorder (OCD), **2**:113, 125, 127, 129, **5**:125–127, 140
Occupational therapy, **1**:36, 65, **2**:131, **5**:145, 147
Oil spills, **1**:21
Oopherectomy, **3**:144
Opiates, **4**:25, 47, 50, 62, **5**:115
Opioids, **1**:164, **3**:197*t*, **4**:25–26, 40, 50, 83, 84, **5**:116
addiction and, **4**:25–26
definition of, **4**:25
pregnancy, risks of using during, **4**:58*t*
risks of using, **4**:26
substances containing, **4**:25
Oppositional defiant disorder (ODD), **5**:101
Optimism, **2**:110, **5**:111
Oral sex, **3**:78–80, 89, 94, 95, 112, 130, 134, 146–147, 152, 156, 157, 160
Organic and natural foods, **1**:19, **2**:40
Orthorexia nervosa, **2**:113, 123, 126–127
Osteoarthritis, **1**:67
Osteoporosis, **1**:109, **2**:45, 129, 149, 176
Outdoor residential fire hazards, **1**:148
Overdose, **1**:65, 164, **4**:10, 23, 25, 110, 114
injuries, **1**:156, **2**:162–163
Overweight, **1**:1, 11
See also Diets, Obesity, Weight management
Ovulation, **3**:21, 133, 134–136, 139, 180, 181*f*
Oxytocin, **5**:79

1: Health Basics
2: Nutrition and Physical Fitness
3: Sexual Health and Development
4: Alcohol, Tobacco, and Other Drugs
5: Mental and Emotional Health

Pandemic, **1**:39, 41
Pansexual, **3**:41, 52
Parenting, **3**:204–206
  child care, **3**:218–220
    carjacking, **3**:219–220
    day care centers or nurseries, **3**:219
    in-home help, **3**:219
    stranger safety, **3**:219–220
  coparenting and family relationships, **3**:206–207
  culture and, **3**:204
  discipline, **3**:102, 106, 205–206, **5**:12, 30
    consequences for behaviors, **3**:206
    consistency and, **3**:206
    punishment, **3**:206
    shaking, **3**:206, **5**:147–148
    spanking, **3**:206
  men and, **3**:204–205
  other responsibilities for parents, **3**:220–221
  single-parent family, **5**:10
  substance use and, **4**:60–61
  teen parents, **3**:220–221
    financial considerations, **3**:220–221
    health insurance, **3**:220
    Single Parent Alliance and Resource Center, **3**:221
    Teen Opinions on parenting challenges, **3**:221
  women and, **3**:204
  See also Baby care; Child health care
Parkinson's disease, **1**:66, **2**:45
Particle pollution, **1**:14–15, 17
Pastoral counselor, **1**:37
Pathological, **2**:115, **5**:99, 107, 153–155
PCP, **4**:17, 23, 40, 48, 51, 60, 62
Peanut allergy, **1**:55, **2**:30, 31
  See also Allergies, Food allergies
Pear shape, **2**:69
Pedestrian safety, **1**:130, 138–139, 162
Pelvic exam, **1**:114, **3**:163
Pelvic inflammatory disease (PID), **3**:137, 156, 159, 161, 163
Performance therapist, **1**:36
Perishable food items, **2**:20
Personal space, **5**:44–45
Personality disorders, **5**:104, 115, 121
Pervasive developmental disorders (PDDs), **5**:100–101, 144
  See also Autism, Autism spectrum disorders (ASD)
Pessimism, **5**:111
Pesticides, **1**:12, 15, 16, 17, 19–20, 26, 27, **2**:21, 36, 38, 40
  pregnancy and, **3**:191
Pesticide Amendment (1954), **2**:21
Pests, **1**:19–20, 26, 94, 101
Pet dander, **1**:13, 24, 25, 26, 55, 56
Pharmacotherapy, **2**:131, **5**:164
Phencyclidine (PCP, angel dust), **4**:17, 23, 40, 48, 51, 60, 62
Phenobarbital, **4**:8
Philtrum, **5**:146
Phlebotomist, **1**:36
Physical Activity Guidelines for Americans, **2**:154–157
  children and adolescents,
    examples of exercise, **2**:155*t*
    exercise recommendations, **2**:154*t*
Physical activity intensity (relative), **2**:150
Physical activity (PA) energy factors, **2**:74*t*
Physical therapist, **1**:36
Physical therapy, **1**:65–68, **5**:145, 147
Physician assistant, **1**:36
Pica, **2**:127–128, **5**:101
Placebo, **2**:97, **5**:60
Plastic surgery, **2**:111, **3**:8, 9, 17, 26, 48, **5**:56
  See also Cosmetic surgery
Pneumonia, **1**:38,40, 42–43, 49, 50, 64, **2**:95, 129, **3**:154, 156, **4**:55
Podiatrist, **1**:36
Poison Squad, **2**:20
Poisoning, **1**:15, 19, 164, 181–182, **2**:127–128, **4**:25, 31, 60
  alcohol poisoning, **4**:6, 114
  food poisoning, **1**:85, **3**:190
  poison control centers, **2**:42, **3**:210

poisons, **1**:3, 15, 60, 164, 176, 181–182, **2**:20, 22, **3**:26, 211, **4**:11, 12, **5**:139
poisonous hallucinogens, **4**:19
poisonous snakes in the United States, **1**:183*f*, 184
See also Toxins
Polyamory, **3**:72–73
Polypharmacy, **5**:168
Pornography, **3**:96–98, **5**:46, 49–53
benefits/harm of, **3**:96–98
forms of, **3**:96
gender and approval of, **3**:97, 98
magazines and comics, **3**:98
sexual violence and, **3**:96, 97–98
sexualized media, **3**:97–98, **5**:49–50
Teen Opinions on, **3**:97
Teens Hooked on Porn (2007), **3**:98
Posttraumatic stress disorder (PTSD), **5**:33, 99, 107, 109, 123, 127–129
causes of, **5**:127
physical integrity, **5**:127–128
proximity, **5**:128–129
recovery rate, **5**:129
resilience, **5**:128
symptoms of, **5**:128
treatment, **5**:129
Potassium
blood levels, **1**:61, **2**:128
deficiencies, **2**:75, 128
dietary sources of, **2**:8, 12, 18, 39, 80*t*
See also Hyperkalemia, Hypokalemia
Practical skills, **5**:143–144
Prader-Willi syndrome, **2**:123, 128–129
Prediabetes, **1**:59
Preejaculate, **3**:13*t*, 133
Prefrontal cortex, **5**:18
Pregnancy
artificial insemination, **3**:177
birth, preparing for, **3**:190, 192–193
Lamaze classes, **3**:193
Braxton Hicks contractions, **3**:189
childbirth health care team, **3**:193–194
chloasma, **3**:188
conception, **3**:177–178, 179*f*
fetal development, **3**:185–186
diagnosing, **3**:178–180
common symptoms of, **3**:178–179
symptoms requiring medical intervention, **3**:179–180
What to Expect When You're Expecting (Murkoff & Mazel), **3**:180
douching, **3**:187
ectopic pregnancy, **3**:161
food and, **3**:190–191
full-term fetus, **3**:190
hemorrhoids, **1**:87, **3**:189, 199
labor and childbirth, **3**:194–201
active labor, **3**:198
breech, **3**:196
C-section (Cesarean section), **3**:196
crowning, **3**:198
delivering alone, **3**:195*t*
dilation, **3**:194, 196, 198
early labor, **3**:195–196
effacement, **3**:196
episiotomy, **3**:198
false labor, **3**:195
hydrotherapy, **3**:196–197
mucous plug, **3**:194
placenta, **3**:183, 186, 195, 198
transverse, **3**:196
types of pain relief for childbirth, **3**:197*t*
water breaking, **3**:194
waterbirthing, **3**:197
linea negra, **3**:188
mask of pregnancy (melisma), **3**:188
measures for a healthy pregnancy, **3**:190
morning sickness, **3**:187
sea bands, **3**:187
periodontitis and, **3**:188
postpartum, **3**:199–200
baby blues, **3**:199, 200
bonding, **3**:200–201
postpartum depression, **3**:199, 200
postpartum psychosis, **3**:200
umbilicus care, **3**:199
WIC program, **3**:204
See also Baby care, Breastfeeding, Circumcision
reducing risks, **3**:190–192
Accutane and Retin-A, **3**:192
extreme noise, **3**:192
folic acid, **1**:109, **2**:10*t*, 45*t*, **3**:192
hair treatments, **3**:191
harmful substances, **3**:190–191

1: Health Basics
2: Nutrition and Physical Fitness
3: Sexual Health and Development
4: Alcohol, Tobacco, and Other Drugs
5: Mental and Emotional Health

Pregnancy (*continued*)
nutrition, **1**:109, **2**:21, 22–23, 27, 44, 71, 176, **3**:192
pollution and, **1**:15
tanning beds, **3**:192
X-rays, **3**:191
responses to pregnancy, **3**:183–185
abandonment, **3**:185
abortion, **3**:183–184
adoption, **3**:184
sexual desire and, **3**:187
sexual intercourse and, **3**:177
stages and symptoms, **3**:187–190
first trimester, **3**:187–188
second trimester, **3**:187
third trimester, **3**:189–190
substance use and, **4**:56–60
alcohol, **3**:191, **4**:61–62
caffeine, **4**:21, 62
depressant drugs, **4**:10
inhalants, **4**:32
methamphetamine, **4**:20
smoking, **3**:191, **4**:13, 60, 191
tests, **3**:180–182
amniocentesis, **3**:181–182
Doppler, **3**:186
group B streptococcus (GBS), **3**:182
home pregnancy test, **3**:180–181
human chorionic gonadotropin (HcG), **3**:180
ultrasound, **3**:181
trimesters, **3**:186
in vitro fertilization, **3**:177, **3**:178*f*
See also Amniotic fluid, Fetal alcohol spectrum disorders (FASD), Gestational diabetes, Ovulation
Premature ejaculation, **3**:133
Premenstrual syndrome (PMS), **3**:22–23
Prescription medications, **4**:2–3
abuse of, **4**:3
antibiotics, **4**:2
aspirin, **4**:1
dispensing, **4**:1, 2
disposal of, **4**:3
over-the-counter (OTC), **4**:1
opiates, **4**:25, 50
psychotropic drugs, **4**:2, **5**:164–166
side effects, **4**:2, 3
weight-loss drugs, **2**:92*t*
Prevention
ear health, **1**:90–91
hair, **1**:99–101
levels of prevention
primary, **1**:85
secondary, **1**:85
tertiary, **1**:85
nutrition and, **1**:109
skin cancers, **1**:23, 69, 95–97, 111, **2**:28
sunburn, **1**:22, 95, 97
sunscreen, **1**:95–96
tattoos and body piercings, **1**:97–99, **3**:26–30, 152, 155, **5**:2, 114
UV index forecast, **1**:96*f*
vaccinations (immunizations), **1**:105–109
schedule for children/teens, **1**:108*f*
for tetanus, **1**:108–109
See also Acne, Dental health, Fungal infections, Health screenings and medical visits, Hearing, Heart disease, Hygiene, Lice, Scabies, Swimmer's ear
Prions, **2**:22–23
See also Creutzfeldt-Jakob (mad cow) disease
Pro-anorexia (pro-an) websites, **2**:119
Problem-solving skills, **3**:25, **5**:41
Produce, **2**:38–38
Progression principle, **2**:151, 153, 155
Prospective study, **5**:60
Protozoa, **1**:17, 39, 69
giardia, **1**:17
malaria, **1**:69–70
trichomoniasis, **3**:162–163
See also Sickle cell disease
Psychiatrists, **1**:36, **2**:130, **4**:80, **5**:100, 122, 136, 161, 162
Psychodynamic therapy, **5**:116, 156, 159

Psychoeducation, **4**:79
Psychologists, **1**:36, **2**:131, **4**:1, 80, 82, 104, **5**:33, 83, 100, 136, 139, 151, 153, 161–162
Psychosis, **4**:9
Psychotherapy, **2**:118, 121, 133, **5**:113, 123, 129, 160–161, 164
 See also Cognitive-behavioral therapy, Dialectical behavior therapy (DBT), Psychodynamic psychotherapy
Psychotropic medications, **4**:2, **5**:164–166
Public opinion/media and wellness, **1**:4–6
Public transportation safety, **1**:141–142, 162
Pure Food and Drug Act (1906), **2**:20, 21

Radioactive pollution, **1**:20–21, 24, 176
Radiotherapy, **1**:68–69
Radon, **1**:14, 24
Randomized study, **5**:60
Rape/sexual assault, **3**:102, 109–115, 131
 acquaintance or date rape, **3**:110–112, **4**:10, 23
 alcohol/drugs and, **3**:112
 consent and, **3**:111–112, 150
 date rape drugs, **3**:112, **4**:8, 10, 23
 dealing with, **3**: 108, 113–114
 familial rape, **3**:110
 gang rape, **3**:110–111
 pornography and, **3**:96–98, **5**:50
 preventing, **3**:112–113
 provocative clothing and, **3**:109
 rape myth, **3**:98, **5**:50
 reporting, **3**:108, 114
 responsibility for, **3**:109
 spousal rape, **3**:110
 statutory rape, **3**:82, 109, 150, **5**:31
Rapid eye movement (REM), **1**:6*t*, 8
Refeeding syndrome, **2**:129, 132–133
Rehabilitation, **1**:36, 58, 65, **2**:131, 164, **4**:80
Reinforcers, **3**:218, **4**:41, 82, **5**:157–158, 167
Remission, **1**:66
Research studies
 critical thinking and media, **5**:57–61
 conflict of interest, **5**:58, 59
 control group, **5**:60
 health quizzes, **5**:61
 placebo, **2**:97, **5**:60
 research
  design, **5**:60
  participants or subjects, **5**:59–60
  results, **5**:60–61
 researchers and funding sources, **5**:57–59
 types of studies
  blind, **5**:60
  controlled, **5**:60
  double-blind, **5**:60
  prospective, **5**:60
  randomized, **5**:60
  retrospective, **5**:60
 valid information, **5**:57
Relationships, family and peer
 adjusting to a new home, **5**:14
 families, **5**:9
  blended (stepfamily), **5**:9–10, 12–13
  custody, **5**:12
  divorce, **5**:10–12, 13–14
  extended, **5**:9
  half sibling, **5**:12
  households with no father, **5**:20–21
  nontraditional, **5**:9, 10, 21
  nuclear (traditional), **5**:9, 10
  same-sex parents, **3**:36, **5**:9, 10, 15, 17, 21
  separation, **5**:11
  single-parent, **5**:10
  stepfamilies, **5**:12–13
   stepparent, **5**:12
   stepsiblings, **5**:12
 family roles, shifting, **5**:17–18
 father-adolescent relationship, **5**:20
 friendships, growing within the context of, **5**:22
 healthy relationships with family and friends, **5**:17
 mother-adolescent relationship, **5**:19
 parent-teen communication, **5**:18–19
 peer pressure, **5**:23–24
 peer relationships, challenging, **5**:22–23
  See also Adoption, Bullying, Foster care, Gangs, Social networking, Violence

1: Health Basics
2: Nutrition and Physical Fitness
3: Sexual Health and Development
4: Alcohol, Tobacco, and Other Drugs
5: Mental and Emotional Health

Relationships
abusive relationships, **3**:101–109
causes of abuse, **3**:102–103
cycle of abuse, **3**:105, 106*f*
effects of abuse, **3**:105–108
emotional, **3**:101
help options, **3**:108–109
myths about, **3**:107
neglect, **3**:102
physical, **3**:101
sexual, **3**:102
statistics, **3**:104
stopping abuse, **3**:109
teen dating violence, **3**:103*t*
tips for abusive teens, **3**:110
warning signs of, **3**:103–105
breakups, dealing with, **3**:75–76
commitment, **3**:71–73, 74
dating
blind, **3**:70
casual, **3**:70
double , **3**:70–71
group, **3**:70–71
online, **3**:71, **3**:72
serious, **3**:71
speed, **3**:71
difficult relationships, **3**:100–101
falling in love, **3**:73–75
attraction and, **3**:74
closeness and, **3**:74
commitment and, **3**:74
infatuation, **3**:74, 75
romantic love, **3**:74–75
true love, **3**:75
healthy/unhealthy relationships, **3**:99–100
sex, **3**:76–78
age of consent, **3**:82–84
questions about, **3**:78
readiness for, **3**:77–78, 77*t*
sexual consent, **3**:111–112
types of relationships
casual, **3**:69
closed, **3**:73
family, **3**:67–68
friends, **3**:68–69
intimate, **3**:69–70
monogamous, **3**:72
open, **3**:73
polyamorous, **3**:72–73
See also Rape/sexual assault; Safe sex; Sexual harassment
Relaxation, **1**:9, 10, 54, 87, **3**:196, **4**:109–110, **5**:88, 115, 158
relaxation strategies, **5**:84–86
See also Stress and coping
Reparative (orientation change) therapy, **3**:36–37
Residential/Health care options for the elderly, **1**:63–64
Resistance
ability to stop electrical current, **1**:179
to infections/disease, **1**:68, 69, 108
to insulin, **1**:59
to medication, **3**:157
resistance exercises, **2**:148–149, 153, 155
Respiratory
diseases, **1**: 39–44, 54–58, **2**:44, 66, **4**:10, 15, 16, 55, 62
failure, **1**:47, 57, **4**:10, 19, 23, 26
infections, **1**:38, 39–44, 48, 103, 107, **5**:146
system, **1**:54, **2**:152, 155, **4**:49–50
See also Allergies, Anaphylaxis, Asthma, Chronic obstructive pulmonary disease (COPD), Cystic fibrosis, Emphysema
Respite care, **1**:63
Rest, **1**:9–10, 40, 42, 43, 47, 158, 159, 180, **2**:124, 165, **3**:161, 187, 190, 196, 203, **5**:88, 125
Resting metabolic rate (RMR), **2**:71
RMR of body organs, **2**:71*t*
Restlessness, **4**:13, 19, 21, 22, 62, **5**:108, 136
Retinopathy, **1**:97
Retrospective study, **5**:60
Rett's disorder, **5**:100
Rheumatoid arthritis (RA), **1**:67

Risk-taking behavior, **1:**137, **3:**32, **4:**108, **5:**24, 35, 44, 109, 114, 117–119
  choking game, **5:**117–118
  getting help for, **5:**118–119
Ritalin (methylphenidate), **4:**20–21
Rohypnol (roofies), **3:**112, **4:**10, 22–23, 51
Rosenberg Self-Esteem Scale, **5:**7*t*
Roux-en-Y bypass (RNY), **2:**94, 95
Runner's diarrhea, **2:**170–171
Ryan, Monique, **2:**82

Safe sex, **3:**77, 87, 129–175, **5:**52
  abstinence, **3:**129–132
  communicating about, **3:**90–95
  contraception (birth control), **3:**132–146
  HIV/AIDS, **3:**146, 148, 152–155
  importance of, **3:**90
  relationships and environmental influences, **3:**76–78
  practices, **3:**90, 94
  safer sex, **3:**146
    measures for, **3:**147–149
  STD (sexually transmitted disease), **3:**129–130, 155–163
  sexually transmitted infection (STI), **3:**129–130
  strategies for talking about safe sex, **3:**93–95
  Teen Opinions on talking about, **3:**92
  unsafe sex, **1:**2, **3:**37, 91, 93, 146, **4:**49, 54, 56, **5:**61
  See also Condoms; Contraception; HIV/AIDS; Oral sex; Sexual activity, legal issues pertaining to; STDs (sexually transmitted diseases)
Safety
  bicycle, **1:**85, 140–141, **3:**208
  fall precautions, **1:**160–161
  food, **1:**164–165
  school, **1:**50–51, 162–163
  skateboards, **1:** 140–141, 155
  sports, **1:**154–160, **2:**157–166
  workplace, **1:**24, 50–51, 150–151, 161–162
  See also Disasters, safety during; Fire safety, Motor vehicle safety; Poisoning, Public transportation safety, Water safety
Saliva, **1:**56, 103, **4:**14
Satiety, **2:**92
Scabies, **1:**94–95
Schizophrenia
  causes, **5:**151
  dealing with, **5:**152–153
  delusions, **5:**149–150, 152–153
  hallucinations, **5:**150
  negative symptoms, **5:**149
  other psychotic disorders, **5:**105, 151–152
  positive symptoms, **5:**149
  schizoaffective disorder, **5:**152
  schizophreniform disorder, **5:**152
  subtypes, **5:**150–151
School safety, **1:**162–163, **5:**38–39
  after-school activities, **1:**163–164
  in school building, **1:**162
  sport activities, **1:**163–164
  travelling to school, **1:**162
  violence and, **1:**163
School-based mental health professionals, **1:**12, 37, 163, **3:**51, 86, 109, 114, 117, **4:**79, 100, 103, 104, 115, **5:**15, 33, 38, 125, 157, 163–164
Seasonal affective disorder (SAD), **5:**108
Sedative-hypnotics, **4:**8, 10, 40, **5:**166
Seizure disorder (epilepsy), **1:**47, 48, 59, 60, 65–66, 179, 180, 181, **2:**42, 44, 97, **3:**24, 208, **4:**6, 8–10, 19, 44, 51, 60, 84, 97, **5:**109, 117, 143, 147, 166
Selenium toxicity, **2:**43
  Marco Polo, and, **2:**43
  selenosis, **2:**43
Self-image and self-esteem
  self-image, **3:**8, 25–26, 33, 40, **5:**1–2, 8, 40
  self-efficacy, **5:**3
  self-esteem, **1:**10–12, 91, 154, **2:**107, 109, 110, 113, 120, 122, 125, 134, 135, 161, **3:**25–26, 37, 40, 74, 100, 101, 107, **5:**2–9, 21, 27, 33, 110, 111, 115, 143
    ethnic identity and, **5:**5
    extracurricular activities and, **5:**4–5
    family and, **5:**4
    formation of, **5:**3–5
    low self-esteem, **5:**6

1: Health Basics
2: Nutrition and Physical Fitness
3: Sexual Health and Development
4: Alcohol, Tobacco, and Other Drugs
5: Mental and Emotional Health

Self-image and self-esteem (*continued*)
media influences and, **5**:5
peers and, **5**:4
questionnaire, **5**:7*t*
religion and, **5**:5
Rosenberg Self-Esteem Scale, **5**:7*t*
school and, **5**:4
ways to improve, **5**:6–8
Self-destructive behaviors, **2**:116, **3**:76, **5**:107, 114–116
Freedom from Harm (Gratz & Chapman) on, **5**:114, **5**:115
treatments for self-harming behavior, **5**:115–116, 118
Semivegetarians, **2**:176
Sensation
loss of, **3**:16
strange/unusual, **1**:65, **4**:17, **5**:124
Separation anxiety disorder, **5**:101
Separation/divorce, **5**:11
See also Divorce
Sex at parties, **3**:95–96
regret or remorse, **3**:96
Sexting, **5**:51–54
case study, **5**:53
dangers of, **5**:51–52
prevalence, **5**:51
Teen Opinions on, **5**:52
Sexual abstinence, **3**:95, 129–132
Teen Opinions on, **3**:130
teen sexual intercourse myths, **3**:131
See also STDs (sexually transmitted diseases), Virginity and abstinence
Sexual activity, legal issues pertaining to, **3**:149–152
age of consent, **3**:150
confidentiality, minors and health care, **1**:113, **3**:150–152, **5**:157
legal ages for sexual participants, **3**:150
mandatory reporting, **3**:150
minors' right to consent to health care, **3**:151
statutory rape, **3**:82, 109, 150, **5**:31
STDs (sexually transmitted diseases), **3**:148, 151
Sexual abuse. *See* Abusive relationships, Incest
Sexual assault. *See* Rape, Statutory rape
Sexual behavior, **1**:2, **3**:67, 77, 79, 84–98, 111, 114, 115, **4**:44, 53, 56, **5**:40, 44, 46, 47, 49, 103, 112, 117, 167
activities and, **3**:78, 84–98
physical development and, **3**:84
respecting boundaries around, **3**:89–90
sex versus sexuality, **3**:85
See also Masturbation, Pornography, Sex at parties
Sexual and gender identity disorders, **5**:103
Sexual expression, **3**:85, 129
Sexual harassment, **3**:98, 114–118, **5**:38, 42–43
dealing with, **3**:117–118
examples of, **3**:114–115
flirting, **3**:116–117
helping a victim of, **3**:118
illegality of, **3**:117
innuendo, **3**:115
of LGBTQI individuals, **3**:115
statistics, **3**:115
Title IX of the Education Amendments of 1972, **3**:117
workplace, **5**:42–43
Sexual or gender minority, **3**:42, **5**:46
See also LGBTQI
Sexual orientation, **2**:113, **3**:31, 32, 34–42, 51–53, 85–87, 95
bisexuality, **2**:113, **3**:34–36, 38, 49, 51, 85
bullying and, **3**:42, 51, 53, 85, **5**:27
choice and, **3**:35–36, 86
definition, **3**:34
versus gender identity, **3**:40, 41
gender roles and socialization, **3**:38, 39–40, 43, 85, 129, **5**:1, 36, 40, 46
hate incident/hate crimes and, **3**:36, 42, 50, 51,53, 101, **5**:27, 30,
heterosexism, **3**:35–36, 50

heterosexuality defined, **3**:34, 85
homophobia, **3**:35–37, 50, 86
internalized homophobia, **3**:37
homosexuality, **2**:113, **3**:34–38, 50, 85–86, 155
versus intersex, **3**:48
media and, **3**:35, 85–86, **5**:40
"metrosexual," **3**:38
spectrum, **3**:34, 51, 52
reparative therapy and, **3**:36–37
sexual harassment and, **3**:114, 115
Teen Opinions on, **3**:36
See also Kinsey Heterosexual-Homosexual Rating Scale, LGBTQI
Shaken baby syndrome, **3**:206, **5**:147–148
Shaman, **1**:2
Sickle cell disease, **1**:3, 69–71, 70*f*, **3**:182
Simple carbohydrate, **2**:3, 170–171
Single Parent Alliance and Resource Center, **3**:221
Sinus infection, **1**:39–40, 103
Skateboard safety, **1**:141
Skin cancer, **1**:23, 69, 95–97, 111, **2**:28
Sleep, **1**:6–9
sleep disorders, **5**:102
types of, **1**:6*t*, 8
Sleeve gastrectomy, **2**: 93–95
Smog, **1**:14, 22
Smoking, **4**:55
baby safety and, **3**:211
breastfeeding and, **4**:62
cancer and, **1**:68
carcinogens, **4**:12
CDC report on, **4**:113
health problems associated with, **4**:12
heart disease and, **1**:52
during pregnancy, **4**:13, 60
respiratory system and, **4**:49–50
safety, **1**:150
secondhand smoke, **1**:57, **3**:191, **4**:13, 16, 49, 55, 60, 62, 67
social implications of tobacco use, **4**:68
withdrawal from, **4**:13
See also Nicotine
Snake, animal, and insect bites, **1**:182–185, 183*f*
Social environment, effects on well-being
cultural influences, **5**:44–46
cybersex, **5**:50–54
media
sexualized, **5**:49–50
media influences, **5**:46–49
phone sex, **5**:50
school life, **5**:40
self-defense, **3**:113, **5**:39
work life, **5**:40–42
part-time employment, **5**:41–42
relationships with supervisors and coworkers, **5**:42
See also Acculturation, Body image, Cliques, Consumerism, Personal space, School safety, Sexting, Social norms, Workplace sexual harassment
Social networking, **3**:115, **5**:24–29, 46, 49, 51, 55
dangers of, **5**:26
cyberbullying, **5**:2, 27–29
image and, **5**:25–26
percentage of people using, **5**:25
popular activities on, **5**:25
Teen Opinions on, **5**:25
Social norms, **1**:2, **3**:67, 129, **5**:35, 40, 43–46, 81
Social skills, **5**:116, 143, 145, 158
Social support, **1**:2, **2**:135, **3**:50–51, 69, **4**:74,79, 102, 110, **5**:13, 19, 20, 80, 83 85, 92, 93, 111, 120, 144
Social worker, **1**:36, **2**:131, **3**:194, **4**:80, 104, **5**:15, 161–163
Soil pollution, **1**:12, 14, 18–19
Solar eclipse, **1**:23
Somatoform and factitious disorders, **2**:125, **5**:107
Sore throats, **1**:39
Speech
pathologist, **1**:36
therapy, **1**:65, **5**:145, 147
Spinal tap. *See* Lumbar puncture
Sports injuries, **1**:155–158, **2**:162–166, **3**:208
acute injuries, **1**:156, **2**:162
back injuries, **1**:157
concussion, **1**:157–158, **2**:164–166
neck injuries, **1**:157
overuse injuries, **1**:156, **2**:162–163
pain medication, **1**:158
recovering from, **1**:158

1: Health Basics
2: Nutrition and Physical Fitness
3: Sexual Health and Development
4: Alcohol, Tobacco, and Other Drugs
5: Mental and Emotional Health

Sports injuries (*continued*)
  spinal fracture, **1**:157
  sport with highest percentage, **1**:156
  strains/sprains, **1**:156–157
    lateral ankle sprain, **1**:157*f*
  stress fractures, **1**:156
  See also Sports safety, Tendonitis, Traumatic brain injuries (TBI), Whiplash
Sports nutrition, **2**:167–177
  carbohydrates, **2**:170–173
  fats, **2**:173
  hydration, **2**:167–168
    overhydration, **2**:168
    rehydration, **2**:169–170
    tips for athletes, **2**:168–170
    USATF hydration guidelines, **2**:167*t*
  low-fat chocolate milk, **2**:172
  Sports Nutrition for Endurance Athletes, **2**:82, 172
  Sports Nutrition Guidebook (Clark), **2**:172
  protein, **2**:173–175
  timing/recommended foods before competition, **2**:174*t*
  urine color, **2**:167, 169
  vegetarian athletes, **2**:175–177
  vitamins and minerals, **2**:175
  See also Runner's diarrhea
Sports safety, **1**:154–160
  advice for, **1**:159–160*t*
  cell phones and, **1**:156
  equipment and protection, **1**:155
  practicing, **1**:156
  preparations for exercise or sports, **1**:155–156
  warming up, **1**:155–156
  See also Sports injuries
Sports supplements, **2**:125, 175, 177–184, **4**:30
  claims, evidence, and safety, **2**:180–182
  efficacy of, **2**:179–183, 180–182*t*
  MVM dietary supplements, **2**:182–183
  popular supplements used by athletes, **2**:177–178
  safety of, **2**:177, 179, 180–182*t*
  See also Dietary supplements
Sprains, **1**:156–157
Staph infections, **1**:49
Statutory rape, **3**:82, 109, 150, **5**:31
STDs (sexually transmitted diseases), **3**:129–130, 155–163
  condoms and, **3**:139, 149
  InSPOT website and, **3**:148
  legal considerations, **3**:148, 151
  oral sex and, **3**:130, 146
  sexual intercourse and, **3**:130
  talking about, **3**:91–93, 147–149
  testing for, **3**:163
  See also Chlamydia, Genital candidiasis, Genital warts, Gonorrhea, Human papillomavirus (HPV), Pelvic inflammatory disease (PID), Syphilis, Trichomoniasis
Stereotypic movement disorder, **5**:101
Steroids, **1**:66, **2**:179, 182, **3**:6, 49, 25, **4**:26–31
  anabolic steroids, **2**:179, **4**:27–28
    side effects, **3**:6, **4**:29–30, 51
  cancer and, **4**:55
  cardiovascular system and, **4**:50
  corticosteroids, **4**:2, 27
    side effects, **4**:28–29
  cortisone, **3**:45
  effects on
    fetus and newborn, **4**:59
    liver, **5**:50–51
    musculoskeletal system, **4**:51
    skin, **4**:51
  hormonal effects, **4**:53
  mental health and, **4**:30–31
  misuse of, **4**:40, **5**:56
  neurological (nervous) system and, **4**:51
  to reduce inflammation, **1**:91
  risks of steroid use, **2**:182, **3**:157, **4**:31
  weight gain and, **1**:11, **5**:56
Stethoscope, **1**:112
Stigma
  associated with mental health disorders, **2**:63, 116, **3**:49, **4**:109, **5**:110, 140, 141, 142
    Teen Opinions on, **5**:142

Stimulants, **4:**19–22
  ADHD medications, **4:**20–21
  amphetamines, **4:**19–20
  cocaine, **4:**19
  diet pills, **4:**20
  khat, **4:**21–22
  methamphetamine, **4:**19–20
  minor stimulants
    caffeine, **4:**21
    ephedra, **2:**97, 98, 184, **4:**21
    guarana, **4:**21
    theobromine, **4:**21
    theophylline, **4:**21
  nicotine, **4:**22
Stomach flu, **1:**40–42
STP, **4:**17
Stress and coping
  causes of stress, **5:**79–82
  communication styles, **5:**89–91
    aggressive, **5:**89
    assertive, **5:**91
    behavior and communication styles, **5:**90*t*
    passive, **5:**89
  effects of stress, **5:**79
  fight-or-flight system, **5:**77
  hostility, **5:**80
  perceived stress, **5:**77
  relaxation strategies, **5:**84–86
    biofeedback, **5:**84, 86
    cognitive-behavioral therapy (CBT), **5:**84, 85–86
    deep breathing, **5:**85
    hypnosis and meditation, **5:**85
    physical exercise, **5:**85
    progressive muscle relaxation, **5:**85
    relaxation responses, **5:**85
    supportive counseling, **5:**85
    time management, **5:**84–85
  stress, **5:**77–78
  stress management skills, **4:**82, **5:**15–16, 158
  stressors
    family, **5:**80–81
    personal, **5:**80
    social, **5:**81
  tend and befriend, **5:**79
  Type A behavior, **5:**79–80
  Type B behavior, **5:**80
  workplace stress, **5:**81–82
  See also Anger, Anger management, Adrenaline (epinephrine), Coping, Endorphins, Oxytocin, Venting
Stress fracture, **1:**156, **2:**162
Stroke (cerebrovascular accident), **1:**22, 52–54, 64–65, 70, 104, 109, **2:**24, 64, 65, 69, 75, 97, 160, **4:**12, 19, 50, 51, 53, 67, **5:**109, 117
Stye, **1:**49
Subcultures, **1:**2
Substance misuse, abuse, and dependence, **4:**39–44
  abuse
    chronic misuse, **4:**48–49
    defined, **4:**43
    diagnostic criteria, **4:**42
  dependence
    defined, **4:**43
    diagnostic criteria, **4:**42, 44
    health problems, **4:**44
    symptoms, **4:**43–44
    tolerance, **4:**43
    withdrawal, **4:**43–44
  prevention, **4:**74–79
    benefits of, **4:**76–77
    early intervention, **4:**78–79
    risk factors, **4:**75–76
    prevention strategies
      targeted, **4:**75–76
      universal, **4:**75, **4:**76
  social implications of, **4:**66–68
    alcohol abuse, **4:**66–67
    other drugs, **4:**68
    tobacco, **4:**67
  treatment, **4:**79–84
    12-step groups, **3:**36, **4:**81, 106
    agonist-antagonist drug treatment, **4:**84
    approaches
      harm reduction, **4:**105–107
      abstinence, **4:**106–107
    behavioral therapy (BT), **4:**82
    Buprenorphine, **4:**84
    cognitive-behavioral therapy (CBT), **4:**82
    contingency management, **4:**82
    continuum of care, **4:**79
      detoxification (detox), **4:**80–81
      inpatient treatment, **4:**80–81

1: Health Basics
2: Nutrition and Physical Fitness
3: Sexual Health and Development
4: Alcohol, Tobacco, and Other Drugs
5: Mental and Emotional Health

Substance misuse, abuse, and dependence (*continued*)
intensive outpatient therapy (IOP), **4**:80
medically managed treatment, **4**:80
outpatient treatment, **4**:79–80
psychoeducation, **4**:79
denial (failure of problem recognition) and, **4**:81
disulfrum (Antabuse), **4**:83–84
drug screening and, **4**:81
medication therapy, **4**:83–84
motivational interviewing, **4**:82–83
nicotine replacement therapy for teens, **4**:83
referrals for, **4**:82
support groups, **4**:81
treatment for withdrawal, **4**:84
See also Alcoholics Anonymous (AA), Al-Anon, Alateen, Nar-Anon, Narcotics Anonymous
Substance use, **4**:41–42
body temperature and, **4**:53
cardiovascular system and, **4**:50
during pregnancy and nursing, **4**:56–60
alcohol, **3**:191, **4**:61–62
amphetamines, **4**:59
barbiturates, **4**:62
birth defects, **4**:57
breastfeeding, **4**:61–63
club drugs, **4**:60
cocaine, **4**:59
coffee drinking, **4**:21, 62
depressant drugs, **4**:10
drug withdrawal, **4**:57–58
effects on fetus and newborn, **4**:59–60
fetal alcohol spectrum disorders (FASDs), **4**:61
heroin, **4**:59–60, 62
inhalants, **4**:32
marijuana, **4**:59, 62
methamphetamine, **4**:20, 62
risk categories of prescription medications, **4**:57
risks of medication use during pregnancy, **4**:58*t*
smoking/secondhand smoke, **1**:57, **3**:191, **4**:13, 16, 49, 55, 60, 62, 67
teratogenicity, **4**:57
effects on
brain chemistry, **4**:45–47, 46*f*
brain function
alcohol, **4**:47
depressants, **4**:47
hallucinogens, **4**:48
stimulants, **4**:47–48
See also MDMA (Ecstasy)
emotions and behavior, **4**:48–49
gastrointestinal (digestive) system and, **4**:50
HIV/AIDS, and, **4**:54, 55–56
hormones and, **4**:53
impact on
community, **4**:65–66
family, **4**:64–65
personal relationships, **4**:66
infectious diseases and, **4**:54
influences on, **4**:69–73
access to substances, **4**:70
location and, **4**:69
personal influences, **4**:72–73
regional laws and regulations, **4**:70
social and media influences, **4**:70–71
kidneys and, **4**:51
legal implications of, **4**:68–69
controlled substances, **4**:69
minimum drinking age, **4**:69
Teen Opinions on, **4**:68
tobacco use, **4**:68, 69
liver and, **4**:50–51
metabolic and endocrine effects, **4**:53–54
musculoskeletal system and, **4**:51
myths about, **4**:73–74
nasal lining damage, **4**:52
neurological (nervous) system and, **4**:51

oral health and, **4:**52
parenting and, **4:**60–61
problematic substance use, **4:**42
respiratory system and, **4:**49–50
routes of administration, **4:**54–56
ingestion, **4:**2, 54
inhalation, **4:**55
injection, **4:**2, 55–56
intramuscular (IM), **4:**2
intravenous (IV), **4:**2
intranasal, **4:**2
oral, **4:**2, 54
rectal **4:**2
subcutaneous, **4:**2, 55
sublingual, **4:**2, 56
transdermal, **4:**2, 56
topical, **4:**2
the skin and, **4:**51–52
smoking, **4:**49, **4:**55
See also Granuloma
Substance use, coping with, **4:**102–115
asking for help, **4:**104–105
resources, **4:**105
tips, **4:**105
determining if someone has a substance use problem, **4:**103–104
friends or family members using, **4:**107–114
outward signs, **4:**107–108
Teen Opinions on friends or family who misuse substances, **4:**111
helping a friend with a substance use problem, **4:**111–114
finding the right time and place, **4:**112
making decisions in the moment, **4:**113–114
setting limits, **4:**112–113
starting a conversation, **4:**112
using I-statements, **4:**112
helping a relative with a substance use problem, **4:**114–115
key points to remember, **4:**115
NIDA for Teens website, **4:**104
resources for, **4:**104
Rethinking Drinking (NIAAA), **4:**104
how substance use affects others, **4:**109
myth about sobering up, **4:**114
peer and family pressure, **4:**102–103
risk taking and other dangerous behaviors, **4:**108–109
self-care, support, and safety, **4:**109–111
self-care plan, **4:**109–110
staying safe, **4:**110–111
support from others, **4:**110
things not to do, **4:**115
Substance use, making choices about, **4:**95–102
choices importance of, **4:**95–96
decision-making, **4:**100–102
sticking with a decision, **4:**102
worksheet for, **4:**99
knowing what to say, **4:**96
negative consequences of substance use , **4:**97–98
potential benefits of substance use, **4:**96
values and, **4:**98–100
values exploration exercise, **4:**100
values exploration worksheet, **4:**101
Substance-related disorders, **5:**106
Sudden infant death syndrome (SIDS), **1:**107, **3:**192–193, 203, 214, **4:**55, 60
Sugar alcohol, **2:**3*t*
Suicide, **5:**119–123
assisted, **5:**120, 122
cluster, **5:**121
culture and, **5:**120, 122
myths, **5:**122
pact, **5:**121
prevention of, **5:**121–123
rates of, **5:**119–120
rational suicide, **5:**120
reasons for, **5:**120
treatment of, **5:**123
warning signs, **5:**122–123
Sunburns, **1:**22, 95, 97
Sun protective factor (SPF), **1:**95, 97
Sunscreen, **1:**95–96
Surgical interventions for weight loss, **2:**93–96
Survey of Activity, Fitness, and Exercise (SAFE), **2:**153
Sutures, **1:**181, 183
Swimmer's ear, **1:**90–91, 91*f*
Syphilis, **3:**146, 161–162
Systemic diseases, **1:**67–71

1: Health Basics
2: Nutrition and Physical Fitness
3: Sexual Health and Development
4: Alcohol, Tobacco, and Other Drugs
5: Mental and Emotional Health

Tanning bed, **1**:97
Tattoo and body piercing, **1**:97–99, **3**:26–30, 152, 155, **5**:2, 114
  Association of Professional Piercers (APP), **3**:29
  photographs of, **3**:28
  Teen Opinions on, **3**:27
  See also: Allergies, Infection, Body piercings
Teen dating violence, **3**:103*t*
Teen Opinions on
  body modifications, **3**:27
  cyberbullying, **5**:29
  eating disorders, **2**:111, 119
  mental health disorders, **5**:142, 160
  minimum drinking age, **4**:68
  parenting, **3**:221
  pornography, **3**:97
  pro-anorexia (pro-an) websites, **2**:119
  safe sex, **3**:92, 130
  sexting, **5**:52
  sexual orientation, **3**:36
  social networking, **5**:25
  substance misuse, **4**:111
  tattoos and body piercings, **3**:27
  virginity and abstinence, **3**:82
  virginity and oral sex, **3**:80
Tendonitis, **1**:156, **2**:162
Teratogenicity, **4**:57
  behavioral, **4**:57
  medication risks, **4**:58*t*
morphologic, **4**:57
Terrorist attacks, **1**:165, 175, 176, **5**:127
Tetanus vaccinations, **1**:108–109
Thermal pollution, **1**:21–22
Thunderstorms and lightning, **1**:152, 169, 173–174
Tic disorders, **5**:101
Tinea cruris. *See* Jock itch
Title IX of the Education Amendments of 1972, **3**:117
Tobacco
  carcinogens, **4**:12, 14
  cigarettes, **1**:4, 15, 27, 107, 150, **2**:110, 127, 130, 179, 182, **3**:193, **4**:11, 12–16, 32, 42, 49, 55, 62, 67, 70, 71, 72, 76, 82–83, 96, 113, **5**:115, 167
  graphic warning labels, **4**:11*f*
  health problems associated with, **4**:12
  secondhand smoke, **1**:57, **3**:191, **4**:13, 49, 55, 60, 62, 67
  smokeless (chewing and snuff), **4**:13–14
  See also Nicotine, Smoking, Sudden infant death syndrome (SIDS)
Tooth injury or loss (accidental), **1**:185
Tornadoes, **1**:165, 166, 169, 173
  tornado warning, **1**:173
  tornado watch, **1**:173
Tourette's disorder, **5**:101, 126
Toxic shock syndrome (TSS), **3**:24
Toxins, **1**:3, 17, 19, 56, 60, 61, 162, 181, **2**:91, **3**:24, 26, 191, 212–213, **5**:139
  See also Poisoning
Toxoplasma gondii, **2**:22–23, **3**:154
Tranquilizer, **5**:166
Transgender, **3**:40–42
  challenges and support, **3**:42, 43
  See also Development, Gender identity, Hormones, LGBTQI
Transient ischemic attack (TIA), **1**:64
Transphobia, **3**:41
Transplant, **2**:23, **4**:27
  bone marrow, **1**:69, 71
  heart, **1**:52
  kidney, **1**:62
  liver, **1**:46, 47
Transvestite, **3**:40
Traumatic brain injuries (TBI), **2**:164–165
  See also Concussion
Tremors, **1**:47, 66, **4**:9, 21, 23, **5**:147, 167
Trichomoniasis, **3**:162–163
Trichotillomania, **5**:104
Tsunami, **1**: 165, 166, 174
Tubal ligation, **3**:144
Tuberculosis (TB), **1**:43–44
  BCG vaccine, **1**:44

rates of TB cases in U.S, **1**:44*f*
Type A behavior, **5**:79–80
Type B behavior, **5**:80
Typhoid, **1**:17

Ulcers, **1**:45, 58, 70, **2**:94–95, **3**:157, **4**:6, 21, 22, 52, 55, **5**:79
Ultrasound, **1**:61, **3**:181
Ultraviolet radiation, **1**:22–23
damage from, **1**:23
UVA, **1**:22–23, 97
UVB, **1**:22–23, 97
UVC, **1**:22–23
UV index forecast, **1**:96*f*
Upper respiratory infection (URI), **1**:39–42
humidifiers and, **1**:40
See also Bronchitis, Ear infection, H1N1 virus, Influenza (flue), Pneumonia, Sinus infection, Sore throats, Tuberculosis (TB), Walking pneumonia
Uranium, **1**:14
Urinary system, **1**:58
cystitis, **1**:44
urethra, **1**:44
Urinary tract infections (UTI), **1**:44–45, 64, **2**:129, **3**:141, 153, **5**;152
Urticaria. *See* Hives
U.S. Food and Drug Administration (FDA), **2**:20–21, **5**:59
U.S Pharmacopeia (USP), **2**:44
USA Today, **5**:57

Vaccinations. *See* Immunization (vaccinations)
Vaccine, **1**:41–44, 46, 49, 105–107, 116, **3**:154, 160
Valid information, **2**:18, **5**:1, 57, 59, 60, 61
Valium, **4**:8
Values, **1**:1, 2, **2**:115, **3**:30–33, 37, 50, 72, 77, 79, 84, 90, 129, **4**:95, 96, 97, 98–101, **5**:8, 9, 21, 22, 44, 46, 81, 185
social values, **1**:1
Varicoceles, **1**:112
Vasectomy, **3**:144
Vegetarian
diet, **2**:17, 26, 44, 46, 119, 175–177
lacto-ovo vegetarian, **2**:176
semivegetarian, **2**:176
Vegan, **2**:176
Vegetarian athletes, **2**:175–177
Gonzalez, Tony, **2**:176
Vegetarian Starter Kit, **2**:176
Venereal disease (VD). *See* STDs (sexually transmitted diseases)
Venom, **1**:183–184
Venting, **5**:88
Vertical banded gastroplasty, **2**:95
Violence, **1**:127, 175, **3**:16–17, 33, 96–98, 104, **5**:30, 32–33, 49, 50, 131, 154
anger and, **5**:87
depression and, **5**:33
exposure to, **5**:32
help, how to get, **5**:33
impact of, **5**:33
myth, **5**:32
National Center for Victims of Crime (NCVC), **5**:33
pornography and sexual violence, **3**:96, 97–98
prevalence, **5**:32
school safety and, **1**:163, **5**:38–39
substance use and, **4**:6, 18, 31, 64, 65, 115, **5**:80*f*
teen dating, **3**:103*t*
workplace, **1**:161
See also Bullying, Domestic violence, Gangs, Rape/sexual assault, Relationships/Abusive relationships
Virginity and abstinence, **3**:78–84
Abstinence (definition), **3**:79
deciding not to have sex, **3**:80–82
hymen and virginity, **3**:78–79
legality and appropriateness of sex, **3**:82–84
religion and, **3**:79
Teen Opinions on telling someone you don't want to have sex, **3**:82
Teen Opinions on virginity and oral sex, **3**:80
virgin, definition of, **3**:131
what counts as sex?, survey, **3**:79*t*
Virilization, **3**:44, 47
Viruses, **1**:26, 38

1: Health Basics
2: Nutrition and Physical Fitness
3: Sexual Health and Development
4: Alcohol, Tobacco, and Other Drugs
5: Mental and Emotional Health

Vision
  blurred or double, **1**:8, 47, 60, 66, **2**:166, **3**:112, 182, **4**:20, 24
  impairment/problems, **1**:60, 64, **3**:180, **4**:8, **5**:118, 146, 147
  loss, **1**:109, 114
  night, **2**:9
Vitamins, **1**:10, 58, 89, **2**:1, 3, 7–8, 28, 39, 42, 44, 45–46*t*, 81, 88, 89, 93–95, 128, 175–176, 182–183, **3**:190, 191, 192
  deficiency, **2**:15, 16, 18
  fat-soluble, **2**:8, 9*t*, 92
  vitamin B complex, **2**:8
  vitamin D, **1**:22–23, **2**:19, 28, 75, 175–176, 179, **4**:26
    dietary sources of, **2**:78*t*
    myth, **2**:28
  water-soluble, **2**:8, 10–11*t*
Volatile organic compound (VOC), **1**:27
Voltage, **1**:178

Waist circumference, **2**:67, 68
Waist-to-hip ratio, **2**:68
Walking pneumonia, **1**:43
Washing
  athletic clothes/uniforms, and MRSA, **1**:50
  babies, **3**:209
  bedding, **1**:26, 101, **3**:209
  clothing, **1**:94, 101, 176, **3**:209
  body, **1**:86–88, 100, 176
  face, **1**:88–89, 92
  fruits and vegetables, **1**:19, 165, **3**:154
  hands, **1**:39, 50, 85–86, 89, 93, **3**:209, **5**:126
  hair, **1**:99, 100, 176
Water (drinking), **1**:45, 103, 156, 166, **2**:6–7, 29, 41, 167, 171, 173, **4**:40
  See also Dehydration, Hydration
Water intoxication, **2**:168
Water pollution, **1**:14, 15, 17–18, 20, 21
Water safety, **1**:151–154
  alcohol and, **1**:153, 154
  animals and swimming, **1**:151–152
  boater's fatigue, **1**:154
  boating safety, **1**:152–154
  currents and, **1**:153
  diving and, **1**:152
  drowning, **1**:151
  flotation devices or life jackets, **1**:153, 154*f*
  hyperthermia, **1**:152
  lifeguard, **1**:151, 152
  lightning and, **1**:152
  swimming lessons, **1**:151
  waterskiing, **1**:153
  See also Motor vehicle safety
Waterbirthing, **3**:197
Waxing, **1**:88
Weight management
  American Personal Responsibility in Food Consumption Act (2005), **2**:62
  appearance and weight, **2**:64–65
  body shapes, **2**:68–69
    ectomorph, **2**:69
    endomorph, **2**:69
    mesomorph, **2**:69
  calorie needs, daily, **2**:72*t*
  controversy, **2**:61
    body weight and health debate, **2**:75
  diet, meanings of, **2**:83
  dietary sources of
    potassium, **2**:80*t*
    calcium, **2**:77*t*
    vitamin D, **2**:78*t*
  doctor prescribed weight-loss methods and surgical interventions, **2**:91–96
    adolescents and, **2**:96
    complications, **2**:95, **2**:96
    surgical interventions for weight loss, **2**:93–94
    weight-loss drugs, **2**:92–93, 92*t*
      See also Gastric bypass procedures
  fad diets and weight-loss aids, **2**:87–91
  gain or lose weight safely, **2**:78–81

500-calorie rule, **2**:81
gaining weight, **2**:81–83
factors influencing, **2**:81
nutrient-dense food ideas for, **2**:82–83*t*
menu plans, **2**:82
tips and strategies for, **2**:81–82, 84–86
standard formula for, **2**:79–81
healthy weight, **2**:66–69
lifestyle choices and, **2**:84, 86
losing weight, **2**:83–87
calorie count for, **2**:86
keys to losing weight, **2**:84–86
permanent weight loss statistics, **2**:86
maintaining a healthy weight, **2**:69–78
"10 Tips Nutrition Education Series," **2**:73
Choose MyPlate Interactive Tool link, **2**:73
daily eating plan design, **2**:73
Dietary Guidelines for Americans, **2**:16–19, 74–76
recommendations for children and teens, **2**:76–78
estimated energy requirement (EER), **2**:71
food portion sizes, **2**:74, 76
formulas for, **2**:70–71
My Food-a-Pedia, **2**:73
MyPlate guidelines, **2**:73
MyPyramid Food Tracker, **2**:73
MyPyramid/MyPlate and, **2**:74
"Nutrition Essentials," **2**:76
nutrition websites, **2**:74
snacking and, **2**:76–77
sources of excessive calories, **2**:75
maintaining lost weight, **2**:86
satiety, **2**:92
serving size, **2**:76
underweight, **2**:64
video games and, **2**:70
weight loss industry, **2**:64
weight measurement tools, **2**:68*t*
weight-loss supplements and gadgets, **2**:97–99
safety and effectiveness, **2**:98*t*
studies of, **2**:97
See also Basal metabolic rate (BMR), Body mass index (BMI), Dietary supplements, Diets, Ephedra, Gastric bypass procedures, Nutritional comparison of fast foods, Physical activity (PA) energy factors, Resting metabolic rate (RMR)
Weis, Charlie, **2**:95
Wellness
culture and family influences, **1**:2
environment and, **1**:3–4
exercise and, **1**:11–12
factors affecting, **1**:1–6
friends and associates, **1**:2
genetics and, **1**:3
public opinion and the media, **1**:4–6
rest, **1**:9–10
society and, **1**:1
See also Eating habits, Environmental fitness, Insomnia, Relaxation, Sleep
Whiplash, **1**:157
Wildfire, **1**:14, 22, 148, 165, 166, 173–175
Winter storm, **1**:175
Work or study environment pollution, **1**:24
Workplace safety, **1**:161–162
Workplace sexual harassment, **5**:42–43
Workplace stress, **5**:81–82
World Health Organization (WHO), **2**:22, 61, **3**:15, 16

Xanax, **4**:8
X-rays, **3**:191
diagnostic, **1**:43, 45, 57, 111, 113, **3**:7
mammograms, **1**:111, **3**:7
pregnancy and, **3**:191
radiotherapy, **1**:68

Zygote, **3**:178, 185–186